DEPRESSION
IN THE ELDERLY

DEPRESSION IN THE ELDERLY
An Interdisciplinary Approach

Edited by

G. Maureen Chaisson-Stewart, R.N., Ph.D.

Adjunct Faculty
Department of Psychiatry
University of Arizona Health Sciences Center
Tucson, Arizona
Consultant/Psychotherapist in Private Practice
Tempe, Arizona
Behavioral Health Nursing Clinical Specialist/Consultant
Veterans Administration Medical Center
Phoenix, Arizona

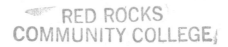
A WILEY MEDICAL PUBLICATION
JOHN WILEY & SONS
New York · Chichester · Brisbane · Toronto · Singapore

Library of Congress Cataloging in Publication Data:

Main Entry under title:

Depression in the elderly.

  (A Wiley medical publication)
  Includes index.
  1. Depression, Mental. 2. Geriatric psychiatry.
I. Chaisson-Stewart, G. Maureen (Grace Maureen)
II. Series. [DNLM: 1. Depression—in old age.
WM 171 D42417]
RC537.D4434 1985   618.97'68527   84-26952
ISBN 0-471-87059-5

Printed in the United States of America

10 9 8 7 6 5 4 3 2 1

To Grace Turecan Forsythe, my mother, who showed me a good old age

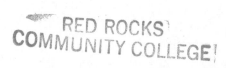

Contributors

James Allender, M.A.
Psychology Assistant
Department of Psychiatry
University of Arizona Health Sciences Center
Tucson, Arizona

G. Maureen Chaisson-Stewart, R.N., Ph.D.
Adjunct Faculty
Department of Psychiatry
University of Arizona Health Sciences Center
Tucson, Arizona
Consultant/Psychotherapist in Private Practice
Tempe, Arizona
Behavioral Health Nursing Clinical Specialist/Consultant
Veterans Administration Medical Center
Phoenix, Arizona

M. Anne Corbishley, M.Ed.
Doctoral Candidate
College of Education
Department of Counseling and Guidance
University of Arizona Health Sciences Center
Tucson, Arizona

Marian Emr, B.A.
Public Affairs Specialist
National Institute on Aging
National Institutes of Health
Bethesda, Maryland

Arthur J. Engler, R.N., B.S.
Research Assistant
School of Nursing
University of Maryland
Baltimore, Maryland

Barbara R. Heller, R.N., Ed.D., F.A.A.N.
Associate Professor
Graduate Faculty
School of Nursing
University of Maryland
Baltimore, Maryland
Consultant, Research and Education Clinical Center
National Institutes of Health
Bethesda, Maryland

Alfred W. Kaszniak, Ph.D.
Associate Professor
Department of Psychiatry
University of Arizona Health Sciences Center
Tucson, Arizona

Edith Kettel, B.A.
Consultant, History of Art and Environmental Planning
Wantagh, New York

Menachem Sadeh, M.D.
Post-Doctoral Fellow
Department of Internal Medicine
University of Arizona Health Sciences Center
Tucson, Arizona

Catherine M. Shisslak, Ph.D.
Assistant Professor
College of Medicine
Department of Psychiatry
Psychology Programs
University of Arizona Health Sciences Center
Tucson, Arizona

James E. Spar, M.D.
Assistant Professor in Residence
Department of Psychiatry and Biobehavioral Sciences
UCLA School of Medicine
Director, Geriatric Psychiatry Inpatient Unit
UCLA Neuropsychiatric Institute
Los Angeles, California

Lawrence Z. Stern, M.D.
Associate Professor
Department of Internal Medicine
University of Arizona Health Sciences Center
Tucson, Arizona

James Utic, Ph.D.
Clinical Psychologist in Private Practice
Mesa, Arizona

Ruth B. Weg, Ph.D.
Associate Professor of Biology/Gerontology
Ethel Percy Andrus Gerontology Center
University of Southern California
Los Angeles, California

Elizabeth B. Yost, Ph.D.
Associate Professor
College of Education
Department of Counseling and Guidance
University of Arizona Health Sciences Center
Tucson, Arizona

Foreword

The depressed elderly need an advocate. An undetermined but definitely substantial number of elderly are depressed. Yet countless numbers go untreated because of deficient information, improper diagnosis, or unavailability of the full range of treatment modalities.

Over the past six years, the Alzheimer's Disease and Related Diseases Association has raised the level of American consciousness about dementia. This laudable effort is in direct contrast to the minimal effort to increase knowledge about depression, a condition with a markedly better prognosis.

Ironically, many continue to believe that Alzheimer's Disease and depression usually overlap and are often identical. Still others believe that clinical depression is normal in later life.

Mourning and sadness are common states in later life, but they are not indicative of clinical depression. On the other hand, depression in late life can present in a variety of subtle and sometimes confusing ways: somatic complaints, such as pain; apathy and withdrawal; panic states with exaggerated sense of helplessness; or pseudodementia.

Proper diagnosis and assessment followed by appropriate treatment usually result in significant improvement or reversal of depression. *Depression in the Elderly: An Interdisciplinary Approach* emphasizes the importance of early detection and prevention of depression by presenting an integrated, multidisciplinary approach to a complex subject. It focuses on problem-oriented interventions within a holistic framework. The text avocates for the depressed elderly.

This book can be used as a reference for older people, their families and friends, and professionals. It provides basic information and a variety of viewpoints on this common and potentially fatal condition. If this information can permeate our society and become general knowledge, the lives of many of our aging people will clearly benefit.

Sanford I. Finkel, M.D.
Medical Director
Charter/Barclay Hospital
Chicago, Illinois

Preface

Estimates of prevalence of depression symptoms in the over-65 population vary as much as the theories about their cause. No doubt the confusion that exists about the identification and proper treatment of this major health problem is largely related to the rudimentary literature that existed on this topic before the 1960's. Since then, scientific investigations in both gerontology and depression have increased in proportion to the increase of both elderly and depressed people in our population. Today the literature on these two subjects is so vast and scattered that it is difficult for the busy professional to access and assimilate into daily clinical practice. In this book, a multidisciplinary panel of contributors describe the scientific advances in gerontology and depression, synthesizing from the conclusions in both these areas of investigation to create a useful guide for busy practitioners who confront this difficult problem everyday.

Depression in the Elderly is intended to serve as a reference source. It is thorough and provides both details and practical tools. The book should be a continuing source of information for the practitioner and researcher.

Select chapters will be of special interest to the members of particular disciplines—nurses, social workers, family physicians, internists, psychologists, psychiatrists, social scientists, gerontologists, nursing home administrators, the clergy, case workers, environmental planners, activity therapists, volunteer coordinators, and nutritionists—because they represent the specialized knowledge of the respective disciplines. However, by also reviewing the other chapters, readers will increase their awareness and appreciation of the complementary expertise available from their professional teammates.

In the past, professionals have had blind spots in recognizing and accurately diagnosing depression in those over 65. In this book, the authors advocate early detection and prevention, providing information to meet these goals as well as secondary and tertiary care goals. Chapters 1–5 focus on identification, an integrated theory of depression in the elderly, psychological assessment, and differential diagnosis from organic brain syndrome.

Our inability to identify depression in its early stages has often left us with tertiary interventions that have been largely drug-oriented and designed as palliatives to reduce discomfort and disability. Thus, the services rendered have often been unidisciplinary and have focused on a single cause and cure. In reality, as we can see from Chapter 4, depresion is usually multifaceted in origin. Also, the longer it is neglected, the more complex it becomes, continually generating new problems. Often problems are labeled "medical" by the physician, "neurological" by the neurologist, "economic" by the case worker, "social" by the director of a senior center, or "spiritual" by the minister. Each may be correct but each is identifying only a piece of the whole. If these viewpoints and attendant specialized expertise are not shared in a team approach to treatment of a complex problem, the patient may drift unrelieved for an extended period in the health care system. This book, through its multidisciplinary authorship and holistic orientation, espouses and demonstrates the need for an interdisciplinary approach. The authors advocate collaboration based upon clear communication and mutual respect for the contributions of each discipline in jointly planning assessment and interventions. Without such an integrated approach, the risk of missing important puzzle pieces that set all of the others in place or awry is greatly increased.

Although the research on treatment of depression in the elderly is still far from complete, Chapters 6–13 describe current and developing intervention methods. Of special note are chapters that discuss promising areas underestimated in their therapeutic potential: nutrition, exercise, voluntarism, and environmental planning.

Recognizing the multiplicity of causes and the broad scope of problems that give rise to the alarmingly high incidence of depression in the elderly and the great inter-individual differences in this population, it seems appropriate and economically sound to custom design individualized, holistic, problem-focused interventions rather than to depend upon one type of intervention to meet the needs of all. This book supplies a wealth of information needed by the involved disciplines to design such individualized treatment plans.

G. Maureen Chaisson-Stewart

Acknowledgments

Though writing is a solitary activity, a book is never a solitary endeavor. So it is with this book, which merely marks the end of a process of development and conception, a process greatly influenced and supported by numerous people. Each deserves recognition and thanks for his or her unique and important contributions.

I am especially grateful to those who supported the idea and day-by-day struggles to bring the book to completion: my husband, Fred, and my teenage children, Monique and Paul; my sister, Edith; my good friend, typist, and fellow author, Donna Goodrich; Jean Crosier, the librarian at the Phoenix Veterans Administration Medical Center; and Janet Foltin, Associate Nursing Editor at John Wiley & Sons, Inc.

Those who provided me the impetus to study and write about depression in the elderly were Eleanor Bauwens and Sandra Anderson, who invited me to contribute a chapter on the subject for their book, *Chronic Illness: Concepts and Application.* They stimulated my appetite. Katherine Young, Project Director of a Nursing Research Development Grant awarded to the University of Arizona College of Nursing by the Division of Nursing of the Department of Health and Human Services, garnered the funds to conduct a limited but pioneering pilot study on the use of cognitive behavioral group therapy as a treatment for depression in this age group. For the success of that project and the stimulus that it provided for the writing of this text, I am indebted to Larry Beutler, Ph.D., Professor and Director of Research in the Department of Psychiatry, Arizona Health Sciences Center, University of Arizona, consultant to the project; Elizabeth Yost, Ph.D., trainer of the cognitive therapists in the project; and Jim Allender, faithful and diligent research assistant to the end.

Perhaps my best teachers were elderly patients and research subjects, who allowed me to enter the private world of their hidden thoughts and feelings about the past, present, and future. Then there were professional colleagues from a variety of disciplines, tutors in their own right, who demonstrated both effective and ineffective methods of diagnosing and treating the problem. Published authors and researchers who spoke to me from the written page about concepts and research findings fed my hunger for solutions and new knowledge. Finally, when all was digested and integrated, the nursing staff of the Nursing Home Care Unit of the Veterans Administration Medical Center in Phoenix, Arizona gave the book's content its first audience. Their enthusiastic response cheered me on to the finish line.

The book is special because of its contributors, each expert in a component of clinical practice vital to the treatment of depression in the elderly.

Finally, I would like to thank those who reviewed the manuscript and offered special insights from their daily clinical expertise in caring for the depressed elderly. From the Veterans Administration Medical Center in Phoenix, Arizona they are Jack Harrington, M.D., psychiatrist; Michael Tidwell, M.S.N., staff nurse in psychiatry; and Karen Walenga, R.N., supervisor of the Nursing Home Care Unit. Other reviewers were Eldonna Shields, M.S.N., Gerontological Nurse Specialist, Vermillion, Ohio; Helene Finnegan, M.S.W., and Phillip Halpern, M.D., both members of mobile geropsychiatric teams on Long Island, New York.

G. Maureen Chaisson-Stewart

Contents

DEPRESSION
IN THE ELDERLY

Concepts

1

Depression Incidence: Past, Present, and Future

G. Maureen Chaisson-Stewart

Depression is the most prevalent mental disorder of late life. Yet, it is the most overlooked, misdiagnosed, and inadequately treated illness. Left untreated, depression prevents those over 65 from enjoying the satisfactions and involvements unique to the autumn of life. When neglected and allowed to run its course, depression is an emotional and financial drain, not only for the elderly person but for society as well. In too many cases, its ending is suicide. But perhaps the greatest tragedy is that while depression is generally ignored, it remains the most treatable mental health problem in the elderly.

Depression, in all age groups, is the most common psychiatric disorder treated in office practice and in outpatient clinics (Beck, 1967). It is so pervasive in the final quarter of the twentieth century that it seems as if the age of anxiety is giving way to the age of depression (Renshaw, 1973).

Data indicate that depression was epidemic in other periods of Western history, usually eras of societal unrest and social repression. During the Peloponnesian War, Athens was besieged, and the population, despairing of victory and dreading the plague, experienced an epidemic of depression. As described by Thucydides (Brock, 1929): "the most terrible feature of the whole trouble was the depression which seized all who knew themselves attacked; giving way forthwith to despair, they involved themselves still further, and made no resistance." Again, as the great Hellenistic Age drew to a close in the third century B.C., an epidemic of suicide occurred in Alexandria.

Melancholia had become prevalent again in Europe in the half-century following 1586, when Timothy Bright published *A Treatise on Melancholie*, the first writing on this subject in English. According to J. J. Schwab (1971),

3

The epidemic apparently extended into the middle of the next century, a few decades after the publication of Burton's *Anatomy of Melancholy* in 1621. Evidence of the pervasiveness of melancholia comes from the drama of the day and other literature, as well as from medical sources . . . depression was known as the Elizabethan malady or the English sickness.

The social experiences of that time parallel the present era. It was a period of very little security. In England, for example, the great victory over the Armada produced few, if any, immediate gains. The populace lived for the next two decades in fear of invasion, and the balance of power was shifting against the English. The economy was seriously inflated to meet defense demands. There was increasing secularization and religious upheaval. Rival factions were on the point of open warfare.

The contemporary scene is similar in many ways. There is fear of international communism and the nuclear bomb. Vietnam and other unresolved military conflicts haunt our memories, evoking feelings of helplessness and futility. The complexity of modern life and rapidity of change overwhelms the individual. Secularization, including widespread resignation of clergy, is a fact of the day. We are in a time of transition, when social forms that have outworn their usefulness are being rejected. In times like these, when the threat of loss and attack seems pervasive and imminent, depression is a likely response.

Current estimates are that 7–15 percent of the U.S. population suffer with treatable and unrecognized depression on any one day (Cohen, 1977). The world incidence of depression, according to the World Health Organization, is 3 percent of the world's population or about 100 million people (Freyhan, 1979). Given that depression is the number one mental health problem worldwide and given that the elderly comprise a rapidly expanding segment of the population, judging by population trends alone, we can expect that as the numbers of elderly increase, so will they represent an increasing proportion of the depressed population.

Estimates of the incidence of depression among the elderly range from 20 percent (Weissman, 1978) to 50 percent (Rosenfeld, 1978), with 25 percent the commonly accepted estimate of self-report of dysphoric mood in this age group (Bettis, 1979). The wide variance of estimated incidence is partially related to the fact that early epidemiological studies emphasized the etiology of psychiatric disorders rather than specific diagnostic criteria. Yet, if we set aside studies of the incidence of depression and merely look at population trends, reported prevalence of psychiatric illness in the general population, and risk factors in the elderly, it seems logical to conclude that depression must be excessive in this age group.

It is estimated that eight million elderly in the United States live in conditions conducive to the development of mental illness (National

Council on Aging, 1978). Five million, or 25 percent, of older people live in conditions of poverty or near poverty. Another million are estimated to have serious physical illness, and still another million are socially isolated. Approximately one million, or 5 percent, reside in long-term care facilities, mostly nursing homes. Deprived of good nutrition, social interaction, exercise, and emotional support, oversedated and treated as nonpersons they are subject to the same factors that contribute to the development of pseudodementia in institutionalized Soviet dissidents. In similar situations, when the elderly person becomes increasingly confused and debilitated, the basic cause of the deteriorated mental state and/or physical state—depression—is apt to get lost in forgotten documents or memories. Understanding the factors that contribute to the development of depression in the elderly, identifying it early, and treating it appropriately are the subjects of this text.

POPULATION TRENDS

The elderly population of the United States will expand from 25 million today to about 55 million in 2050 (Fahey, 1981). The big jump in the proportion of the population over 65 will come between 2010 and 2020, when the post-World War II baby boom generation passes 65. At that time, an estimated 1 in every 7 Americans will be over 65, compared to about 1 in 10 today. By 2030, the ratio will be one in six (Bureau of the Census, 1976). Especially significant is the fact that the greatest percentage of increase in the elderly population will be in the over-75 age group (33 percent). The group aged 65 to 75, or "young-old," will increase only 15 percent (*Newsweek*, 1982). "I view this as one of the most important demographic issues of our time," commented Jacob S. Siegel, a senior statistician in the Census Bureau's population division.

Theodore Lidz (1968) calls the increasing size of the aged population one of the major social problems of contemporary society. Above all, this group will place increasing demands on health professionals to care for their members who are suffering from chronic conditions and depression. To meet these demands, we will need to expand our knowledge base in geriatrics and geropsychiatry and the corps of specialists trained in these areas.

If the present disproportionate geographic distribution of elderly continues, some states will be forced to bear a larger portion of the responsibility and costs than other states. For example, the census report shows that in 1975 New York and California had the greatest number of people over 65, with nearly two million each. They were followed by Pennsylvania, Florida, Illinois, Texas, and Ohio, each of which had more than one million persons over 65. Also, the growth in the number of elderly between 1970 and 1980 in Arizona (91 percent), Nevada (113 percent), Hawaii (73 percent), and Florida (106 percent) was nearly triple (30 percent) the increase for the country as a whole (12 percent).

SUICIDE IN THE ELDERLY

Although the elderly constitute 10 percent of the population in this country, they account for 25 percent of the total number of reported suicides (National Center for Health Statistics, 1977). Thus, suicide among the elderly occurs at rates more than triple those experienced in the general population (Schaie and Birren, 1977). In old age, the ratio for suicides in males and females is 10 to 1. In males, peak rates occur among old people in their 70s and 80s, not only in the United States but also in 18 of 23 other countries reporting data to the World Health Organization (WHO, 1961).

Although the suicide rate with associated depression is particularly high in elderly white males, women have shown higher depression scores than men at every age, in every country where these studies have been made, and in every time period over the past 40 years (Freedman, et al. 1982). Older women suffer from a "triple jeopardy" of being older, female, and members of a minority group, (Jackson, 1972).

Suicides in the elderly are more violent and dangerous than in any other age group and attempts are rarely gestures (Gage, 1971). Depressed men in the over-50 age group have the most successful record for carrying out suicidal thought (Whybrow, 1978).

In categorizing suicides according to intention and outcome, Farber (1968) developed a model that also can be used to compare the suicides according to sex and age. As displayed in Table 1.1, more older males intend to die and do die following a suicidal act. In fact, between the ages of 65 and 69, male suicides outnumber female suicides by 4 to 1, but by age 85, the ratio increases to about 12 to 1 (Bromley, 1966; Weiss, 1968).

While the suicide statistics in the elderly are alarming, it is important to recognize that these figures are derived only from reported suicides, and since suicides are under-reported in the United States (Miller, 1978), we can conclude that the suicide rate in the elderly is even higher than the data reveal. Allen Wellner, a psychologist at the Long Island Jewish Hillside Medical Center in New York, estimates that for every reported suicide there is an unreported one.

Furthermore, reported suicides do not include those elderly whose suicide ideas take the form of relatively passive wishes for death. Very often, when people feel trapped, depressed, or constricted, but not altogether hopeless or helpless, they choose an alternative to suicide in the form of risk-taking behaviors (Litman, 1981) such as neglecting to take prescribed medications, eating inadequately in quantity and quality, overindulging in food or drinks, not complying with physicians' instructions, or engaging in activities with a high risk for injury.

Table 1.1
SUICIDE ACCORDING TO INTENTION,
OUTCOME, AGE, AND SEX.

Intention	Outcome	
	Death	Survival
To die	More Older Males	
Not to die		More Younger Females

Because "depression prior to suicide is probably universal" (Levitt and Lubin, 1975), we can expect the suicide rate to be a good indicator of the prevalence of depression in a particular age group or population. When Robert Litman (1981) divided suicides into subgroups according to their underlying psychiatric pathology, he estimated that 40 percent had a primary affective disorder of a depressive nature, 20–25 percent were alcoholic with evidence of secondary depression, and 10–12 percent were diagnosed as schizophrenic. Accordingly, since suicide rates increase with age, so too must the rate of depression.

Unless factors that contribute to depression change appreciably in the future, the incidence of depression in a graying America is likely to increase.

COST TO ELDERLY AND SOCIETY

If the present high incidence of depression among the elderly continues, it will ultimately result in increasing pressure on the health care delivery system. Depressed elderly neglect their health: they get insufficient sleep and eat poorly. In an effort to have their mental anguish relieved in ways that are less stigmatizing than admitting to difficulty in coping, they often somatize their problems and become frequent visitors to doctors' offices, running up bills for diagnostic studies and turning into hypochondriacs whose problems are never completely resolved.

Many finally become lifetime residents of nursing homes because they are too mentally distraught or dependent to care for their own basic needs. When elderly depressed persons live in a community with minimal social service resources and no intermediate living arrangements, their residential choices are limited to two polarities: home or nursing home. Depression and inadequate coping increases their risk for a premature admission to a nursing home. A nursing home placement constricts their world and life options and leaves them feeling trapped and neglected, feelings that further exacerbate the depression and accelerate their mental and physical decline.

The resulting costs to society are high. Conservative projections are that if we continue our present course, by the year 2030 we will be spending $30 billion (1978-value dollars) for the care of elderly patients with chronic neurological and psychiatric infirmities. This sum exceeds our present or projected allocations for *all* health care. Estimates of health care utilization by depressed patients in industrialized Western nations indicate that for every depressed patient in a psychiatric hospital, there will be four in a psychiatric ambulatory clinic, eight in touch with a general practitioner, and 50 in the general population (Lehman, 1971). However, future costs may not be so exorbitant if social trends improve so as to reduce or eliminate the factors that contribute to a high incidence of depression.

THE ELDERLY OF THE FUTURE

We can predict fairly accurately the characteristics of those who will be old in the year 2055, because most of them were already born by 1985. Also, based upon beginning social trends, we can project a picture of a future society's attitudes and expectations of its older citizens.

The elderly of the future are expected to be different from the elderly of today in several ways. There will be increasing numbers of the "young-old," persons in their late 50s and 60s and in their early 70s, who are retired, healthy, and vigorous, and who will be seeking meaningful ways to use their time (National Institute on Aging, 1977). These people will be seeking opportunities in society for enriching their lives and improving society at large. They will be less likely to accept the stereotypic thinking about the roles and abilities of old people. Instead, they will challenge those stereotypes by pressing themselves toward greater achievements and by pressing society toward greater acceptance of them.

Perception of the aging process is, at least in part, a residue of immemorial myths and social prejudices that propel people into decline (*Newsweek*, 1982). Future elderly, however, will disprove long-held myths about old age. According to Joseph Campbell, a world authority on mythology, myths are public dreams or vehicles of communication between the conscious and the unconscious. He reports that this form of communication has broken down in the modern Western world and old myths are no longer operative (*Time*, 1972). One of the most important functions of mythology is to guide the individual, stage by stage, through the psychological crises of a useful life. As such, they greatly influence attitudes and expectations about roles and behaviors appropriate to each stage and the timing of life events, such as, when to work, marry, go to school, or retire. The breakdown of these myths can be expected to bring with it an expansion of options for the elderly: fewer role constrictions, more ambiguity, and increasing latitude with regard to age-appropriate behavior in dress, work, leisure, and other dimensions of life-style.

There are already signs that traditional notions about which activities are appropriate to which age in the life cycle (that youth is the time for education; adulthood and middle age the time for work, and old age the time for leisure) are dying. Economic and technological changes in society are shaking up these traditional expectations of age-appropriate behavior. Already one-third of institutions of higher education are involved in teaching older persons. More than two million persons over 55 years of age have returned to school. Bernice Neugarten (1970) predicts

The future will probably see greater experimentation and greater flexibility in the time of education, work, and leisure, with more middle-aged and older people being retrained for new jobs or engaged in formal education as the means to self-fulfillment; with more leisure spread throughout adulthood; with long work sabbaticals; and with periods in and out of the workplace. Women are already entering and leaving the labor market at various points in their lives--the same may become true for men who may study for a few years, work for a few years, return for more education, and so on.

Age-role stereotyping that has restricted the options of the aged, just as sex-role stereotyping restricted the options of women before the women's liberation movement, will be greatly reduced and, with it, the associated depression. Once again, Neugarten (1970) looked into the future to describe this aspect.

Chronological age may become less important in the future, with young, middle-aged, and old participating in the society according to each person's special abilities and special experience. With greater physical vigor in the middle-aged and old, with mass education and communication influencing the old as well as the young, with the young maturing more quickly, and the old aging less quickly, with political and economic rights being more evenly distributed across age groups, the result is likely to be a society in which age categories and age restrictions will be relaxed.

If Neugarten's predictions come true, tomorrow's elderly will enter their senior years with a lifetime of change in roles and activities behind them. As such, they are likely to be a group with a higher level of flexibility and adaptability than the present generation of elderly. Presumably, those characteristics will greatly enhance their mental health status and reduce their vulnerability to depression in old age.

The "empty nest syndrome," which precipitates a developmental, reactive depression in aging women, will probably be less common in the future. According to Gordon Streib (1970),

The fact that more women will be employed outside the home suggests that their lives will have other foci than child rearing. Furthermore, the increasing emphasis on the the dangers of overpopulation and the desirability of small families, coupled with the pronouncements from women's liberation groups that women have a destiny other than as breeding machines, will encourage women to have broader interests. Opportunities for travel and other leisure pursuits also suggest that parents will be able to find substitute interests for family-centered activities. With the problems of the "generation gap" and the increasing cost of higher education for children, many families will find the "empty nest" period a time of contentment and fulfillment.

The status of the elderly in America has already improved greatly, according to the final report of the 1981 White House Conference on Aging, (Federal Council on Aging, 1980). The report concludes that America now has "the wealthiest, best-fed, best-housed, healthiest, most self-reliant older population in our history." Although there are, no doubt, millions who do not fit that rosy picture, it has evidently become more possible than ever before to grow old gracefully in America. Ninety-five percent of those over 65 are capable of living productive, self-fulfilling lives (Galton, 1975).

The demographic characteristics of future populations of young-old and old-old will be different in several ways. Their residences may be different. Recent studies indicate that the older population living in metropolitan areas will be dispersed over increasingly large suburban areas in the next two decades.

They will be better educated and will have received better medical care throughout their lives. They will be a fairly sophisticated group who matured in an era in which psychological help was thought desirable rather than taboo. With an increase in education and appreciation of psychology and psychiatry, it is likely that they will seek counseling early for mental health problems and will expect and accept more help from the mental health system.

The "old-old" persons (over 75) will show the greatest increase in numbers and they will have different problems. An increasing minority of them will remain vigorous and active, but the majority will need a range of supportive and restorative health and social services. They will be a disproportionately disadvantaged group, as the National Institute on Aging (1977) has pointed out, explaining that

The reasons are several, including the fact that this group includes many immigrants who were poorly educated and who have spent their working years at low-paying jobs. Many have been unable to accumulate savings or to build up sufficient equity in the social security system to sustain them adequately through their years of retirement.

Many of the factors influencing the future status and well-being of the elderly are neither predictable nor controllable. A sudden increase in the birth rate can drain economic resources from the old and concentrate them on the young, who always command a higher priority. The viability of the social security system or some substitute form of medical and financial care for the retired will determine the economic welfare of future elderly.

The politics of expansion have always, in all societies, meant choices in favor of youth. When population growth is high and economic resources are limited, the young are usually served first. Even though the elderly of tomorrow are likely to be more political in voicing their needs, their present average low income is likely to persist within the foreseeable future. Retirement is necessary in a technological society with an expanding labor force. With inflation, the real income of retirees, based upon earlier work experience, decreases. This situation will probably continue; therefore, the stress of economic insecurity, which puts the elderly at risk for depression, is not likely to abate.

The actual effect that changing characteristics of future elderly cohorts and their future society will have upon the incidence of depression in this population will be determined in time or through research. Cohort analysis research directed at answering questions about the influence of history and social trends upon the characteristics of an age cluster or group is particularly needed. An example of questions to be answered by this type of analysis are these: Does the aging cohort that lived through the depression display a different social and behavioral pattern from a cohort that did not? How are different work histories reflected in financial security (or lack of it) in retirement? What are the effects of changing patterns of work and leisure on the lives of different cohorts? Answers to these questions should help us anticipate how future cohorts are apt to deal with crises in their lives, the stereotypes they will hold about age-appropriate roles, behavior, and life styles, and the type of social and economic support they will expect and receive from family.

NEED FOR MORE RESEARCH

Even though 25 percent of admissions into public mental hospitals is of persons aged 65 or over, less than 1 percent of the federal mental health budget goes to research on aging or the aged (Neugarten, 1970). The need for research related to the mental health of the elderly has been clearly stated by the Committee on Mental Health and Illness of the Elderly of the President's Commission on Mental Health (Federal Council on Aging, 1980). The two recommendations of the committee that are relevant to this discussion are as follows:

> Recommendation II. Research on depression. An expanded effort to determine the causes, treatment and prevention of depression in older persons including investigations of the relationships of depression to suicide, alcoholism and other symptomatic and behavioral disorders should be initiated.
>
> Recommendation III. Actions to develop a national data base on the epidemiology and demography of mental disorders of the elderly must be undertaken.

The importance of epidemiological and demographic studies of the elderly and their health status is explained in the report as follows:

> If we are to serve the mental health needs of our older population well, we need to understand who and where they are, the particular mental health problems to which they are prone, the numbers affected, the long-term course and changing incidence of particular disorders, and the relation of mental health and illness patterns to service, manpower, training and research needs.
>
> Such data are vital to the development of informed national policy, to provide a basis for meaningful manpower planning and deployment, and for sound evaluation of our service delivery systems. If such data-gathering is sustained consistently over a relatively long period of time, we may gain some clues from the past that may help us to anticipate future needs.

Without a data base derived from epidemiological studies, we are left with population trends alone as a means of predicting the future prevalence of depression in the elderly and the consequent future demands for mental health care. Because epidemiological studies of depression to date have differed greatly—in their definition of a case of mental disorder, diagnostic procedures, the classification of the mental disorder, and the measures of prevalence used (Redick, et al. 1972) and, consequently, in their results—it has been difficult to draw any conclusions.

These differences across studies are well illustrated in Table 1.2, which compares some of the most frequently cited U.S. incident studies according to diagnostic criteria, method of sample selection, and age of sample. The information in Table 1.2 confirms what Busse and Pfeiffer (1969) noted about prevalence studies: "Different diagnostic criteria are used in different studies, and the cut-off between what is seen as still within normal limits and what is seen as pathological is by no means uniform."

Referring to Table 1.2, in the study by Weissman and Myer (1978), the sample included 511 subjects between the ages of 26 and 66. The rates

TABLE 1.2
PREVALENCE STUDIES OF DEPRESSION IN THE ELDERLY

Year	Authors	Sample Size	Age	Population Pool	Selection Method	Operational Definition	Incidence (%)
1961	Whittier and Korenyi	540	60+	State hospital admissions	Systematic	1952 APA nomenclature	38
1965	Kreitman et al.	21	35–74	Referrals to hypochondriasis clinic	Convenience, sequential	Self-report of depression in response to questioning	50
1978	Weissman and Myer	511	26–66	Community survey of households	Systematic household survey, adults in household selected at random	SADS-RDC[a] RDS DSM III	8.1 (current) ≥ 66 yrs 18.9 (lifetime) ≥ 66 yrs
1980	Blazer and Williams	997	65+	Community survey, including homes and institutions	Stratified random	DSM III	3.7 Major Depressive Disorder 4.7 Dysphoria
1982	Freedman et al.	166	60–86	Patients with arthritis or hypertension in family physician's office	Sequential—during selected time period	Zung DSI[b] score of 60+	25

[a] Schedule for Affective Disorders and Schizophrenia Diagnostic Research Criteria.
[b] Zung Depression Status Inventory.

13

of depression noted in those over 65 are only a subsample of the group. Unfortunately, since the oldest subjects in the Weissman study were 66, it cannot be considered to reflect accurately the prevalence of depression in the elderly group (65–85).

Nevertheless, Weissman's study as well as that of Blazer and Williams (1980) are the only U.S. studies that were based on a community sample. The Committee on Mental Health and Illness in the elderly have already voiced their concern about this lack of community surveys:

> At present, our available data on the mental health and illness patterns among the elderly are sketchy at best. We know most about those who have already come in contact with the formal mental health system, particularly the institutionalized; we know relatively little about the community dwelling and those we most need to understand—older people who are now out of contact with the system, but in need of help.
>
> While some community surveys have been conducted, we do not have a national data base on our community-dwelling elderly. Important geographic distinctions remain unknown, as do possible variances associated with economic, social, racial and ethnic factors.

The main advantage of a community sample over an in-treatment sample is that the former has greater external validity and includes 75 percent of the population who never seek treatment. For, as Weissman discovered in his study, only approximately one-quarter of his community sample with current psychiatric diagnoses actually sought professional help during the previous year. Another advantage of these two community surveys is that they use new improved diagnostic techniques and criterion—structured questionnaires, operational definitions, and the Diagnostic and Statistical Manual of Mental Disorders (DSM III)—which handle "criterion, subject, occasion, and information variance of discrete psychiatric disorders" (Weissman, 1978). It is noteworthy that in the survey by Weissman and the survey by Blazer and Williams, both of which use DSM III criteria for operationally defining depression, the resulting incidence rates for depression in the elderly are considerably lower than the results obtained from studies of in-treatment populations using other less well-developed diagnostic criteria. Reviewing these American studies and the European prevalence studies summarized by B. J. Gurland (1976), one must conclude with G. Klerman (1971) that "relatively few American studies on incidence and prevalence approach the sophistication and quality of the Scandinavian and British studies." Certainly, it is clear that we need more community surveys because they can reveal important geographic distinctions and possible variances associated with economic, social, racial, and ethnic factors now unknown.

By acknowledging the methodological weaknesses of past epidemiological studies, we can begin the process of correcting them. The work must continue because incidence studies of depression do more than inform us of the extent of the problem. According to Gurland (1976), they serve to 1) draw attention to the problem; 2) aid in recognition of age-specific forms of the illness; and 3) provide data for examination of causes. By identifying causative factors, incidence studies provide the data needed to develop risk profiles, which can serve as aids to early identification and treatment.

Also, in future studies we need to make finer distinctions in age classifications between the "young-old" and the "old-old" rather than lumping all the elderly into an over-65 category. By using such categories, we will be able to detect important differences in mental health status at varying stages of the old age continuum. Without such fine age distinctions, it is difficult to identify many age-related changes of importance to researchers and clinicians alike.

Longitudinal studies that trace depression through successive age groups are needed also. Such studies would allow us to evaluate and compare the following alternative hypotheses concerning variations in depression levels with age: 1) depression remains at a constant, high level in some persons throughout life; 2) depression levels increase with age; and 3) depression levels peak and then abate or show some other variant of a wave-like curve (Freedman et al., 1982).

In conclusion, as stated in Recommendation III of the Task Panel of the President's Commission on Mental Health: "Actions to develop a national data base on the epidemiology and demography of mental disorders of the elderly must be undertaken" (Federal Council on Aging, 1980). As explained by the panel, these data are vital for relating mental health and illness patterns to service, manpower, training, and research needs. When such data are gathered over a relatively long period, it helps policy makers gain clues from the past that help in determining if an age of depression is likely to pass with the times or linger as one of the most costly and tragic public health problems of this era.

REFERENCES

Beck, A.J. *The Diagnosis and Management of Depression*. Philadelphia: University of Pennsylvania Press, 1967.

Bettis, S. Depression: the "common cold" of the elderly. *Generations*, Spring 1979, III:4, 15.

Blazer, D., and Williams, C. Epidemiology of dysphoria and depression in an elderly population. *American Journal of Psychiatry*, April 1980, 137:4, 439–44.

Brock, A. *Greek Medicine*. New York: E.P. Dutton, 1929.

Bureau of the Census. *Demographic Aspects of Aging and the Older Population in the United States.* Current Population Reports: Special Studies, Series 23, No. 59. Washington, D.C.: U.S. Government Printing Office, 1976.

Busse, E. W., and Pfeiffer, E. (Eds.). *Behavior and Adaptation in Late Life.* Boston: Little, Brown, 1969.

Cohen, G.D. Approach to the geriatric patient. *Medical Clinics of North America,* July 1977, 61:4, 855–66.

Fahey, C.J. *Annual Report to the President—1981.* Washington, D.C.: Federal Council on Aging, 1981.

Farber, M.L. *Theory of Suicide.* New York: Funk & Wagnalls, 1968.

Federal Council on Aging. *Mental Health and the Elderly Recommendations for Action.* DHEW Publication No. (OHDS) 80-20960. Washington, D.C.: U.S. Government Printing Office, 1980.

Freedman, N., Bucci, W., and Elkawitz, E. Depression in a family practice elderly population. *Journal of the American Geriatric Society,* June 1982, 30(6):372–77.

Freyhan, F. *Letter to Readers.* Bulletin No. 1. International Committee for Prevention and Treatment of Depression, Washington, D.C., May 1979.

Gage, F.B. Suicide in the aged. *American Journal of Nursing,* November 1971, 71:2153–55.

Galton, L. *Don't Give Up on an Aging Parent.* New York: Crown 1975.

Gurland, B.J. The comparative frequency of depression in various adult age groups. *Journal of Gerontology,* 1976, 31:283–91.

Klerman, G. Clinical research in depression. *Archives of General Psychiatry,* 1971, 24:305–19.

Kreitman, N, Sainsbury, P, Pearce, K, and Costain, W.R. Hypochondriasis and depression in out-patients at a general hospital. *British Journal of Psychiatry,* 1965, 111:607.

Lehman, H. Epidemiology of depressive disorders. In Fieve, R. (Ed.), *Depression in the 70's.* Princeton, N.J.: Excerpta Medica, 1971.

Levitt, E.E., and Lubin, B. *Depression: Concepts, Controversies and Some New Facts.* New York: Springer, 1975.

Lidz, T. *The Person.* New York: Basic Books, 1968.

Litman, R.E. The depressed and suicidal patient. Keynote address, proceedings of a Symposium presented by the University of Arkansas for Medical Sciences. Nutley, N.J., Roche Labs: 1981.

Miller, M. Geriatric suicide: The Arizona study. *Gerontologist,* 1978, 18:488–95.

National Center for Health Statistics. *Advance Report, Final Mortality Statistics, 1975,* February 11, 1977.

National Council on Aging. *Fact Book on Aging.* Washington, D.C.: National Council on Aging, 1978.

National Institute on Aging. *Our Future Selves, a Research Plan Toward Understanding Aging.* DHEW Publication No. 77-1096. Washington, D.C.: U.S. Government Printing Office, 1977.

Neugarten, B. *The Old and the Young in Modern Societies.* In, Shanas, E. (Ed.), *Aging in Contemporary Society.* Beverly Hills, Calif.: Sage, 1970.

Newsweek. Growing old, feeling young. November 1, 1982.

Redick, R.W., Kramer, M., and Taube, C.A. Epidemiology of mental illness and utilization of psychiatric facilities among older persons. In Busse, R.W., and Pfeiffer, E. (Eds.), *Mental Illness in Later Life.* New York: American Psychiatry Association, 1972.

Renshaw, D.C. Depression in the 1970's. *Diseases of the Nervous System,* June–July 1973, 34:244.

Rosenfeld, A.H. *New Views on Older Lives,* DHEW Publication No. (ADM) 78-687. Washington, D.C.: U.S. Government Printing Office, 1978.

Schaie, K.W., and Birren, J.E. *Handbook of the Psychology of Aging.* New York: Van Nostrand Reinhold 1977.

Schwab, J.J. Psychosocial medicine and the contemporary scene. *Comprehensive Psychiatry,* 1971, 12(1):19–26.

Streib, G. *Old Age and the Family: Facts and Forecasts.* In Shanas (Ed.) *Aging in Contemporary Society.* Beverly Hills, Calif.: Sage, 1970.

Time. The need for new myths. January 17, 1972, p. 34.

Weissman, M.M., and Myer, J.K. Affective disorders in a U.S. community: the use of research diagnostic criteria in an epidemiologic survey. *Archives of General Psychiatry,* November 1978, 35:1304–11.

Whittier, J.R., and Korenyi, C. Selected characteristics of aged patients: a study of mental hospital admissions. *Comprehensive Psychiatry,* 1961, 2:113.

Whybrow, P.C. Evaluating and treating severe depression. *Consultant,* January 1978, 18:134–39.

World Health Organization. *Mental Health Problems of Aging and the Aged.* Sixth Report of the Expert Committee on Mental Health, World Health Organization Technical Report Series, No. 171. Geneva, Switzerland: World Health Organization, 1961.

2

The Diagnostic Dilemma

G. Maureen Chaisson-Stewart

There are many reasons why depression is difficult to diagnose. The constellation and severity of its symptoms vary from one person to the next. Its vegetative symptoms mimic other physical ailments with which it is often confused. Sometimes it can be a precursor of a genuine physical illness, and often it accompanies illness as a psychological reaction to perceived losses in physical health. The psychological tests used to identify and measure the severity of depression have inherent and sometimes unavoidable weaknesses in structure, validity, and reliability. Until recently there have been no objective laboratory tests that could be used to assess the physiological changes uniquely manifest in depression. Still, tests like the dexamethasone suppression test (DST) and the thyroid releasing hormone (TRH) stimulation test are new and not widely known or utilized (see Chapter 5).

In the absence of definitive signs and unambiguous data, the diagnostician must rely heavily upon the patient's report of psychological as well as physical discomfort. However, many depressed individuals do not recognize their depression and, therefore, are unable to report it. Even significant others may misperceive it and view it simplistically and judgmentally. Dysphoria is called "grouchiness," "hostility," or "ill-humor." The depressively fatigued person is considered lazy or unmotivated. The person who speaks too often about the persistent, discomforting physical components of depression is thought to be a bore, a chronic complainer, or a hypochondriac.

Rarely do the depressed elderly recognize their depression for what it is and report it as such. Yet, some who do recognize it are reluctant to report it because of the stigma that they associate with any mental weakness. Consequently, when the data are absent, withheld, or skewed in the patient's historical reporting, it is only a professional's perceptive and

18

persistent searching for clues within the context of a trusting therapeutic relationship that will uncover a hidden and unrecognized depression.

This chapter reviews a few of the problems of diagnosis that have caused depression to be the most prevalent yet most missed or inaccurately diagnosed problem in the elderly. By being forewarned, it is hoped, professionals will be better able to avoid these pitfalls in the future. Misdiagnosis leads to mistreatment and, unfortunately, a tragic and needless decline in the mental health status of the elderly. What we need instead is accurate and early diagnosis.

PSYCHOLOGICAL TESTING METHODS

Psychological methods used in assessing and diagnosing depression have their own inherent problems. Commonly used psychological assessment tools include symptom checklists, structured and unstructured psychiatric interviews, and even computerized interview techniques. A major use of these instruments, especially in research settings, is for evaluating the effects and impact of various treatments (Raskin, 1979). They can also be used in clinical practice to determine the existence and extent of depression in the client. No matter which assessment method is used, the clinician and researcher ought to consider the unique weaknesses and strengths of each instrument before deciding which one to use and how to interpret the results. This section will include a brief overview of some of the problems with the most frequently used measures of depression—self-report inventories and interviews—with special emphasis on the special problems that occur when they are used with an elderly population.

For a more thorough discussion of the assets and liabilities of the major classes of depression measures, see Table 2.1 and Chapter 5, which provides a detailed and thorough analysis of current neuropsychological tools for assessing psychological dysfunction in the elderly.

Self-Report Inventories

Self-report inventories have an inherent, unavoidable liability: a tendency to induce a negative response set (Hughes et al., 1982). The patient may purposely deceive the tester with socially desirable or otherwise erroneous answers: "Denial of symptoms, especially feelings of depression, anxiety and hostility is quite common in older persons" (Raskin, 1979). For this reason, some testers use ratings by significant others (Katz and Lyerly, 1963) or tests that measure an individual's tendency to give socially desirable responses (Crowne and Marlowe, 1959) to assess the reliability and validity of the respondent's answers.

Some elderly people may be confused by some of the terms used in rating scales. If someone is not readily available to clarify the meanings intended or to answer their questions about particular items, they are

TABLE 2.1

EXAMPLE INSTRUMENTS, ASSETS AND LIABILITIES OF THE MAJOR CLASSES OF
DEPRESSION MEASURES

Class	Example Instrument	Assets	Liabilities
Self-report inventories	Beck Depression Inventory	Inexpensive Ease of administration Assessment of subjective symptoms	Cultural and subjective response bias Voluntary deception
Self-monitoring	Hersen and Bellack	Multiple assessment of target behaviors	Reactivity Selection effects
Ratings by significant others	Katz Adjustment Scale	Naturalistic observation of functional and interpersonal behavior	Reliable raters often unavailable Deception and/or bias by raters
Clinician ratings	Hamilton Rating Scale	Sensitivity Professional knowledge utilized	Interrater reliability poor Generalization outside interview questionable
Ward observations	Brief Psychiatric Rating Scale	Seminaturalistic observation by paraprofessionals	Generalization questionable Inadequate description of depressive behavior

Source: Hughes, J.R., O'Hara, M.W., and Rehm, L.P. Measurement of depression in clinical trials: an overview. *Journal of Clinical Psychiatry*, March 1982, 43:3, 85–88.

likely to leave the item blank or may respond on the basis of an inaccurate assumption about its intended meaning. As John Hughes and his colleagues (1982) noted:

> Self-report tests rely on the assumption that the definitions of terms such as "mood," "guilt," and "pessimism" are stable across subjects. The definitions of many psychological terms vary across groups of different cultures and socioeconomic status (and age cohort). Even within sociological groups, personal definitions of psychological terms change across time both quantitatively and qualitatively as a person becomes more depressed.

Sometimes the instruments used to assess depression in the elderly were standardized on a young adult population and never validated on an older age group. For example, the original Beck Depression Inventory (BDI) was validated on subjects ranging in age from 15 to 44 years (Beck et al., 1961).

To compound the problem, many of the self-report inventories used to identify and quantify the severity of depression include items inquiring

TABLE 2.2

SOME EFFECTS OF PHYSICAL ILLNESS SYMPTOMATOLOGY ON RESPONSES TO BDI

BDI Item			Characteristic of Illnesses That May Inflate Score
J.	(Self-image Change)		Disfiguring illness
	3 ___ ×	I feel that I am ugly or repulsive looking.	
	2 ___	I feel that there are permanent changes in my appearance and they make me look unattractive.	
	1 ___	I am worried that I am looking old or unattractive.	
	0 ___	I don't feel I look any worse than I used to.	
K.	(Work-Difficulty)		Painful illness
	3 ___	I can't do any work at all.	Debilitating illness
	2 ___ ×	I have to push myself very hard to do anything.	
	1 ___	It takes extra effort to get started at doing something.	
	0 ___	I can work about as well as before.	
L.	(Fatigability)		Debilitating illness
	3 ___	I get too tired to do anything.	
	2 ___	I get tired from doing anything.	
	1 ___ ×	I get tired more easily than I used to.	
	0 ___	I don't get any more tired than usual.	
M.	(Anorexia)		Painful illness
	3 ___ ×	I have no appetite at all any more.	Debilitating illness
	2 ___	My appetite is much worse now.	
	1 ___	My appetite is not as good as it used to be.	
	0 ___	My appetite is no worse than usual.	

about physical symptoms or vegetative signs of depression. Given that this population has a high incidence of chronic health problems, an item related to physical manifestations of disease can inflate figures falsely. For example, in the Zung Depression Status Inventory (DSI) a patient who has experienced recent weight loss due to a physical illness might receive a higher depression score on item 7 (weight loss) if the nature of the weight loss was not explored with the patient in a supplementary interview. Also, while either weight loss or weight gain (in short, any recent change in weight) can be a symptom of depression, the DSI only allows for weight loss.

People experiencing disfiguring, debilitating, and painful illnesses are apt to score high on the last four items in the BDI (short-form), which relate to self-image, work-difficulty, fatigability, and anorexia. As shown in Table 2.2, their answers to these items may be more a measure of the effects of their physical illness than of depressive symptomatology.

In criticizing the somatic skewness of self-report inventories, Zemore (1979) went so far as to conclude that the aged were no more depressed than young adults. He drew this conclusion because, when he extracted somatic complaints from the BDI in his study of a depressed elderly sample, the young adult scores on the remaining items were not statistically different from the scores of the aged.

While the problems of detecting and measuring depression with rating scales are many, they can be exceedingly useful screening devices to obtain preliminary data about the overall mood state of the patient. The proper and appropriate use of these and other tests to measure depression and differentiate from organic brain disease are covered thoroughly in Chapter 5.

Interviews

When depression is rated in a structured interview, which suggests structured questions to be addressed to the patient but leaves the final rating to the judgment of the interviewer, the biases of the interviewer are likely to distort his or her ratings of the patient. Also, no matter how structured the interview, the interviewer's style of interaction and expertise as an interviewer can affect the results. Or there may be interviewer-interviewee interaction distortions—the interviewer unknowingly cueing the patient to respond in a certain way, for example. The interviewer's sex, age, and appearance can either discourage or encourage self-disclosure on the part of the interviewee, depending upon the patient's preconceived notions and personal biases. Age of the interviewer especially may evoke emotionally skewed responses in the elderly subject, depending upon their personal biases related to generational differences.

Sometimes interviewers find it difficult to establish and maintain rapport with an elderly depressed patient, a prerequisite for a successful interview. As Allen Raskin (1979) has explained:

> It has been demonstrated that elderly individuals often have limited attention spans, decreased tolerance for ambiguity, a distaste for mechanical gadgetry, such as stop watches, and impatience or anger with test items or questions that they view as irrelevant to their daily lives.

Elderly patients can be offended by the intrusive nature of items that inquire about their libido and current enjoyment of sex, especially if they have never been married or are widowed.

The aged who have sensory losses in hearing and sight may have special difficulty in responding accurately to questions in written or verbal form, yet test constructors often fail to take this factor into account. For this reason it is advisable to redo all questionnaires and self-report inventories in large type and have a resource person available at the time of testing to answer the respondent's questions or even read items to the respondent. Even with this precaution, some elderly people who have difficulty accepting their hearing loss may 1) deny that they have one and 2) respond in the affirmative to questions rather than reveal their hearing deficit and lack of understanding. To avoid this likelihood, hearing tests are often requested as part of a recommended preliminary complete physical examination.

Finally, since the elderly tend to show a considerable amount of variability in their level of functioning and performance from day to day, depending upon the day, a sole testing may not be valid. For this reason, multiple testings over time are recommended (Raskin, 1979) to establish true deficits and to get some fix on intraindividual differences in test performance.

DIAGNOSTIC DISCREPANCY

"The intriguing differences in the incidence of depression and schizophrenia in the United States and the United Kingdom have been known for many years," Levitt and Lubin (1975) commented in citing the research of Kramer (1965). The question of whether the differences between the two countries in their reported rates of depression are the result of actual differences or a function of systematic, cross-national variations in diagnostic practices waited until 1964 to be addressed in the project titled "Diagnosis of Mental Disorder in the United States and United Kingdom," funded by the National Institute of Mental Health. The project's director was the distinguished emeritus professor of psychology at Columbia University and chief of psychiatric research for the New York State Department of Mental Hygiene, Joseph Zubin.

To quote B. J. Gurland's (1976) report of the study:

> The Cross-National Project for the Study of the Mental Disorders in the United States and the United Kingdom has studied and compared diagnoses made by some American and British psychiatrists on patients in the adult and elderly age range. The clinical conditions of the patients were held constant between the two countries (1) by classifying the patients into diagnostic or symptom categories based on cross-nationally reliable assessments by project staff, or (2) by showing videotapes of the same series of patients to audiences of psychiatrists in the two countries. There were substantial cross-national disagreements on the diagnosis of many of the patients studied, including the fact that the [*British psychiatrists were more likely to diagnose affective disorders than were their American colleagues.*] . . . A further analysis of age and diagnoses along the same lines showed that even when the clinical condition of the patients was held constant across the

age groups, the public hospital psychiatrists in both countries [*tended to diagnose affective disorders more often in the middle age range (35–59 years) than in older or younger patients.*] In the younger age group there was a bias in favor of the diagnosis of schizophrenia and [*in the older age group this bias was in favor of a diagnosis of organic disorder.*] The latter bias may be compounded by the tendency of the elderly depressed subject to readily admit to difficulty with his memory, even when formal testing of memory functions shows no impairment.

In summary, this study reveals that, compared to their London counterparts, psychiatrists in New York hospitals had a much narrower concept of depression. In addition, they discovered that the rate of chronic organic brain syndrome diagnosed among elderly first admissions to mental hospitals in the United States was almost twice that reported in the United Kingdom. However, when consistent classification methods were used cross-culturally, the incidence of depression in the U.S. increased. These results indicate that the diagnostic discrepancy between the two countries was an artifact resulting from divergent diagnostic practices (Rosenfeld, 1978), with hospital psychiatrists in the U.S. tending to misdiagnose depression (Levitt and Lubin 1975).

PHYSICAL OR PSYCHOLOGICAL PROBLEM

Because of the overlap in symptom constellations and the frequent coexistence of depression and physical illness, it sometimes can be difficult to distinguish between the two or determine which is the root problem. Differential diagnosis becomes a real dilemma.

Research reveals that 20–50 percent of medical patients with the constellation of somatic symptoms of insomnia, anorexia, decreased libido, and constipation were found to have depressive illness (Kreitman et al., 1965; Pilowsky et al. 1969). Burvill (1971) estimates that a psychopathological disturbance is present but is overlooked in as many as 50 percent of any group of medical and surgical patients. This situation is especially prevalent in the geriatric population.

According to Schwab et al. (1965, 1966), hospitalized patients frequently manifest symptoms of depression. This conclusion resulted from a study of unselected general hospital admissions whose depression was measured with five indexes: the clinicians' diagnosis, the psychiatrists' ratings of the patient's protocols, the scores on the Beck Depression Inventory, the Hamilton Rating Scale, and the Affective Statement Index. Nearly all of these general medical patients reported the presence of one or more of the psychological symptoms usually included in the depression syndrome, as shown in Table 2.3 (Schwab et al., 1966) as well as somatic symptoms of depression, as shown in Table 2.4 (Schwab et al., 1965). Of the 153

TABLE 2.3

PSYCHOLOGICAL SYMPTOMS OF
DEPRESSION FOUND IN GENERAL
MEDICAL PATIENTS

Symptom	Percentage of Patients
Irritability	78
Anxiety	75
Depressed mood	50
Crying	36
Loneliness	36
Guilt	31
Feelings of dissatisfaction	29
Pessimism	25
Indecisiveness	22
Helplessness	22
Self-hate	18
Feelings of failure	15
Suicidal thoughts	14
Feelings of being punished	10
Hopelessness	7

Source: Schwab, J.J., Bialow, M.R., Clemmons, R.S., and Holzer, C.E. The affective symptomatology of depression in medical in-patients. *Psychosomatics*, August 1966, 7:214–17.

hospitalized subjects in the study, 29 patients were found to be in the positive range for depression on at least three of the five indexes.

When the somatic symptomatology of the 29 clinically depressed patients was compared with the somatic symptomatology of the remaining 124 patients, significant differences between the depressed and nondepressed group emerged. In the depressed group, six of the somatic complaints (fatigue, insomnia, upper gastrointestinal distress, anorexia, lower gastrointestinal complaints, and headaches) tended to appear in clusters; at least 80 percent of the depressed patients had at least four of the six complaints as shown in Table 2.5. However, the most striking differences between the depressed and nondepressed groups were found for severe insomnia and severe anorexia, making these two symptoms of particular value in differentially diagnosing a true depression from symptoms of physical illness.

Just as physical illness can mimic depression and vice versa, physical illness may also cause a depression-like syndrome. Depression that is organic in origin can originate with a full-blown illness or just a chemical imbalance in the body. A number of temporary reversible disorders may precipitate a depressive syndrome. These illnesses include malnutrition,

TABLE 2.4

OCCURRENCE OF PHYSICAL SYMPTOMS OF DEPRESSION
AMONG GENERAL MEDICAL PATIENTS

Symptoms	Percentage of Patients
Fatigue, lethargy	70
Insomia	68
Upper gastrointestinal disturbances (indigestion, etc.)	52
Headache	42
Anorexia	40
Lower gastrointestinal disturbances (constipation)	39
Recent weight loss	32
Chest tightness or pain	29
Tachycardia	29
Generalized pain	22
Recent loss of libido	21
Urinary disturbances (frequency, dysuria)	21

Source: Schwab, J.J., Clemmons, R.I., Bialow, M., Duggan, V., and Davis, B. A study of somatic symptomatology of depression in medical in-patients. *Psychosomatics,* 1965, 6:273–77.

anemia, diabetes, generalized infection, myocardial infarction, and thyroid disorder (Jacobson, 1968).

Depression can also be a response to the loss perceived to accompany illness, hospitalization, and/or an unfavorable diagnosis. Also, "A disabled person may be a depressed patient whose illness and impairment is aggravated and exaggerated by the mental disorder it evokes" (Goldfarb,

TABLE 2.5

SOMATIC SYMPTOMS CLUSTERED

Number of the Most Common Symptoms	Depressed, N = 29 (%)	Nondepressed, N = 124 (%)
6	21	4
5	35	12
4	24	15
3	14	31
2	0	16
1	3	16
0	3	6

Source: Schwab, J.J., Clemmons, R.I., Bialow, M., Duggan, V., and Davis, B. A study of somatic symptomatology of depression in medical in-patients. *Psychosomatics,* 1965, 6:273–77.

1967). Nevertheless, the basic diagnostic question remains: Which came first?, or, what is the basic cause of the depression? The answer to this question dictates the treatment.

The basic diagnostic question about causation is further complicated by new research findings that indicate that whereas physical illness can precipitate a depression, the converse can also be true: depression can be the precursor of a physical illness (see Chapter 4). Ultimately, perhaps the only answer to the similarities and close causative links between depression and physical illnesses is to *consider depression as a potential aggravating factor or underlying cause in every physical illness.*

DEPRESSION IN THE DIAGNOSTIC WORK UP

There are other confounding elements in diagnosing depression in the elderly. Like many chronic illnesses and organic brain syndromes (OBS), depression is an age-related illness—that is, the incidence of depression increases with age. Consequently, diagnosticians who exclude depression in their lists of potential diagnoses in an elderly patient, either because they are unaware of its prevalence or because they consider it to be a normal characteristic of senesence, are bound to misdiagnose depression as either organic brain syndrome or some other known or unknown chronic physical ailment.

When the elderly are viewed stereotypically, other symptoms that are diagnostic of depression, such as constipation, insomnia, fatigue, and decreased libido, are written off as problems of advancing age. Irritability can be viewed as "cantankerousness" in an older person.

One physician, who did not consider depression in his diagnostic work-up, informed a depressed 73-year-old man that the results of the extensive laboratory and x-ray tests he had undergone were negative. In interpreting these negative results to the patient, the physician stated that there were two possible explanations for his symptoms of weakness, lethargy, and poor appetite—either there was absolutely nothing wrong with him or, more likely, his physical illness was not yet severe enough to manifest clear symptoms that would differentiate it from other similar illnesses. In other words, the patient was told to go home and either believe that he was physically well or wait to get sicker—a depressing prospect for a depressed and anxious man. Those alternatives are likely to convert a depressed patient with a pessimistic outlook into a hypochondriac. Such patients vigilantly monitor their every body function lest they miss the allusive identifying sign of a masked or rare illness.

TERMINOLOGY OF DEPRESSION

The terminology of depression can be confusing. A person who reports feeling "depressed" may be describing any or all of the following: a

TABLE 2.6
CHANGES FROM NORMAL TO DEPRESSED STATE

Items	Changes	
	Normal State	Depressed State
Stimulus	Response	
Loved object	Affection	Loss of feeling, revulsion
Favorite activities	Pleasure	Boredom
New opportunities	Enthusiasm	Indifference
Humor	Amusement	Mirthlessness
Novel stimuli	Curiosity	Lack of interest
Abuse	Anger	Self-criticism, sadness
Goal or drive	Direction	
Gratification	Pleasure	Avoidance
Welfare	Self-care	Self-neglect
Self-preservation	Survival	Suicide
Achievement	Success	Withdrawal
Thinking	Appraisal	
About self	Realistic	Self-devaluating
About future	Hopeful	Hopeless
About environment	Realistic	Overwhelming
Biological and physiological activities	Symptom	
Appetite	Spontaneous hunger	Loss of appetite
Sexuality	Spontaneous desire	Loss of desire
Sleep	Restful	Disturbed
Energy	Spontaneous	Fatigued

Source: Beck, A.T., The development of depression: a cognitive model. In Friedman, R., and Katz, M., The Psychology of Depression, Washington, D.C.: Hemisphere, 1974.

temporary mood state, a psychological illness, or a retardation of motor activity. Each use of the term is accurate. However, when one term is used for multiple and differing manifestations of the same problem, it does not allow differentiation of degree or nature of the problem.

It is important at the outset to establish a working definition of depression. Everyone occasionally feels depressed, experiencing a mood of vague dissatisfaction, sadness, boredom, and lethargy. When this mood persists or recurs often to a degree that disrupts normal life, work, and relationships with others, the individual can be considered to be suffering from depression, an affective illness (Mendel, 1972). The specific changes from the normal state that are present in depression have been contrasted by Beck (1974) in a table, reproduced here as Table 2.6.

A person who is truly depressed requires professional help. Self-directed treatment, such as increasing activity or ventilating feelings to others, may effectively bury the depression for a period of time but is hardly a cure. Depression left untreated tends to persist, draining the coping energies not only of the depressed person but also of those with whom he lives, works, and associates.

Grief may be considered to be a subtype of depression but even the categorizing of types of depression has proceeded slowly and with considerable controversy. If grief is incapacitating and abnormally prolonged (beyond six to eight weeks of the acute symptoms), it can progress to a chronic reactive depression. Grief that is of normal duration can help the individual to face a loss and experience and accept feelings of anger and resentment associated with a loss (Mitchell, 1974). According to Alex Comfort (1978), grief is a "common feature of old age. It requires no medication, but support."

The meaning of the term *depression* first evolved at the end of the nineteenth century, when it was primarily applied to psychotic states, then called "melancholia." Both Freud (1856–1939) and Emil Kraepelin (1856–1926) derived their observations from patients who were both depressed and psychotic. In their formulations, they tried to contrast normal sadness from the psychotic depression they called melancholia. The primary symptom of melancholia was agitation. It was an illness that occurred most often in women of menopausal age. In making these distinctions, the main nosological effort in the early twentieth century was aimed at distinguishing psychotic states from nonpsychotic states and then dividing the larger group of psychotic conditions into categories such as schizophrenia and affective disorders.

Over the years the incidence of involutional melancholia has declined either because it never existed as a clinical phenomenon in the first place or, due to shifting theoretical orientations, the classification is no longer useful (Rosenthal, 1968; Beck, 1967). It has also disappeared under the impact of electroconvulsive therapy (ECT) and antidepressant drugs administered at earlier ages (Rosenthal, 1968).

During the 1930s and 40s, according to G. Klerman (1971), there was considerable controversy between the two theoretical schools of depression, the dualists and the unitarists. Because the controversy became so extreme and acrimonious, there was a general reaction to classification systems during the era of World War II. Classification efforts were subsequently revised and in the 1970s that diagnostic criteria for depression were established and incorporated into the Diagnostic and Statistical Manual of Mental Disorders—III (DSM III) of the American Psychiatric Association (1978), which did not take effect as a diagnostic guide until January 1980.

This protracted history of controversy about the most accurate definition of depression may be related to the vague nature of depressive symptoms and the fact that they vary in their clustering from one person to another. After a thorough review and evaluation of both the tested and untested schemas for defining and classifying depression, Levitt and Lubin (1975) concluded that the diagnosis of depression should rest on a primary subjective symptom of expressed mood. They stated: "There may or may

TABLE 2.7
ENDOGENOUS vs. REACTIVE DEPRESSION

Factor	Endogenous	Reactive
Identifiable precipitating stressor	Lacking	Present
Vegetative symptoms	More severe	Less severe
Response to pharmacotherapy and ECT	More responsive	Less responsive
Response to psychotherapy	Less responsive	More responsive

not be associated symptoms, but a case is not diagnosed as depression unless an *expressed mood of depression* is the major symptom." This conception and definition of depression, which depends more upon the individual's felt and expressed mood state than upon other associated or vegetative symptoms, follows the lead of the theoreticians of the U.S.–U.K. project (Gurland, 1976). When depressed mood is not expressed, the diagnosis rests upon symptoms of depressed function, such as physical symptoms, which can be confused with genuine physical illnesses.

The Meyerian or unitary view of depression (Meyer, 1905) is that it varies in degree according to the severity of the symptoms, indications for hospitalization, and legal requirements for commitment (Klerman, 1971). It differs from the dualistic or binary view of depression as an illness of two distinct subtypes: endogenous and reactive, a distinction that was derived from a 1929 paper by Gillespie (1948). These two subtypes have been differentiated according to the factors of 1) degree of vegetative symptoms; 2) presence of a precipitating environmental stressor; and 3) differential response to somatic therapies as shown in Table 2.7 (Rush, 1979).

Another dualistic distinction of types of depression, such as neurotic-psychotic, is unfortunately "often used interchangeably with the endogenous-reactive dichotomy, although psychosis is not the necessary criteria for the endogenous depressive type" (Klerman, 1971, p. 311).

Levitt and Lubin (1975) and others rejected the endogenous-reactive dualistic conceptualization of depression because "there is insufficient empirical data to support the perceived differential response to somatic vs psychotherapy" (p. 135). The main distinguishing factors of vegetative symptoms and precipitating factors, they concluded, may be more related to continuous variables of chronicity and degree of occurrence than to discrete categories or subtypes. These conclusions are compatible with the unitary view of depression, which emphasizes the underlying unity and common features of the illness. It is the view that has been associated with Adolf Meyer and his school of psychiatry and by Menninger in his book, *The Vital Balance* (Klerman, 1971). There is more discussion about the unitary view in Chapter 4.

When they were developing the DSM-III, researchers discovered that certain signs and symptoms clustered together with a high frequency in different groups of patients. These symptom constellations then became the basis for the DSM-III diagnostic categories of depression. R. L. Spitzer, Chief of Psychiatric Research at the New York State Psychiatric Institute, was the chairman of the task force to develop the DSM-III. According to Spitzer (1980), the advantages of the DSM-III over the previous DSM-II are that it 1) uses a descriptive rather than a theoretical approach, 2) uses a multiaxial approach, 3) contains new categories, and 4) deletes outdated categories. Other advantages of this diagnostic system that are especially relevant to the diagnosis of depression in the elderly are 1) it permits the consideration of organic etiology, which as mentioned earlier, is so relevant in depression in an elderly population, 2) it allows for disorders that may coexist or be superimposed upon a depression (such as organic brain syndrome), and 3) it provides a workable definition of grief as an uncomplicated bereavement, not a mental disorder, which can become malignant or dysfunctional if it increases in severity or is overly prolonged.

In the DSM-III, depression appears in three main sections under 1) affective disorders, 2) organic affective syndrome, and 3) adjustment disorders with depressed mood. Of these three sections, the affective disorder section is the largest.

Freedman et al. (1982) have suggested that we go one step beyond the DSM-III classifications for depression and, through research, identify symptom clusters characteristic of depression in the aged. Such data could uncover finer distinctions in the depressive syndrome as it is uniquely manifested in old age in comparison with other age groups. It could potentially differentiate forms of depression unique to specific periods in the aging cycle and, by so doing, yield additional age-related subcategories of depression. With more precise age-related diagnostic schema, one would then be better able to study the evolution of depression during specific periods of the aging cycle. Research by Freedman and colleagues indicates that indeed there are finer distinctions between symptom clusters or superordinate factors in the manifestation of depression in the elderly.

The sample in the Freedman study consisted of 166 patients who visited a family practice clinic for regular examinations. There were 108 women and 58 men ranging in age from 60 to 86, all of whom had a major diagnosis of either arthritis or hypertension, the two most frequent diagnoses in the elderly. The degree of depression that the subjects experienced was measured by the Zung Depression or Status Inventory and a semi structured interviewer-rated inventory administered by the physician. Using Zung's degree-of-depression categories, derived from studies of the general population, one-fourth of the elderly sample in Freedman's study were moderately to severely depressed.

Using factor analysis of the responses to the items on the Zung inventory, Freedman and colleagues found a characteristic depressive syndrome afflicting the elderly subjects only. The syndrome was marked by feelings of emptiness and meaninglessness and was associated with reduced metabolic function. The shape of the curve on this characteristic depressive syndrome suggests the possibility of a developmental geriatric depressive crisis peaking in women between 65 and 69 years of age and in men between 70 and 74. Such a crisis would parallel the emotional crisis of adolescence. More research is needed to determine if such developmental crises do occur at predictable ages in the elderly. If so, they may deserve a separate subclassification under depression. Also, if future research validates these initial findings, one will need to teach the elderly and their caregivers to detect the signs of impending developmental crises and strengthen the person's ability to cope with them.

Despite the new clarity of diagnostic classification schema, the symptoms of depression still remain analagous and confused with other illnesses in the elderly, particularly organic brain syndrome. Differentiation of depression from senile dementia is the last and perhaps the most difficult diagnostic dilemma of the primary care physician or mental health practitioner who lacks both the specialized neurological and psychological testing skill and equipment to definitively distinguish one from the other.

DEPRESSION VS ORGANIC BRAIN SYNDROME

In differentially diagnosing depression and organic brain syndrome, interpretation of diagnostic tests has been a major source of diagnostic error. Scores on the Mental Status Questionnaire (MSQ) (Perlen & Butler, 1971; Kahn et al., 1960), which is the test most frequently used to assess memory and orientation (diagnostic factors in senile dementia) are apt to be either misinterpreted or weighted too heavily as a definitive sign of organically based cognitive dysfunction. According to Strain (1975), a low score on the MSQ does not help differentiate central nervous system disease. Rather, it identifies diminished cognitive capacity, which can be caused by one or a combination of the following:

1. Organic brain syndrome
2. Mental retardation
3. Low intelligence quotient
4. Minimal education
5. Cultural deprivation
6. Poor hearing
7. Myxedema

Short-term memory deficits, revealed in the MSQ and often considered diagnostic of OBS, are frequently exaggerated in depressed persons with normal brain function and minimized in non-depressed persons with altered brain function. In fact, Kahn et al. (1975) reported that the belief that recent memory is more impaired than remote memory in organic brain syndrome is not substantiated empirically. Instead, it is part of the stereotyped thinking that results in inaccurate diagnoses.

The symptoms of disorientation and deficient short-term memory, which many consider to be diagnostic of OBS, may also be present in severe depression and, therefore, provide insufficient evidence to rule out depression. Decreased intellectual functioning to the point where the patient is unable to perform activities of daily living and communicate thoughts in an organized manner is often cited as a distinguishing symptom of OBS. However, cognitive functioning can also be impaired in severe depression. Incidences of poor judgment and shallowness of affect that have been cited as key signs of OBS are also present in the severely depressed. Therefore, any of the aforementioned symptoms that are identified in the interview or from MSQ results and observations are inadequate to differentiate depression from OBS definitively.

The MSQ, although relied upon so heavily in differentiating depression from OBS, oversimplifies; it only measures basic areas of mentation. The modified MSQ (Pfeiffer, 1975), by incorporating consideration of the cultural background and educational attainment of the examiner, reduces some of the bias in the test.

Libow (1977) developed an approach to assessing mental state in the elderly that includes factors such as reasoning, judgment, emotional state, and overall social functions. The technique, which utilizes a mnemonic device FROMAJE (Function, Reasoning, Orientation, Memory, Arithmetic, Judgment, Emotional State), with each letter representing one aspect of mental function, takes a little longer to administer (20 minutes for the unexperienced interviewer and 10–15 minutes for the experienced clinician) than other mental status tests. As a global interview, it yields a global judgment about the patient's overall social function and emotional state which Libow claims is useful. Numerical ratings are included but not generally applied in using the test. Despite improved, more sensitive forms of the MSQ, it still remains inadequate for declaring a diagnostic verdict.

Even tests of cerebral blood flow, which have been used to assess organic brain disease and differentiate it from depression, provide only a rough indication of changes in the brain. Essentially, it is not clear if reduced cerebral blood flow is a sign that either the brain lacks sufficient blood, blood flow is hampered, or the brain has reduced its metabolic demand (e.g., through degenerative loss of neurons) and hence requires less blood flow. Clearly, neither the MSQ nor the cerebral blood flow test is precise enough to discriminate between functional and organic mental processes.

The following case will illustrate the common and inappropriate use and reliance on the MSQ as a diagnostic tool in differentiating depression from organic brain syndrome. The patient was a 73-year-old female who was admitted to the community hospital at her daughter's request by her family physician to ascertain, through a diagnostic work up, the cause for her mother's mental confusion.

Mrs. M was a widow whose husband had managed all of their affairs. She had only household chores and a hobby of painting from which to draw her identity, self-confidence and purpose in life. Each morning on his hospital rounds, the attending physician would enter her room, greet her briefly and, in his usual hurried manner, immediately begin his daily interrogatory routine by repeating in the same staccato sequence: "Where are you? What day of the week is this? Who was the president in 1974?" Already bereft of husband and confidence, her responses to his questions were hesitant, timid, uncertain and, worse, for her diagnosis, incorrect. Her emotional reaction to the questions and the manner of the examining physician as she described it later was, "I dread his visit. I get so nervous when he fires those questions at me that I forget everything and can't think clearly. Sometimes it's just easier to say, 'I don't know'."

Little did this patient know that "I don't know" provided an ounce of data in the search for differentiating diagnostic clues, a search that is extremely difficult when, as in this case, it does not include the probing and more refined neurological and psychological tests that are explained in Chapter 5. The diagnosis in this case was determined from history, the daily MSQ checks, a computerized axial transverse tomography (CT scan), and blood work. After all these costly tests, the final diagnosis remained tentative: OBS. This diagnosis dictated a discharge plan of transferring her to a nursing home on the grounds that her mental confusion was too great to allow her to live independently. Once the diagnosis had been "confirmed," her daughter and son-in-law, whom she described as "greedy," were empowered to declare her incompetent, assume control over her financial affairs, sell her home and belongings, and settle her into a nursing home. With neither money, confidence, nor prior experience at living independently, and bearing a label of "OBS," her chances of ever leaving the nursing home without her daughter's consent and assistance were almost nil.

According to Barry Lebowitz, an expert on psychiatric problems of the aged at the National Institute of Mental Health, some American doctors jump much too quickly to a diagnosis of dementia. Lebowitz collaborated with Robert Hoffman, chief of the medical-psychiatric unit at St. Mary's Hospital in San Francisco, in reassessing 215 elderly patients who were admitted to the hospital between May 1980 and July 1981 with a diagnosis of dementia. They found that 63 percent of the patients were victims of hormonal imbalance, toxic drug reactions or other mental disorders such as depression. Forty-one percent were wrongly diagnosed. Ten of 18 patients with major depression were rediagnosed as suffering from delirium due to such causes as "drug toxicity," cancer, and dementia. The researchers concluded that greater education of physicians in differential diagnosis of these problems in the elderly and a greater use of neurological and psychiatric consultants would help remedy the problem (Hoffman, 1982).

The tragedy of misdiagnosing depression as OBS is that the treatment plan (maintenance of organic function, reality orientation, and prevention of further regression) and caretaker expectations (increasing deterioration and dependency) that follow a diagnosis of OBS can be antitherapeutic for depression. As Leslie S. Libow (1977) has said "One way to insure senility is to misdiagnose a case of reversible cognitive disorder and consequently treat the patient as a case of chronic brain syndrome."

Elderly patients who are depressed require quite the opposite in treatment (vigorous, active structured therapy, socialization, anti-depressant medication) and caretaker expectations (increasing level of performance and independence) if they are to recuperate. Rather than being restricted in their choices and experiencing despair of a better future (inherent with most organic brain syndromes in older age), they need expanded options, strengthened coping skills, and hope for recovery. Essential to their receiving what helps rather than what harms them is a rigorous and scientifically based diagnostic work up. Anne Rosenfeld (1978), in a federal report on this subject, observed,

> Too little time is spent in diagnosing and classifying the mental changes in the elderly. This frequently leads to incorrect categorization of changes as "senility." When the patient has this diagnosis he experiences loss of rights and liberties and is treated as "incompetent." Permanent institutionalization is a likely result.

The alert diagnostician will also be aware that symptoms of both depression and OBS can also be induced by medication. Tricyclic antidepressants can precipitate pseudodimentia. Likewise, reserpine, methyldopa (aldomet), antihistamines, corticosteroids, female hormones, anticancer drugs (e.g., vincristine and vinblastine), antituberculous agents (cycloserine) and minor tranquilizers such as diazapam (Valium) have been implicated as a cause of depression (Strain, 1975). Mild to severe depressive states are also common after withdrawal of amphetamines and other stimulant drugs. A fuller discussion of drugs that may cause rather than cure depression is presented in Chapter 6.

MASKED DEPRESSION

Of all the reasons for a missed diagnosis of depression in the elderly, perhaps the main one is the failure on the part of the physician to keep depression in mind as a diagnostic possibility. Usually depression is only considered if the patient freely verbalizes severe depressive or suicidal thoughts. Most depressed patients will only reveal these thoughts within the context of a secure and trusting relationship, the type of relationship that takes time to develop and is seldom achieved in a cursory examination at the doctor's office. Without such verbalization, it is hard to recognize an older person who is depressed.

Few depressed old people are immediately recognized as depressed by professionals. M. Miller (1978) reported that three-fourths of the men in his sample who killed themselves had visited a physician within the month before their suicides. The results of another study indicate that one in four elderly patients with hypochondriacal symptoms were entertaining suicidal ideas at the time of their admission to the hospital (Garrard, 1973). As Sidney Levin (1963) has noted, "It is not uncommon for relatives or friends of an extremely depressed person who has committed or attempted suicide to remark: 'I didn't even know he was depressed.'" The worst of a hidden depression is when these individuals hide their depression from themselves. A number of factors can encourage the denial process, as described by A. I. Goldfarb (1967):

> This masking may be favored by psychodynamic mechanisms which lead to a variety of complex behavioral patterns categorized as "denial"; by culturally determined excessive tolerance of personal suffering in oneself and others; by ignorance or lack of "sophistication"; by absence of funds, facilities, and personnel for proper care or treatment; and because the community is not ready to acknowledge the sociomedical nature of certain problems.

When these denial processes are in effect, detection of depression is doubly difficult. "Sadness or depressed feelings may be expressed only as feelings of emptiness, as an envy of others, or—frustrating to many a clinician—as preoccupation with not feeling well" (Goldfarb, 1967). Even these vague comments of dissatisfaction can be an expression of an underlying depression. Most people do not appreciate how physically debilitating depression can be. They tend to view their physical decline as a purely physical problem and, therefore, need the help of an alert clinician to identify and label the problem for what it is.

In short, "considerable experience is often required before the psychiatrist in training is able to recognize and evaluate the underlying depressive feelings of his patients" (Goldfarb, 1967). If this ability to detect a hidden depression is difficult for the psychiatrist, we must not minimize how difficult it may be for other professionals with less training in the field of mental health. Depressed old persons frequently dress well and neatly, they smile and respond as expected in social situations. In short, they have a lifetime of rehearsing a facade of well-being while underneath they may be aching with a depression that drains their energy and will to live.

Some professionals who recognize the signs of depression in the elderly may be unable to initiate discussion of the problem with the person because of their own prejudices or fears. If they view the elderly person as a parent figure, they may fear that the reaction to discussion of mental problems may be anger, a reaction expected from their own parents if they were to suggest that they had a mental health problem. Questioning the life-satisfaction of parent-figures may be as delicate or taboo a subject to the professional as questioning the sexual satisfaction of their parents. Their fear is that the elderly will take offense or misinterpret their comments as an accusation that they are crazy or cannot handle life. Yet, by not encouraging the old person to recognize depression for what it is, such professionals reinforce the greatest obstacle toward resolution of the problem—denial. By hesitating to suggest to elderly patients the same type of counseling assistance that they would favor for a young adult who is depressed, they deny them the help they need to resolve the problem.

In a study of 50 moderately depressed elderly people (Chaisson, 1984), it was found that the subjects' reaction to the recognition and labeling of their depression was quite the opposite of what many professionals fear. When the problem was openly identified and discussed, most experienced great relief in 1) understanding the nature of their discomfort; 2) knowing there was something they could do about it; and 3) realizing there was some hope for resolution.

HYPOCHONDRIASIS—A SMOKE SCREEN

Depressed patients who ground their depression in somatization are even less likely to appear depressed than the nonsomatizing patient. Following the patient's lead, physicians are apt to accept physical symptoms as pointers to an obscure disease, and the depressed mood, if it is noticed, is considered secondary to a physical illness or indeterminate diagnosis (Krietman et al., 1965).

If the elderly follow the patterns of hypochondriacs in the study by Krietman et al., one can expect that the most common sites of their distress will be the head, abdomen, and chest and the most common complaints will relate to the alimentary and musculoskeletal system. The subjects in the study were 21 patients with depressive disorders who were referred to a special hypochondriasis clinic after prolonged general medical investigation. They were compared with a matched control group of patients with the same diagnosis but with no somatic symptoms, and the differences between the groups were analyzed in an attempt to ascertain the factors responsible for the somatizing process. For some, the statement, "I am ill," seemed to signify, "I am in some kind of distress, but have learned no language other than my body by which to convey this."

The elderly frequently describe their discomfort as a physical rather than a mental or emotional problem. The present cohort of elderly grew up in an era in which psychological problems or treatments were not in vogue. In fact, many elderly who have not been educated to know otherwise still believe that psychological problems are a sign of weakness and may be hereditary. As such, these problems are stigmatizing and shameful. Those who have this attitude are more apt to focus on the physical symptoms of depression, which are usually present in some form, and seek a medical cure for their discomfort. Consequently, a large proportion of the depressed elderly population truly believe and want to be told that their problem is physical rather than psychological.

In some cases, somatic symptoms may provide the mechanism, for an old person who fears being alone, to lock a spouse or other family members through guilt into unhappy, neurotically dependent relationships. Many go to great lengths to deny or hide their psychological distress from an unsympathetic spouse. Their fear is that, once exposed, their psychological problems may give their spouse a reason for discounting their worth or, even worse, rejecting them as a worthwhile companion.

Family members of an elderly hypochondriac are likely to be more fearful of ignoring their physical complaints than are family members of younger hypochondriacs, because the risk that a symptom will ultimately prove to be the "real thing" is greater. Consequently, the family may attend to their elders out of duty and guilt, rather than out of real concern (Herr, 1979). Since the quality of interaction with family tends to be so disease-oriented, relatives are apt to abbreviate the time they spend with them. Aware of the family's withdrawal and fearful of complete abandonment, elderly hypochondriacs are likely to escalate their physical complaints and, with it, their demand for attention. In such cases, aggravated symptoms presented to the diagnosing physician may be more a symptom of dysfunctional family relationships than of an exacerbation of illness. Accordingly, treating physicians will be better able to interpret exaggerated, repetitive physical complaints that lack identifiable organic causes if they are either very well acquainted with the family and its dynamics or if they have data from a behavioral health assessment.

Consultation-liaison or behavioral health services are available in some hospital settings to provide such assessments of hospitalized patients. The advantage of requesting such an assessment during hospitalization is threefold. First, the probability that elderly patients will agree to meet and cooperate with a mental health professional is much greater when they are inpatients than when they are outpatients. Second, hospitalization of patients provides the behavioral health specialist with an opportunity to arrange meetings with family members during their visits and to observe family dynamics, communication patterns, and problem-solving behaviors in vivo. Data derived from such behavioral health assessments can help the physician to achieve a comprehensive understanding of possible motivators and reinforcers in the family that encourage hyponchondriacal reactions. Third, the chances that elderly hypochondriacs will accept counseling after hospital discharge are far greater if they have experienced a supportive, satisfying counseling relationship with a mental health professional during hospitalization than if they are told, as an outpatient, that their problems might be psychologically based and, therefore, they ought to schedule an appointment with a mental health practitioner. In the latter case, the typical, immediate reaction of the elderly is to be deeply offended and then, subsequently, to be angry at the physician's lack of sensitivity and sympathy for their suffering.

While physical investigations of somatic complaints cannot be denied to the complaining patient, they give powerful reinforcements to the patient's fears or beliefs about physical illness and often help to perpetuate a previously nebulous and perhaps transitory concern. However, according to Krietman et al. (1965), it is not the actual procedure that causes the psychological harm so much as the way in which it is explained to the patient.

A physician's explanation that the reported symptoms are "in your head" or are "inconsistent with a diagnosis," leave the hypochondriac feeling discounted, invalidated, and confused. Alternatively, a lengthy diagnostic pursuit of phantom symptoms leaves the hypochondriac anxiously awaiting the breakthrough finding and cure, while, at the same time, it delays exploration of the psychological root of the problem. For most somatizing patients, the realization of the psychological origins of their physical discomfort comes slowly, if at all, through counseling or through their personal experimentation with life-style changes that improve their health and thereby prove to them the connection between stress management and physical well-being.

Somatization, whether it is in the form of hypochondriasis or a psychosomatic illness, can be said to be a strategy for coping with stress in the environment. It is as if the mind and the nervous system convert a conflicted response to stress into either an imagined (hypochondriasis) or real (psychosomatic) symptom. In both cases, the physical signs may be inextricably bound with depression.

DEPRESSION AND PSYCHOSOMATIC ILLNESS

In psychosomatic illness, stressors in the environment are transformed by the nervous system into actual physical disease (Herr, 1979). Whereas in hypochondriasis the physician cannot find physical signs to explain the individual's described symptoms, in psychosomatic illness, the symptoms are either observable or verifiable with diagnostic equipment. In the latter case, the illness cannot be thought of as simply "in the mind" because the body is definitely affected in ways that can be seen and measured, such as high blood pressure, ulcer, colitis, or asthma.

Psychosomatic illness is more likely to occur when the individual has a limited repertoire of coping strategies or when his life circumstances delimit his choices for coping, conditions that frequently exist in the lives of the elderly. The following case illustrates this point.

A 75-year-old woman lived alone for over seven years after the death of her spouse. Her financial resources, which included social security payments and a small monthly income from her husband's pension fund, were limited but sufficient to meet her modest lifestyle. Since her husband's death, she had rebuilt her life around both old and new interests. She had several friends with whom she socialized on a regular basis. The high point of her week was Thursday evenings, when she went to the dance at the Senior Citizen's center. While she missed her husband and had periodic episodes of loneliness, she was essentially satisfied with her single life. Her health during this time was very good.

Toward the end of the seventh year of her widowhood, her only daughter, who lived in San Francisco and who had been a highly successful executive secretary, was in a downward spiral of excessive drinking, loss of self-confidence, and deteriorating job performance. Unmarried and without family or close friends, she felt she had no one to turn to for help. Since her mother had always taught her that home was the place you go to when you need help, she returned to the security of her mother's home when she ultimately lost her job and all her possessions. The re-entry of the daughter, now destitute and dependent, into the mother's life not only brought stress but, with it, constricted coping options for the mother. She began a routine of round-the-clock babysitting for her daughter, to provide her with the companionship that she thought her daughter needed and to police her drinking indirectly by her unremitting presence. As the daughter became increasingly dependent upon her mother and as the mother's options for coping with the situation became more constricted, the mother's health began to deteriorate. The mother saw no end to this depressing situation. Her daughter was offended by her mother's suggestions that she go for counseling. The shame that the mother felt over her daughter's failures and intoxication prevented her from inviting her friends to visit. Thursday night dances were out of the question because of her fear of leaving her daughter alone. Since it was impossible for her to kick her daughter out of the house (she had made her child a lifetime contract of providing succor when it was needed) or to confront her (because it was likely to increase problems by increasing the daughter's drinking), she was stuck psychologically. Two months after her daughter's arrival, the patient began to have severe asthma attacks for the first time in her life. Her breathing worsened, despite aggressive medical treatment to the point where she was admitted to the intensive care unit on the verge of cardiovascular collapse.

With her belief system and parenting promise that "mothers care for their children when they need help, no matter how old they are," this patient left herself with only her body as a vehicle for expressing the stress that she experienced.

As Herbert Weiner (1977) stated: "The balance of three variables may determine whether bronchial asthma or some other illness will occur in a stressful situation." The three variables that were present in this case are the nature and strength of the conflict; defense and coping mechanisms available to the patient; and the extent to which these enable concurrent gratification of certain basic human needs.

In this case, as with many elderly people, the stress is not solely related to their own problems but often is a reaction to the problems of their children over which they have little if any control. The only diagnostic work-up that would tap the psychogenic aspect of the illness would be one that included testing for depression and an evaluation of the patient's stressors and their correlation with the onset of the illness. Particularly important in the elderly is the fact that an evaluation of significant stressors needs to include not only the elderly's own perceived problems but the degree of ownership that they feel of the problems of their children.

REFERENCES

American Psychiatric Association. *Diagnostic and Statistical Manual of Mental Disorders*. Third Edition (DSM-III) Washington, D.C.: APA, 1978.

Beck, A.T. *The Diagnosis and Management of Depression*. Philadelphia: University of Pennsylvania Press, 1967.

Beck, A.T. The development of depression: a cognitive model. In Freedman, R., and Katz, M. (Eds.), *The Psychology of Depression*. Washington, D.C.: Winston, 1974.

Beck, A.T., Ward, C.H., Mendelsohn, M., Mock, J.E. and Erbaugh, J.K. An inventory for measuring depression. *Archives of General Psychiatry*, 1961, 4:561–71.

Burville, P.W. Consecutive psychogeriatric admissions to psychiatric and geriatric hospitals. *Geriatrics*, May 1971, 26:156.

Chaisson, G.M. Cognitive group therapy: training therapists and treating depressed elderly. *Journal of Psychosocial Nursing and Mental Health Services*, May 1984, 22(5).

Comfort, A. *A Good Age*. New York: Simon and Schuster, 1978.

Crowne, D.P., and Marlow, D.A. A new scale of social desirability independent of psycho-pathology. *Journal of Consulting Psychology*, 1959, 23:15–20.

Freedman, N., Bucci, W., and Elkowitz, E. Depression in a family practice elderly population. *Journal of the American Geriatric Society*, June 1982, 30(6):372–77.

Freud, S. *Mourning and Melancholia in Collected Papers*, vol. 4. New York: Basic Books, 1959.

Garrard, R.L. Is your elderly patient talking about suicide? *Consultant*, January 1973, 13:40–50.

Gillespie, R.D. The clinical differentiation of types of depression. Quoted in Abraham, K., *Notes on the Psychoanalytic Investigation and Treatment of Manic-Depressive Insanity and Allied Conditions. Selected papers on Psychoanalyses*. London: Hogarth Press, 1948.

Goldfarb, A.I. Masked depression in the old. *American Journal of Psychotherapy*, 1967, 21(4):791–96.

Gurland, B.J. The comparative frequency of depression in various adult age groups. *Journal of Gerontology*, 1976, 31:283–91.

Herr, J.J. *Counseling Elders and Their Families*. Springer Series on Adulthood and Aging. New York: Springer, 1979.

Hoffman, R.S. Diagnostic errors in the evaluation of behavioral disorders. *Journal of the American Medical Association*, August 27, 1982, 248, 8:964–67.

Hughes, J.R., O'Hara, M.W., and Rehm, L.P. Measurement of depression in clinical trials: an overview. *Journal of Clinical Psychiatry*, March 1982, 43:3, 85–88.

Jacobson, S.B. Geriatric psychiatry today. *Bulletin of the New York Academy of Medicine*, June 1968, 54(6):568–72.

Kahn, R.L., Goldfarb, A.I., Pollack, M., and Peck, A. Brief measures for the determination of mental status of the aged. *American Journal of Psychiatry*, 1960, 117:326.

Kahn, R.L., Zarit, S.H., Hilbert, N.M., and Niederehe, G. Memory complaint and impairment in the aged. *Archives of General Psychiatry*, December 1975, 32:1569–73.

Katz, M.M., and Lyerly, S.B. Methods for measuring adjustment and social behavior in the community: I. Rationale, description, discriminative validity and scale development. *Psychological Reports*, 1963, 13:503–35 (Monograph Supplement IV-V13).

Klerman, G. Clinical research in depression. *Archives of General Psychiatry*, 1971, 24:305–319.

Kraepelin, E. *Manic-depressive Insanity and Paranoia* (reprint of 1921 ed.). New York: Arno, 1976.

Kramer, M. Classification of mental disorders for epidemiologic and medical care purposes: current status, problems and needs. In Katz, M.M., Cole, J.O., and Barton, W.E. (Eds.), *The Role and Methodology of Classification in Psychiatry and Psychopathology*. USDHEW PHS Publication No. 1584. Chevy Chase, Md.: National Institute of Mental Health, 1965.

Kreitman, N., Sainsbury, P., Pearce, K., and Costain, W.R. Hypochondriasis and depression in out-patients in a general hospital. *British Journal of Psychiatry*, 1965, 111:607.

Levin, S. Depression in the aged: a study of the salient external factors. *Geriatrics*, April 1963, 28:302–307.

Levitt, E.E., and Lubin, B. *Depression: Concepts, Controversies and Some New Facts.* New York: Springer, 1975.

Libow, L.S. Senile dementia and pseudosenility: clinical diagnosis. In Eisdorfer, C., and Friedel R., (Eds.), *Cognitive and Emotional Disturbance in the Elderly.* Chicago: Year Book Publishers, 1977.

Mendel, W. Depression and suicide . . . treatment and prevention. *Consultant,* January 1972, 12:115–16.

Meyer, A. A discussion on the classification of the melancholies. *Journal of Nervous and Mental Diseases,* 1905, 32:114.

Miller, M. Geriatric suicide: the Arizona study. *Gerontologist,* 1978, 18:488–95.

Mitchell, R. Advances in psychiatry depression, part 3. *Nursing Times,* July 11, 1974, 70:1085–86.

Perlen, S., and Butler, R. M. Psychiatric aspects of adaptation to the aging process. In Birren, J.E., Butler, R.M., Greenhouse, S.W., Sokoloff, L., and Yarrow, M.R. (Eds.), *Human Aging: A Biological and Behavioral Study.* Publication No. HSM 71-9051. Washington, D.C.: U.S. Government Printing Office, 1971.

Pfeiffer, E. A short portable mental status questionnaire for the assessment of organic brain deficit in elderly patients. *Journal of American Geriatric Society,* 1975, 23:433.

Pilowsky, I., Levine, S., and Boulton, D.M. The classification of depression by numerical taxonomy. *British Journal of Psychiatry,* 1969, 115:937–45.

Raskin, A. Assessing mental health in the elderly. *Generations,* Spring 1979, p. 10ff.

Rosenfeld, A.H. *New Views on Older Lives.* DHEW Publication No. (ADM) 78-687. Washington, D.C.: U.S. Government Printing Office, 1978.

Rosenthal, S. H. The involutional depressive syndrome. *American Journal of Psychiatry,* 1968, 124:21.

Rush, J.A. Cognitive therapy for depression. *Australian and New Zealand Journal of Psychiatry,* 1979, 1391:13–16.

Schwab, J.J., Clemmons, R.I., Bialow, M., Duggan, V., and Davis, B., A study of somatic symptomatology of depression in medical in-patients. *Psychosomatics,* 1965, 6:273–77.

Schwab, J.J., Bialow, M.R.; Clemmons, R.S.; and Holzer, C.E. The affective symptomatology of depression in medical in-patients. *Psychosomatics,* August 1966, 7:214–17.

Spitzer, R.L. *DSM III and Depression.* Studies in Psychiatry, No. 14, audiotape. New York: Roerig Pharmaceutical Co., 1980.

Strain, E.J. *Psychological Care of the Medically Ill: A Primer in Liaison Psychiatry.* New York: Appleton-Century-Crofts, 1975.

Weiner, H.M. *Psychobiology and Human Disease.* New York: Elsevier, 1977.

Zemore, R., Eames, N. Psychic and somatic symptoms of depression among young adults, institutionalized aged and non-institutionalized aged. *Journal of Gerontology,* 1979, 34(5):716–22.

3

Tragedies
of Inappropriate or
Inadequate Treatment

G. Maureen Chaisson-Stewart

Depression is very painful and incapacitating. "It is probably more unpleasant than any disease except rabies. There is constant mental pain and often psychogenic physical pain too," commented John Scott Price (1960). Yet, despite this suffering and the erosion of the quality of their lives, present cohorts of the elderly do not appear for treatment in the offices of mental health professionals. While they comprise 10 percent of the population, only 4 percent of the elderly are treated in outpatient mental health agencies and 1–2 percent are seen in private psychiatric practice (Redick et al., 1972).

The exact reasons for this worrisome lack of interface between the high incidence of depression in the elderly and the mental health services available to them are not clear. This chapter will discuss some of the many proposed explanations for this lack of interface. Critical review of present barriers to treatment is an essential first step. For, no matter how expert our professionals and how effective our treatment methods, if the elderly are not willing candidates for help, there will be no progress in addressing the problem of depression in this age group.

THE ELDERLY—RELUCTANT OR UNAWARE

Older people are less inclined than younger people to define their personal problems as suitable for outside help, either informal or professional. Instead, they tend to define difficulties, especially mental health difficulties, as unchangeable and to stress the individual's responsibility to help himself. The fact that these age differences also tend to persist regardless of education indicates that nonuse of services may be related more to attitude than to a lack of insight or knowledge of services available. In their research, Blazer and Williams (1980) found that depressed subjects had a low expressed need to see a counselor despite their symptomology. In their sample, the actual use of counseling was practically nil. Only 1 percent were receiving treatment. Instead, most of the subjects demonstrated a high need for "nerve medication."

It seems that the majority of the elderly view psychotherapeutic services in a psychoanalytic model. So envisioned, they expect it to be expensive and demanding (requiring visits for an indefinite period of time). When mental health professionals do not make home visits and the only treatment available is at facilities that are difficult to access due to their location, building layout, or parking problems, the barriers to service become insurmountable. Additionally, for many elderly people, the admission of mental health problems and acceptance of mental health services is stigmatizing; entering a mental health treatment facility, especially if it is so labeled, is therefore embarrassing.

If the elderly were educated to correct their negatively biased attitudes toward mental health treatment and if the treatment options were greater, more accessible, and effective within a limited period of time, the cost would still remain a deterrent. One-third of the elderly are below or hover at the poverty line (Federal Council on Aging, 1980, p.13). Since the 1965 passage of the Medicare program, most elderly Americans depend upon that source to finance their health care. Unfortunately, Medicare legislation established policies that discriminate against mental health care.

"Current limitations in Medicare-Medicaid benefits for mental health care—both regarding the extent and types of coverage—have proven to be shortsighted, inequitable, and costly" (Federal Council on Aging, 1980, p. 57). Since Medicare benefits are greater for in-patient care, patients are often hospitalized when outpatient services would be more appropriate and less expensive. The coverage of rehabilitation, outpatient, and day care services, which might be sufficient to maintain many elderly in the community, are so limited that admission to a nursing home, for many, is the only pathway to needed help.

Furthermore, even though nurses, social workers, and psychologists are the most accessible, economical, and available (in numbers and in the places where they are likely to work), and even though these disciplines have demonstrated a keen interest in treating the mental health problems of the elderly in their practice and in the volume of literature they have contributed on the subject, Medicare reimbursement discriminates against them. It is only available to psychiatrists.

Yet, according to Fritz Freyhan (1979),". . . in no country is the number of psychiatrists sufficient to treat all patients suffering from depressions." Therefore, psychiatric expertise should really be reserved for "patients with more serious depressions, which, because of diagnostic problems, risk of suicide, or delayed response to drug treatment, require special therapeutic approaches."

The need for financing mental health services for an elderly population with fixed and limited incomes is clear. The greatest hope for addressing this problem is in the revision of Medicare policies. It is for this reason that the 1980 President's Commission on Mental Health recommended: "In order to improve the availability and accessibility of mental health care for elderly persons, coverage for mental health services must be provided on an equal basis with coverage for physical health care services, for both acute and chronic illness" (Federal Council on Aging, 1980). Specifically, the Commission recommended a reduction of the beneficiary coinsurance from 50 percent to 20 percent—in line with standard Medicare coverage—and increase of the maximum allowable reimbursement for mental conditions to $750 in any calendar year.

No doubt the lack of legislative vigor in righting the mental health care financing wrongs stems from fears that the costs would be exorbitant. But, according to the President's Commission on Mental Health, these fears are unfounded because 1) the elderly have demonstrated a high responsiveness to psychotherapeutic intervention and 2) early and appropriate treatment can prevent further deterioration. As long as mental health care remains unfinanced and therefore unavailable to the majority of elderly, further decline, both mental and physical, is bound to result, ultimately necessitating long-term institutionalization—a far more costly alternative than early treatment of the predisposing mental health problem.

However, even if society and the professional community were to eliminate all of the barriers to treatment, there would still remain a group of elderly who would cling to their depression for the secondary gains that it affords and that are hard to replace. Depression, in general, and hypochondriasis, in particular, have undeniable secondary gains. As I have observed before (Chaisson, 1981),

Some . . . will set up a situation in which their depression serves to get the attention and acceptance from others that has been lacking from parents in the past and from significant others in the present. Such individuals try to captivate others with their misery. They even accuse others of having brought about their misery, thereby emotionally blackmailing them for affection by arousing guilt.

In interviews of depressed, hypochondriacal patients, Krietman et al. (1965) found it "striking how often the patients would start to describe their spouse's personality with the phrase, 'He's good to me when I'm ill.'" They also noted that these patients had poorer marital relationships than the controls.

Illness, which elicits interest and the company of physicians, relatives, and friends, is hard for a lonely person to relinquish. Even though their depression may pollute the home environment and strain the lives of those close to them, and even drive some loved ones away, the elderly may be constrained by depressive inertia from changing their situation without the vigorous intervention of an outside party.

Some may exacerbate the problem by turning to alcohol or drugs for temporary relief. In their study of 103 people over age 65 with drinking problems in England, Rosin, and Glatt (1980) found that reactive depression precipitated by bereavement, retirement, loneliness, and, less frequently, physical infirmity and marital stress, was the most important cause for excessive drinking.

A usual but inadequate means of coping for many is through the door of their primary physician, where they solicit sympathy and pills. As B. A. Stotsky (1972) observes,

> When the elderly are depressed, they lead isolated and constricted lives. Their world closes in on them and they self-limit and avoid exposure to new or different people and situations. They are not apt to venture out into a mental health clinic for the first time in their life. Instead, they continue to visit their family doctor.

THE USUAL SCENARIO OF TREATMENT

An alarming 30 percent rate of depression is high on the list of problems that patients who are over 80 fail to report to their physician, according to a British study which was reported by John Roe to the American Medical Association in 1982. Glaucoma, nutritional deficiencies, ear wax, and visceral problems were also underreported.

When depressed old persons are moved to seek relief from their misery, they usually turn to their personal physician for help. "Most of the mental health care of elderly patients is carried out by family physicians, although in an unsystematic way" (Stotsky, 1972). To their personal physicians, elderly patients usually express their discomfort in physical complaints rather than describing their emotional or psychosocial problems. "They are more likely to talk about their body than their mood" (Cohen, 1977). Why these patients develop physical symptoms that are depressive equivalents rather than overt depressive reactions is not always clear. Some plausible reasons for this occurrence have already been mentioned; others have observed that some of these patients have a past history of earlier physical illness or injury or a model of such symptomatology among relatives. "Such patients seem to be generally unable to admit to any fault within themselves, regarding symptoms of emotional disorder as 'moral weakness'"(Pfeiffer, 1977).

The importance of the primary physician as the gatekeeper is evidenced by the report that approximately 75 percent of depressed elderly persons who eventually killed themselves sought help from a physician shortly before their suicide (Grollman, 1971; Litman et al., 1963). At the same time, much to the frustration of mental health professionals, the tendency of the elderly is not to use crisis intervention services or outpatient community health services. Of the 8,000 initial calls to the Los Angeles Suicide Prevention Center in 1973 and 1974, only 2.6 percent were from people 60 and over (Farberow and Moriwaki, 1975).

In the physician's office, unfortunately, the feeling state of the patient is often not assessed until it is apparent that no clear cut physical cause exists for the symptoms described (Schaie and Birren, 1977). Many physicians who do detect signs of depression think of it as an emotion rather than a disease (*Patient Care*, 1977). Signs of self-neglect and alcoholism may not be seen as signs of an underlying depression. So they give the patient what he asks for—a diagnostic work up for a physical illness or medication.

"Mental depression in the elderly is probably the most frequently overlooked diagnosis of all. When it is noted, it is too often treated with antidepressants at dosage levels that are correct for younger patients but toxic for the elderly" (Lebow, 1977).

Since the introduction of ataractics, antidepressants, and psychomotor stimulants in the 1950s, pharmacological treatment has been the most prevalent of the somatic treatment methods used in geriatric patients (Rosenstein and Swenson, 1980). Unfortunately, however, antidepressants have side effects that aggravate preexisting physical conditions commonly found in the older person (glaucoma, heart irregularities, constipation, and urinary retention). These complicating side effects that are likely to accompany treatment with antidepressants are well-explained by Strain (1975).

> While the side effects that occur with the antidepressants are not more serious than those produced by the other psychotropic drugs, they are more diffuse and, above all, they are *more likely to mimic symptoms of medical and psychological dysfunction.* The psychological symptoms that occur with the antidepressants include confusional states, hallucinations, delusions, disorientation, anxiety, and hypomania. In addition, antidepressant medication may produce such neurological symptoms as numbness, tingling, paresthesia, ataxia, tremor, peripheral neuropathy, seizures, alterations in EEG, and tinnitus. The side effects produced by the antidepressants may, as noted above, mimic medical illness as well, specifically, gastrointestinal disorders, such as constipation, paralytic ileus, anorexia, nausea, vomiting, diarrhea, and abdominal cramps. Or they may produce more diffuse physiological symptomatology, such as fluctuations in

weight, dizziness, weakness, fatigue, perspiration, altered blood sugar, and headache. (italics by author)

Consequently, even though the antidepressants may provide some symptomatic relief from the depression, they also create more stress in the form of physical problems in individuals who are already overstressed.

Some elderly people are sufficiently depressed to require institutionalization. However, in the last 25 years, the pattern of institutionalization of the seriously demented elderly has changed. Under a philosophy of "mainstreaming"—an attempt to reintegrate institutionalized persons back into the society—many elderly have been transferred from institutional care settings to community settings. Between 1960 and 1976, there was a 245 percent increase in the number of nursing home residents, while the number of elderly residing in mental hospitals decreased from 37 to 8 percent. Another large percentage live in boarding homes or foster care facilities where little ongoing care is provided and supportive services are rare. Finally, only 15 percent of patients over 65 who are discharged from state mental hospitals are referred to outpatient psychiatric clinics.

This shifting pattern of institutionalization of the elderly with mental disorders placed a new demand upon nursing home personnel to manage a high incidence of psychological problems of their patients, a demand that was not planned for in the original mission of nursing homes. Since the staff in most nursing homes are trained and hired to provide custodial care for patients, few are prepared to individually or programmatically treat the mental health problems of their patients. Consequently, few of the depressed institutionalized elderly, who live in conditions that are conducive to mental illness, will ever receive any form of counseling or treatment.

PROFESSIONALS—BIASED OR UNPREPARED

Physicians, the helpers to whom the elderly reach out most often in their distress, too often underestimate the healing potential of their acceptance, attentive listening, and understanding responses to elderly patients. "Such listening is not only the way to arrive at a proper diagnosis of the problems, but it gains the old person's confidence and thus is the first big step toward solving the problems. . . . Herein lies the quintessence of the art of medicine" (Kern, 1971). "Physicians ought to be more aware that they are themselves powerful remedies, more powerful than any drug in the pharmacopoeia. This is something the old family doctor understood; often having little else to prescribe, he prescribed himself" (Galton, 1975).

Relating therapeutically to a patient takes time, and when time equates with money in a busy somatically oriented medical practice, it is less likely to be a high priority. When physicians lack the time, interest, or skills to intervene psychotherapeutically, it is time for a referral to a mental health professional. However, the usual scenario of current practice seldom ends with a referral of a depressed old person to a mental health professional. Stotsky (1972) noted that most psychological treatment of elderly patients is conducted by family physicians and that psychiatric consultation is sporadic and not highly valued by the nonpsychiatric medical profession. Many authors have suggested that an ageism bias of physicians prevents them from recommending psychiatric or psychological treatment for the elderly.

This referral bias was documented by Ginsburg and Goldstein (1974) when they discovered that medical hospital staff referred younger patients with elevated MMPI profiles to psychiatric wards significantly more often than elderly patients with matched MMPI profiles. In another study, Kucharski, et al., (1979) surveyed 60 physicians who listed their specialty in the local telephone book as family practice, general practice, internal medicine, internist, or general surgery. A comparison of the demographic characteristics of the physician sample with the total pool of possible responders listed in the area's Register of Physicians and Surgeons indicated that the responders were representative of the physician population in the area.

Physicians in the sample were asked to indicate what treatment they would recommend for each of the patients whose history was briefly described in eight vignettes. On alternate forms of the questionnaire, the age of the patient was reversed for each vignette. Content analysis of the physician responses revealed that members of the young group were referred for psychological assistance significantly more often than were members of the old group. Of those who were referred for psychological assistance, almost 74 percent of the old group and 75 percent of the young group were referred to a psychiatrist or psychologist. Community mental health centers and in-patient facilities were seldom used as a source of psychological assistance. Of those not referred, old cases were more likely to be sent to a neurologist or other physician, were given no treatment, or were prescribed psychotropic medications without the concomitant attention of a mental health professional. The results of this research support the position of Hoogerbeets and LaWall (1975) that physician bias against referral of elderly patients for mental health assistance may be a significant contributor to the neglect of psychological problems of this population.

If primary care physicians are disinclined to refer elderly patients for mental health services, who does refer the small percentage of elderly who are on the caseload of mental health agencies? A review of the over 2,300 patients referred to a geriatric outreach program in the Seattle-King County community between 1973 and 1977 revealed that families were significantly more likely than other sources to refer demented elderly patients; over one-third of the referrals were in this category (Reifler and Wu, 1982). Health agencies were significantly more likely to refer depressed patients. Apartment managers, on the other hand, were significantly less likely to refer depressed patients, finding them to be unobtrusive, quiet, and untroublesome tenants. None of the referrals were listed as coming from physicians.

The same stereotypic ideas that infect the primary physician's thinking and cause him to overlook depression in his elderly patients, or accept it as a normal accompaniment of aging, are apt also to influence the mental health provider. Just as geriatrics has been a low-prestige specialty in the medical community, so too mental health professionals have preferred young and middle-aged adults over the elderly as clientele for several reasons. First, they are closer in age and, therefore, their problems are easier to relate to, understand, and, supposedly, do something about. Second, many professionals have unwittingly absorbed a prejudicial expectation that the elderly are rigid or mentally deficient and, therefore, not good candidates for change-oriented therapy. Third, there are few approaches, theories, guidelines, or old-age-specific therapies that have been shown, through research, to be appropriately and uniquely effective in treating an elderly population. As a result, professionals feel uncertain and insecure about how best to treat this population. Fourth, few have received special training in working with the elderly.

Rejecting stereotypic attitudes on the part of professionals have been well documented in the literature (Coe, 1966). No doubt they are a contagion from the larger society that does not automatically love and respect the elderly. The terms "ageism" and "gerontophobia" have been coined to describe this phenomena. Ageism (Butler and Lewis, 1977) is the tendency to see abnormality and depression as a normal and expected component of the aging, degenerative process. "Gerontophobia" is a fear of contact and dealing with aging persons (Bunzel, 1972). These negative, rejecting mind-sets compel society to isolate the aged in remote or sequestered places and force them into dependent roles with minimal challenges or expectations of success and/or valued contributions to society. Any group, treated in such a manner, would have to fight doggedly to combat the depressing and debilitating effects of such a negatively weighted feedback process. The elderly must struggle to maintain their self-worth and to fight forces that contribute to an insidious depression. "Of great significance in the etiology of depression and in its persistence, is the resultant loss of self-esteem and the feelings of helplessness about one's life" (Goldstein, 1979).

In a society that measures the worth of its members by their ability to work and contribute economically to the good of the whole, people who have left the work force, such as the retired worker, are accorded a diminished status. Perhaps the seeming lack of concern about the high suicide rate among the elderly in contrast to the higher concern about a relatively lower incidence of suicide among adolescents is due to an economic orientation that "the deaths of such people do not represent a serious loss to the economy" (Miller, 1978).

An example of just how strong an aversion professionals can have for caring for the elderly is revealed by the fact that in England, in response to a circular, many psychiatrists in training indicated that they would rather emigrate than practice psychogeriatrics (Pitt, 1974).

The concerns that influence therapists' interest and willingness to work with the elderly have been summarized by the Group for the Advancement of Psychiatry as follows (GAP, 1971):

1. The aged stimulate the practitioner's fears about his own old age.
2. Elderly patients arouse the practitioner's conflicts about his relationships with parental figures.
3. The practitioner thinks he has nothing to offer old people because he believes that they cannot change their behavior or that their problems are all due to untreatable organic brain disease.
4. The practitioner believes that his skills will be wasted with the aged because they are near death and not really deserving of attention.
5. The patient might die while in treatment, which could challenge the practitioner's sense of importance.
6. The practitioner's colleagues may be contemptuous of his efforts on behalf of aged patients. One often hears the remark that gerontologists or geriatric specialists have a morbid preoccupation with death; their interest in the elderly is considered "sick" or suspect.
7. As mentioned above, a practitioner's myths, stereotypes, and misinformation regarding older people interfere with the recognition of their problems and may preclude a decision to treat.
8. Economic concerns, both real and exaggerated, have provided explanations and excuses for not treating the elderly.
9. The practitioner may be uneasy about the possibility of being overwhelmed by the diversity of the problems an older individual might present.
10. The elderly patient may have problems getting to the practitioner (e.g., physical limitations and transportation difficulties).
11. Cultural insensitivity has slowed community and societal responsiveness to the aged. It was not that long ago that one heard the phrase, "You can't trust anyone over 40."

While many mental health professionals have shied away from the elderly, nurses and attendants in nursing homes have been left to address all their needs, both mental and physical, when the elderly can no longer maintain themselves in the community. Most of the 1.2 million people, or 5 percent of those over 65, admitted to a nursing home do not require extensive or intensive nursing care. The majority simply have a functional dependency in carrying out their activities of daily living. However, since 50–75 percent have a mental or intellectual impairment, their need for psychosocially oriented nursing care is great.

Our society has not been willing to pay the bill to address the psychosocial needs of nursing home residents. Few nursing homes have any mental health professionals that they can call on for help in either a staff or consultant capacity. In the absence of such expert guidance, the nurses are left, usually in inadequate number, to do the best they can. "As long as there is a shortage of personnel, there is a danger of patient care deteriorating. Overburdened staff lose heart, some leave, making the burden heavier and finally only the basic needs of the patient can be catered to" (Whitehead, 1970).

In focusing on their patients' physical needs, "overcare" results. "Our approaches to caring for the aged have tended to the extremes: too little care or too much, with overmedicated and overbedded patients ending their lives in institutions" (Butler and Lewis, 1977). Overcare tends to increase the patient's dependency and undermine their feelings of self-confidence or hope for the future, thereby increasing their depression and mental decline. "They feed them, wash them and too often purge them, but never treat them like adults. Having reduced them to a state of helpless dependency, they criticize them for their regressed behavior." (Whitehead, 1970)

Although inadequate staffing can contribute to this nontherapeutic situation in nursing homes, it is not the sole and sufficient cause for its existence. Institutions with overcare philosophies can be reoriented to better address the psychosocial needs of their residents if staff are themselves supported in their work through ongoing educational programs in geropsychiatry, consultation from mental health professionals and a progressive administrative philosophy that supports staff's creative efforts to shape a therapeutic milieu and policies that are more facilitative than restrictive. In such an environment, conversation, entertainment, group activities, and the patient's individual goals are considered of equal or more importance than carrying out routine nursing tasks. Such a therapeutic milieu is more than staff numbers; it is an attitude or value system. It believes in flexible visiting hours, stimulating and comfortable decor and furnishings, the provision of newspapers, magazines, and books, conversation, asking not telling, allowing for idiosyncrasies, providing money for patients to spend, spectacles to see, hearing aids to hear, dentures to eat, and, overall, respect.

Sad to say, however, buildings change more rapidly in our society than attitudes or level of knowledge of the people providing the care (Clark,

1969). As long as the psychiatric problems of the elderly can no longer be solved by commitment and hiding them away in state hospitals, community service providers and staff of nursing homes need more training and consultation services to assist them in better meeting the psychosocial needs of the elderly. Also, as long as, on the average, 40 percent of an internist's patients are 65 years of age or older, and he spends 60 percent of his time with them, the education of physicians in geriatric medicine and gero-psychiatry needs to be intensified and expanded.

REFERENCES

Blazer, D., and Williams, C. Epidemiology of dysphoria and depression in an elderly population. *American Journal of Psychiatry*, April 1980, 137:4, 439–44.

Bunzel, J.T. Note on the history of a concept-gerontophobia. *Gerontologist*, 1972, 12:116.

Butler, R.N., and Lewis M.I. *Aging and Mental Health*. St. Louis: C.V. Mosby, 1977.

Chaisson, G.M. Depression in the elderly. In Bauwens, E. and Anderson, S. (Eds.), *Chronic Illness: Concepts and Application*. St. Louis: C.V. Mosby, 1981.

Clark, E. Improving post-hospital care for chronically ill elderly patients. *Social Work*, January 1969, 15(1):62–67.

Coe, R. Professional stereotypes hamper treatment of aged. *Geriatric Focus*, September 15, 1966, 15:1–3.

Cohen, G.D. Approach to the geriatric patient. *Medical Clinics of North America*, July 1977, 61(4):855–66.

Farberow, N., and Moriwaki, S. Self-destructive crises in the older person. *Gerontologist*, August 1975, 15:333–37.

Federal Council on Aging. *Mental Health and the Elderly: Recommendations for Action.* The reports of The President's Commission on Mental Health: Task Panel on the Elderly and the Secretary's Committee on the Mental Health and Illness of the Elderly. DHEW Publication No. (OHDS) 80-20960. Washington, D.C.: U.S. Government Printing Office, 1980.

Freyhan, F.A. *Letter to Readers.* Bulletin No. 1, International Committee for Prevention and Treatment of Depression. Washington, D.C., May 1979.

Galton, L. *Don't Give Up on an Aging Parent.* New York: Crown, 1975.

Ginsburg, A., and Goldstein, S. Age bias in referral for psychological consultation. *Journal of Gerontology*, July 1974, 29(4):410–15.

Goldstein, S.E. Depression in the elderly. *Journal of American Geriatric Society*, January 1979, 27(1):38–42.

Grollman, E.A. *Suicide Prevention, Intervention and Postvention.* Boston: Beacon Press, 1971.

Group for the Advancement of Psychiatry. *The Aged and Community Mental Health: A Guide to Program Development*, vol. 8, Series 81. New York: GAP, 1971.

Hoogerbeets, J.D., and LaWall, J. Changing concepts in psychiatric problems of the aged. *Geriatrics*, 1975, 29:83–87.

Kern, R.A. Emotional problems in relation to aging and old age. *Geriatrics*, June 1971, 26(6):93.

Kreitman, N., Sainsbury, P., Pearce, K., and Costain, W.R. Hypochondriasis and depression in out-patients in a general hospital. *British Journal of Psychiatry*, 1965, 111:607.

Kucharski, L.T., White, R.M., and Schratz, M. Age bias: referral for psychological assistance and the private physician. *Journal of Gerontology*, 1979, 34:423–28.

Lebow, L. Statement at the Hearing before the Special Committee on Aging. U.S. Senate, 94th Congress, October 18, 1976. Washington, D.C.: U.S. Government Printing Office, 1977.

Litman, R.E., Curphey, T., Shneidman, E.S., et al. Investigations of equivocal suicide. *Journal of the American Medical Association*, 1963, 184:924–29.

Miller, M. Toward a profile of the older white male suicide. *Gerontologist*, February 1978, 18:80–82.

Patient Care. Treat depression as the curable disease it is. March 1, 1977, 11:20–21.

Pfeiffer, E. Psychopathology and social pathology. In Birren, James C., and Schaie, K.W. (Eds.), *Handbook of the Psychology of Aging*. New York: Van Nostrand Reinhold, 1977.

Pitt, B. *Psychogeriatrics: An Introduction to the Psychiatry of Old Age*. New York: Churchill, 1974.

Price, J.S. Chronic depressive illness. *British Medical Journal*, May 6, 1960, p. 1200.

Redick, R.W., Kramer, M., and Taube, C.A. Epidemiology of mental illness and utilization of psychiatric facilities among older persons. In Busse, R.W. and Pfeiffer, E. (Eds.)., *Mental Illness in Later Life*. New York: American Psychiatric Association, 1972.

Reifler, B., and Wu, S. Managing families of the demented elderly. *Journal of Family Practice*, June 1982, 14(6):1051–56.

Rosenstein, J.C., and Swenson, E.W. *Behavioral Approaches to Therapy with the Elderly: Non-traditional Therapy and Counseling with the Aging*. S. Stansfeld Sargent (Ed.) New York: Springer, 1980.

Rosin, A., and Glatt, M. Alcohol excess in the elderly. *Quarterly Journal of Studies on Alcohol*, 1980, 191, 32(1-A):53–59.

Schaie, K.W., and Birren, J.E. *Handbook of the Psychology of Aging*. New York: Van Nostrand Reinhold, 1977.

Stotsky, B.A. Social and clinical issues in geriatric psychiatry. *American Journal of Psychiatry*, 1972, 129:117.

Strain, E.J. *Psychological Care of the Medically Ill: A Primer in Liaison Psychiatry*. New York: Appleton-Century-Crofts, 1975.

Whitehead, A., *In the Service of Old Age*. Chevy Chase, Md.: Penguin Books, 1970.

4

An Integrated Theory of Depression

G. Maureen Chaisson-Stewart

Depression is a multifaceted, multi-dimensional, multicausal, complex phenomenon. Numerous theorists have attempted to explain the phenomenon from varying perspectives—psychoanalytic, interpersonal, psychosocial, neurochemical, pharmacological, cognitive and/or behavioral—each making a special contribution to a more comprehensive and deeper understanding of the problem in all its complexity.

In the past, there has been some concern that biological etiology meant the deemphasizing of psychological variables as factors in the causation of depression. Rather than viewing biological and psychological frameworks as antithetical, this chapter will present a comprehensive, integrated, and holistic theory of depression that interrelates multiple concepts and constructs of depression previously identified by the major theorists and researchers in the field.

DEPRESSION, A UNITARY PHENOMENON

As explained in Chapter 2, there is insufficient empirical evidence to support the notion that depression is manifested in two main dichotomous clinical types—one a severe, unmitigated mood change (endogenous) and the other a milder, less sustained, and more variable illness (exogenous or reactive). Known as the *binary* view of depression, this framework has been based primarily upon treatment outcome observations; specifically, endogenous depression seems to be more responsive to the somatic therapies, whereas exogenous or reactive depression appears to be responsive to psychotherapy. An alternate conceptualization of these two subclassifications of depression would be to view them on a continuum of illness with the two syndromes represented at the poles of the spectrum or as a single depressive illness with two main variants.

56

The alternate model follows the theory of Adolf Meyer (1905), which was also espoused by the English, primarily in the writings of Sir Aubrey Lewis. It views depression as a psychobiological reaction of the human organism to life's vicissitudes. As such, this framework tends to minimize the importance of organic, constitutional, and genetic factors (Klerman, 1974). This linear or *unitary* concept of depression is found in many American textbooks and was also supported by Levitt and Lubin (1975) in their critical review of the existing research on the differential response of depressed subjects to electrocon vulsive therapy (ECT) and drug treatment. It was their conclusion that response to ECT was more significantly related to the presence or absence of certain symptoms than to the overall diagnosis. This conclusion still allows for the possibility that the constellation of symptoms most commonly associated with endogenous depression may be simply a more severe form of reactive depression.

In attempting to resolve the unitary-binary controversy, Eysenck (1960) has suggested that the binary theory may be an artifact of the factor analytic method of investigation, which favors a binary model. Specifically, if factor-analytic studies of depression symptoms are scored artificially 1 and 0, or present versus absent, such a scoring method does not permit quantification of degree of symptomatology; severity of symptoms are ignored. In order to capture the contiguous nature of depression, according to Eysenck, we must now reconstitute the symptoms under investigation into a five-point scale. Such a summation of symptom intensity will yield severity scores and thereby permit the testing of the continuum theory of depression.

Since the popular factor-analytic methods of studying depressive symptomatology to date have not permitted a fair test of the continuum theory and since, according to Mendels (1965): "endogenous and reactive syndromes occur in their pure form in a small percentage of cases. . . . The majority present a mixed picture." The integrated theory of depression in this chapter espouses the unitary theory. In so doing, unlike some proponents of the unitary model who have used the word *psychotic* as an index of the depth of depression, the term *endogenous* will be used as the descriptor for the severe end of the continuum of illness and the word *reactive* to describe the milder form of the syndrome.

The fact that the precipitants of a depression may not be clearly identifiable in the endogenous form does not preclude that they may have existed at one time or been so well-internalized over time that they are difficult to identify. Goodwin and Bunney (1973) suggest that the reason we assume there is no precipitating factor in endogenous depression might well be an artifact of data gathering. Severely depressed patients may be less aware of the particular events that relate to the onset of their illness . . . either because of a deep repression or because they have been lost to the memory. Psychic conflict may act as an internal stressor capable of

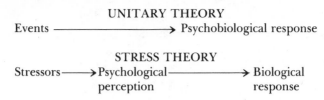

Figure 4.1 Unitary theory.

eliciting a stress response in the absence of an identifiable external social stimulation.

> Frustrated needs and motives, discrepancy between aspiration and achievement, recall of unpleasant past experiences, dreams, and free associations are all examples of internal stressors only indirectly related to the current social interactions or situations. (Pancheri and Benaissa, 1978)

An internal conflict that is not in the conscious awareness of the patient will not be reported by the patient as a stressor. Stressors that are mild or imagined may be overlooked as precipitous of depression. There can also be insidious stresses such as the gradual withdrawal of affection by a spouse (Beck, 1974).

In short, every stimulus, external and internal, in and of itself or by virtue of the symbolic associations it generates in the person, may be a potential precipitant of depression. Along these lines, if one considers precipitative events to include small, internalized, insidious or routine stressors, Peter MacLean (1976a) found that when experiments control for age and disorder severity, cases of endogenous and reactive depression appear indistinguishable.

The unitary theory of depression appears to be compatible with stress theory. The unitary view sees depression as a psychobiological reaction to life events. Similarly, in stress theory, Hans Selye (1978) defines stress as a biological response syndrome that is mediated psychologically by perceptions of stressors (real or imagined agents that stimulate a stress response).

These two theories address the same concepts: A—events, circumstances, or stressors; B—psychological response; and C—biological response in Figure 4.1.

Modern neurobiological findings support the stress model and increasingly emphasize central nervous system (CNS) structures and functions as mediating and integrating the organism's response to its environments. By integrating the two theories, a conceptual framework is proposed, in Figure 4.2, to explain how depression is related to stress.

Depression can be viewed as one type of psychobiological response to stressors that are mediated by the CNS (cognitively and through the

INTEGRATED THEORY

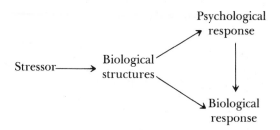

Figure 4.2 Integrated theory.

senses) to produce a syndrome of psychological and somatic symptoms combined.

Commenting upon one of the biological mediators of stress within the central nervous system, Lipton (1976) suggested that the increased depression in the elderly is probably related to biochemical changes resulting in reduced availability of the neurotransmitters that the body needs to adapt to stress. In referring to the stressful stimuli of old age, Epstein (1976) explains that the reason depression is so prevalent in the elderly is that it occurs chiefly as a reaction to age-related stressors. Both appear to be correct. Clearly, with increasing age, the risk for encountering more age-related stressors in greater severity and in more rapid succession increases at a time when biological structures may be diminished in adaptive function, both changes increasing vulnerability for depression.

THE PSYCHOLOGICAL RESPONSE

Depression-Related Stressors

Because the stressors of old age are frequently associated with loss, whether real or perceived, and because loss is a major correlate of depression, one can expect that increased losses in the elderly will increase their risk for depression. "The loss may not be dramatic. . . . As mundane an experience as looking in the mirror while shaving and seeing oneself as old can be disorienting and saddening" (News Journal of AMA, 1979).

Life events in the elderly tend to be associated more with exits than with entrances in the social field. In their research in relating life events to the onset of depression, Myers et al. (1968) found that the onset of depression was related more significantly to the type of life events experienced than to their quantity. Categorizing life events on the basis of entrance or exit of significant people from the patient's social field, they found that exits rather than entrances were followed more frequently by aggravation of symptoms, both of a psychiatric as well as medical nature.

E. S. Paykel's research (1974) supported Meyer's findings that exits are far more likely to be associated with clinical depression requiring treatment, a concept that coincides with the psychiatric concept of separation and loss, and supports the role of these events in clinical depression.

In his research, Paykel (1974) found other characteristics of life events that were related to depression. His sample consisted of 185 depressed patients who were being seen in a variety of treatment facilities in New Haven, Connecticut and an equal number of nondepressed control subjects who were matched for sex, age (in decades), marital status, race, and social class. The control subjects were selected from a total of 938 households that were systematically sampled. One adult was selected at random from each household for an interview. During the interviews, the information collected covered the occurrence of 61 events either six months prior to the interview for the nondepressed subjects or six months prior to the onset of depression for the depressed subjects. Results indicated that the quantity of events is significant in the occurrence of depression. Overall, the depressed subjects reported three times as many events as their matched controls. Also, when events were sorted into two categories, desirable and undesirable (according to cultural norms and social desirability), undesirable events were reported much more frequently by the depressives. Finally, the categorization of life events according to difficulties in interpersonal relations showed a striking difference between the depressed patients and controls: 90 depressed patients reported at least one event from this category as opposed to five controls.

Significant Stressors of Old Age

In conceptualizing the stressors unique to the aged, Sidney Levin (1963) divided them into two broad categories: external and internal. Loss is one of the factors that he cites in the external category. The other external factors are attack, restraint, and threat. The definitions of these factors are

> *Loss* means the loss of a love object or loss of anything in which narcissistic libido is invested, such as a talent or a part of the body.
>
> *Attack* refers to any external force that produces discomfort, pain, or injury. On a physical level, an attack can vary in intensity from a mild pain to extreme, physical violence. On a psychological level, attack can vary in intensity from a mild criticism to severe hostility.
>
> *Restraint* is any external force that restricts those actions that are necessary for the satisfaction of one's basic drives. Freedom from restraint implies the opportunity to find satisfactory outlets for one's drives and, therefore, freedom to be active when one has a need to be active.
>
> *Threat* refers to any event that warns of possible future "loss," "attack," or "restraint."

TABLE 4.1
EXTERNAL STRESSORS OF THE AGED

Loss	Attack	Restraint	Threat
Friends	Stereotypes	Restricted activity	Desertion
Spouse	Illness	Diminished stamina	Disability
Children	Disability	Insufficient finances	Suffering
Role	Pain	Diminished senses	Death
Status		(sight, hearing,	
Income		taste, smell)	
Health		Poor health	
Mobility		Institutionalization	
Body image			
Job			

Using this framework, Table 4.1 catalogs within these subcategories all of the stressors that have been identified in the literature as germane to the elderly population.

Of Levin's four categories of stress factors—loss, attack, restraint, and threat—the one that seems to be a dominant theme of old age is loss. Sixty to 80 percent of depression in the elderly is precipitated by incisive events, almost always losses (Post, 1968). Losses of all kinds are suffered on a scale that few have experienced before.

Fred Charatan (1975) identified the following loss-related stressors of old age:

1. Loss of physical vigor and stamina
2. Loss of mental energy and capacity
3. Loss of sensorial input (sight, hearing, smell, taste)
4. Loss of sources of affection (especially spouse)
5. Loss of peer group
6. Loss of status
7. Loss of income
8. Loss of location
9. Loss of nutrition

Events associated with loss have strong effects on self-esteem and occur more often among depressed than among nondepressed people (Paykel, 1979). Added to the above would be the increasing risk for loss of

10. Memory
11. Sexual satisfaction
12. Health
13. Self-esteem
14. Mobility

15. Safety and security
16. Familiar objects

From this list of loss-related stressors of old age, those that have been identified repeatedly in the literature as the most common precipitators of depression in the elderly will be discussed.

Sexuality

Thwarted sexuality may be a greater contributor to depression in the elderly than previously assumed. Deprived of satisfying sexual intimacy through widowhood, many elderly lose a major source of intimate and empathetic good feelings. "Loneliness and feelings of not being (sexually) attractive or wanted can create depression at any age" (Sviland, 1978). Death of a spouse, especially after a long and happy marriage, can be devastating. "It is doubtful that anyone who has not experienced this tragedy can understand the degree of trauma produced nor the problems of adjustment that must be faced" (Barrett, 1972).

Many of the elderly male callers to the Los Angeles Suicide Prevention Center are still concerned with sexual satisfaction and feel rejected and frustrated because their wives or girlfriends are not responsive enough (Farberow and Moriwaki, 1975).

Women, after reaching menopause and being free of fear of pregnancy, are more desirous of sex than ever before. This need occurs at precisely the time when husbands who are five to ten years older may begin to show impotence (Farberow and Moriwaki, 1975). Many think that there would be less sexual frustration in later years—and perhaps fewer widows—if the chronological trend were reversed so that women married younger men.

Safety and Security

The largest number of elderly people reside in urban areas and the inner city (National Council on Aging, 1975), where the incidence of crime is high. Since women over 65 outnumber men and about 42 percent of them live alone, they are especially vulnerable prey for would-be attackers and robbers. In the 1975 National Council on Aging (NCOA)/Harris Survey, *The Myth and Reality of Aging in America*, fear of crime was one of the "very serious" problems experienced by those over 65.

Threats to safety and security do not all take the form of potential physical injury or harm. A great majority are predicated on trickery and swindling. The New York City newspapers regularly report new scams to separate the elderly from their limited finances. For example, a 78-year-old former city fireman was robbed of $140 by three "nurses" who claimed that they were sent by the hospital to examine him following his discharge. While he was busy in the kitchen making tea for one of the women, the others ransacked his house (Weingrad, 1982). In another case, (Kempton, 1982), a female conartist in New York City would ring the doorbell of an apartment that she knew was occupied by a senior citizen. She would say that she was from the apartment below and that her ceiling was leaking. When she was let in she would rob the occupant.

Living in communities where one's neighbor is a stranger and every shadow, especially if one's vision is limited, poses a potential threat, where attacks on others are a common occurrence, and where police surveillance is limited or over-taxed, weak, isolated, and lonely elderly are in a situation ripe for depression and active paranoia.

Retirement

Retirement often causes a severe loss of self-esteem. Kurt Wolff noted in 1963:

> Among those sociological factors of great influence on the aging process, the factor of retirement is perhaps the most important one. . . . Too much leisure makes [the retired] feel useless and superfluous, causes them to concentrate their interest on their physical status, and gives origin to many psychosomatic complaints (of the worried well) and to depressions.

More recently Diana Woodruff (1977) has observed:

> While we cannot conclusively say that retirement causes death, we do know that life and health are improved in individuals who feel needed, who have adequate financial resources, and who have high social status. The loss of a job resulting from mandatory retirement at the age of 65 deprives individuals of these life-sustaining variables.

One 66-year-old retired refinery worker in New Jersey expressed the feelings of many, "One day you're just like everybody else, and the next day, you're 65 and retired, and you don't belong anymore."

Those who have held positions with high prestige are apt to suffer more from the precipitous decline in their status and attendant self-worth. Whereas, for a blue collar worker, retirement can be a welcome relief from years of dull or tiring work, professionals and executives tend to resist it strongly. However, according to a study conducted in the mid-1970s by sociologists at Duke University, upper level managers, who are used to organizing their own daily routines, recuperate from the initial shock quickly and soon plunge into new careers and other activities (Hanson, 1981). It is the middle level employees—clerks, foremen, semiskilled workers—who suffer most from the "retirement syndrome." Once they have time, they are not sure how to use it. They feel like displaced persons without a place to go or something to do.

To combat the retirement syndrome and the depression that is likely to occur with lowered self-esteem, many over 65 are refusing to stay retired, or are taking advantage of trial retirements that many American businesses and organizations have begun in order to encourage early retirement. Those who refuse to stay retired start new careers or turn old hobbies into new businesses. They act as consultants or join volunteer groups that are so vital to the functioning of many of society's institutions (hospitals, for example). Variations of trial retirements are currently being tested by some employees. In the United States Equal Opportunity Commision employees who have reached the minimum age or years of service to qualify for early retirement can take up to a full year off for a trial retirement to see whether they like it. If they do not, they can return to their old jobs and pay rates. The Polaroid Corporation, based in Cambridge, Massachusetts has launched a similar program, called "rehearsal retirement," but this option offers employees only three months to decide. With an increasing range of retirement alternatives and activities, more retirees are proving that each life stage has its own kind of creativity and worth (Lerner, 1982). With meaningful involvement in society, they continue to live in the present rather than the past and, thereby, they retain enthusiasm, health, vigor and, above all, self-esteem. "When retirement is used as a channel to possibilities never attempted when there was no time, there is every reason for refreshment" (Sheehy, 1981).

Finances

The aged constitute the largest group of poor people in the United States; the income (from all sources) of more than half of all persons over 65 is below the poverty level (Stotsky, 1972). The proportion of elderly blacks who are poor is almost 2.5 times the proportion of elderly whites who are poor. The poorest of the poor are the black aged females living alone, of whom approximately 2 of 3 are officially classified as poor and 78 percent of whom are at least "near poor" (National Council on Aging, 1975).

Although old age brings with it the increased probability of economic hardship, it is also true that people reaching retirement age today are better off than their predecessors. Since 1959, the number of officially counted "poor elderly" has fallen from 33 percent of the elderly to as low as 6 percent when noncash benefits, like home equity, are added to retirement benefits. Fully 70 percent live in their own homes and nearly 9 of every 10 elderly homemakers make no mortgage payments.

However, this improved situation may not continue in the future as it becomes harder to become a homeowner and since it is now much more difficult for the young to purchase their own homes and since one-half of all private sector employees are not covered by any pension plan (*Newsweek*, June 1, 1981). Social Security is the most common source of income for older Americans and it has become the economic mainstay for most. But despite major payroll increases, Social Security trust funds are spending money faster than it comes in, a major concern to the pre- and postretirement population. However, recently enacted legislation has provided a reprieve for the preretirement group who have feared that the Social Security program would not be there when they were ready to retire. The Social Security rescue plan that was signed into law on April 30, 1983 will, it is hoped, solve the system's financial problems for another 35 years, at the least, and 75 years at the most. It increases payroll taxes, delays cost of living increases for six months, and raises the retirement age of the baby boom generation to 67 in the next century, affecting anyone born from 1938 on. Despite these changes to secure the nation's main source of retirement income, inflation still lurks in the wings as the silent villain of retirees on fixed incomes.

Women are the biggest victim of retirement income loss and insecurity. Because of the high mobility of women in the labor force and the fact that many take time off to have children, many women workers are never vested in pension plans even though they work for most of their lives. Other women are excluded from much-needed benefits when their husbands die (*Newsweek*, June 1, 1981).

Reduced income, as in unemployment, has always been among demographic variables, the most highly correlated with the suicide rate (Farber, 1968). Likewise, persons who are most likely to become pathologically depressed have had an inferior educational background which leads to lower annual income plus an inability to improve financial status over the years (Levitt and Lybin, 1975). Also, depression has been shown to be more common among those of lower socioeconomic status (Weissman and Myers, 1978), who also tend to have reduced social support due to relatively small social networks and few confidants (Fischer and Phillips, 1982; Liem and Liem, 1978; Pearlin and Johnson, 1977). The coping responses of people of lower social status are less likely to include active or problem-solving strategies and more likely to involve avoidance responses (Billings and Moos, 1981; Westbrook, 1979).

Poverty underlies poor nutrition and poor health. Poor health and poor nutrition can, by themselves, produce physical symptoms of depression. Without money, it is impossible to purchase legal aid or to pay for mobility and other aids to independence. In short, it seems that for some forms of depression, the therapy of choice may be money.

Health

The great majority of elderly people are healthy enough to lead independent lives. Serious systematic decline in physical capacity typically sets in only after age 75. Medical developments as well as more healthful lifestyles continue to increase and extend good health. Most surveys disclose that fewer than 1 in 5 elderly Americans regard themselves in poor health

(Rabushka and Jacobs, 1980). Yet, older people do suffer disproportionately from a variety of chronic health problems. By the time they are 65, most people are suffering from at least two chronic diseases. These diseases include, but are not limited to, heart disease, emphysema, osteoporosis, kidney disease, glaucoma, bursitis, and arthritis.

For the 80 percent of Americans over 65 (two million) who do have chronic conditions, illness is a fact of life (Eliopoulous, 1981). Of this group, 42 percent find that the chronic condition limits their major activity (U.S. Public Health Service, 1968–1969). With more health problems, they use more health services than the general population: they occupy one-third of hospital beds, use one-fourth of the medications prescribed and 29 cents of each health care expenditure in 1978 was for their care. When they enter hospitals, they stay twice as long as the general population (Fahey, 1981).

When they cannot cope with infirmity and the limitations that it imposes, the stage is set for depression, dependency and institutionalization (Surgeon General, 1979). Suicide often follows a diagnosis of an incurable disease. One man was admitted to a community hospital following an unsuccessful suicide attempt. After learning from his physician that glaucoma was slowly robbing him of the vision that he felt was essential to his retirement avocation—professional golf, he drove his car to an isolated spot in the desert and shot himself in the head. Rather than a slow loss of vision that would have allowed him time to cope and make the necessary life-style changes to accommodate to limited sight, his aborted attempt at self-destruction permanently blinded him in an instant in both eyes and, with no time to adjust, left him a deeply depressed, pathetic figure. Another elderly person who was also suffering from progressive blindness could be heard at the nurses' station shouting in her room to a nurse who was trying to feed her, "Leave me alone. Don't you see, I am trying to die?" For many, physical infirmity, chronic illness, or the diagnosis of an incurable or debilitating disease leads to a deep depression and, for some, suicide.

MEASURING STRESSORS EVENTS IN THE ELDERLY

Knowledge about the relationship between stressful life events and the subsequent onset of psychiatric or physical illness has been derived mainly from research using the Social Readjustment Rating Scale (Holmes and Rahe, 1967). Research results indicate that the higher the score on the scale, the higher the likelihood of developing a wide variety of illnesses—infections, accidents, metabolic dysfunction, mycardial infarctions, and minor health problems (Dohrenwend and Dohrenwend, 1974; Myers et al., 1971; Wyler et al., 1971).

However, no matter how provocative the research seeking to link stress with depression and physical illness, the basic tool upon which the methodology depends, the Social Readjustment Rating Scale, lacks face validity for use on an elderly population. It is not age-specific: the nature of life-events and the social readjustment that they require differ according to age and sex (Lowenthal and Chiriboga, 1973). For young adults, marriage, parenthood, and career development are major concerns; for the postparental age group, men are concerned with work-related problems while women tend to be more concerned with children and their own personal growth; in the postretirement years, according to a survey of letters written to "Dear Abby" (Gaitz and Scott, 1980), loneliness, fear of rejection, interpersonal relationship, and finding a new mate were reported as the most difficult problems faced by the elderly.

Some stressors that seem to plague the elderly, such as threats to safety and security (especially of those who live in high-crime areas), are not included in the Holmes-Rahe Scale. Therefore, in future research about stress in the elderly, new self-report measures of stress must be developed that include age-specific life events and that permit for rating by subjects of the individualized degree of stress associated with specific events.

Life changes should be evaluated to determine the extent to which the individual has control over the event, previous experience in dealing with such changes, resources for coping, health status, and degree of anticipation and preparation (Eisdorfer, 1977; Lowenthal and Chiriboga, 1973; Nelson, 1974). A way also needs to be found to measure the multiple, subtle, unconscious stimuli that operate over long spans of time to produce frequent, intense, and durable stress responses that are the real precursors of disease (Pancheri and Benaissa, 1976).

MEDIATING VARIABLES IN STRESS RESPONSE

Selye (1976) has stated that it is not so much what happens to you as how you perceive it that makes the difference in how much stress one experiences. In other words, stress is subjective and highly individualized. While the body's response to a stressor (described by Selye as the General Adaptation Syndrome) is automatic and the same in each person, it will vary in intensity depending upon each individual's distinct and subjective perception of the stressor. Whereas one person may consider a particular stressor to be a major trauma, another may experience it as an insignificant happening.

The difference in the psychological and biological response in two individuals to the very same phenomena seems to be mediated by other factors besides perception which Selye mentioned. The following additional mediating factors have been mentioned in the literature and will be discussed in greater detail below. They are timing, sensorial input (hearing, sight, smell, taste, kinesthesis, touch, body rhythm), and the "adaptive capacity" of the individual (Jarvik, 1976). Adaptive capacity includes thoughts, perceptions, and support systems. As illustrated in Figure 4.3, thoughts identified as "internal mediators" and social supports or resources identified as "external mediators" interactively mediate the person's perception of an event. When the resultant perception is one of loss and helplessness/hopelessness, depression results.

The theoretical framework in this chapter is intended to explain hypothetically the relationship between mediating factors and their ultimate effect upon the psychological and biological responses to stress. Empirical evidence for the linking of many of the variables with outcome responses is not available, but the concepts have been previously identified by others in the literature in an effort to explain the genesis of depression (Akiskal and McKinney, 1975; Depue, 1979; Billings and Moos, 1982).

Referring to Figure 4.4, when *unrealistic* optimism, resulting from feelings of omnipotence and excessive hope is present, the person seems to act out his feelings without restraint. On the other hand, when *unrealistic* pessimism, resulting from low self-esteem and hopelessness, constrain the person, he represses, denies, and internalizes his feelings, resulting in depression. But the psychodynamic response to stress may not be consistently in one form, either acting out or depression; it can vacillate between the two extremes. Extreme vacillation can be compared to a bipolar depression. A nonvacillating depressive response can be viewed as an analog of unipolar depression that as shown in Figure 4.4, is seen on a continuum of severity, with endogenous depression being the most severe and somatically disruptive ɪᴜrm of the illness. In this model, as depression becomes more severe and moves closer to the endogenous pole, it is expected that the vegetative symptoms will increase and, with it, a tendency toward somatic disorders and ultimately death. By the same token, extreme forms of acting out can lead to behavioral disorders and, ultimately, suicide.

The following sections will discuss in greater detail the significance of the mediating variables mentioned above, that is, timing, sensorial input, thoughts, and support systems. Relevant aspects of the concepts of esteem and hope will be reviewed since they are influenced by the aforementioned mediating factors. All these, in turn, ultimately trigger psychological and biological responses to stress, of which depression is one type.

Timing of Stressors

The timing of stressful life events—how rapidly in succession and at what age they occur as well as their long-term effects—seems to be a critical factor in how well one copes and the likelihood of a resulting depression. Miller (1978) asserts,

> As people grow older they naturally incur more and more significant losses. These losses then "gang up" on them and may result in a cumulative effect much greater than any one of them might have

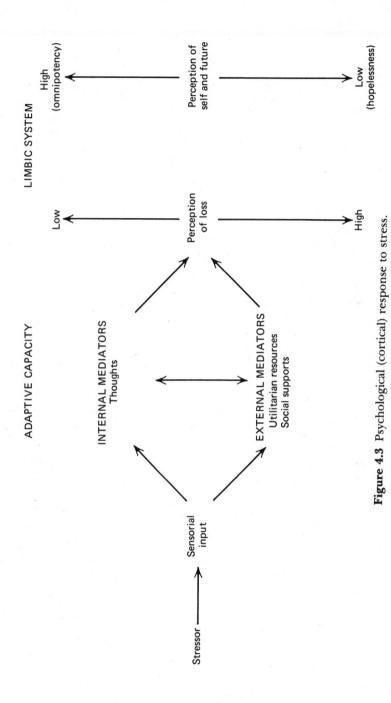

Figure 4.3 Psychological (cortical) response to stress.

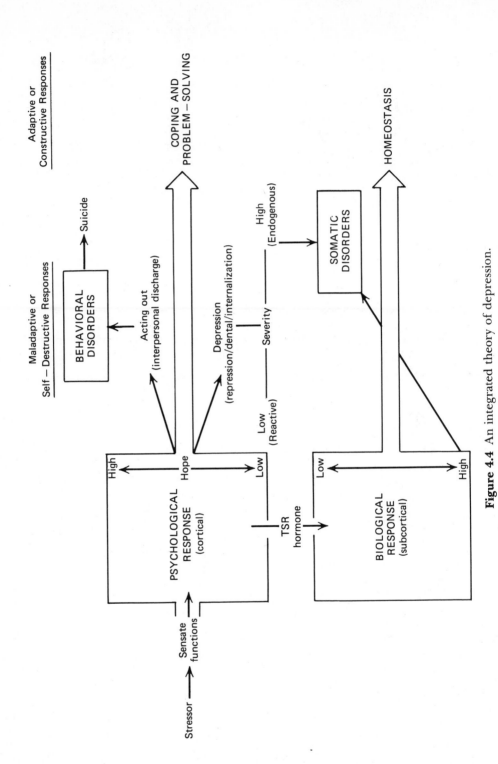

Figure 4.4 An integrated theory of depression.

exerted individually. . . . What is important is not any one loss in particular, but the unexpectedness and swiftness of its onset, the sufferer's reaction to it, and its synergistic effect when combined with extant problems.

In such a situation, one hardly has the time or energy to adjust to one loss before another looms on the horizon. Because it is more difficult to replace losses in later life—a new wife, a better job—one is more apt to feel bereft and hopeless about the future.

Bernice Neugarten (1970) suggests that life events may not constitute as severe a stress if they occur in an appropriate time of life. When they occur at perceived inappropriate times—heart attack at age 30 or death of spouse at age 22—acceptance and coping are usually protracted. Perception of age-appropriateness may also be related to a realistic acceptance and anticipation of all of life's changes, not just the ones associated with youth and middle-age.

Finally, if an event has inherently undesirable long-term consequences, such as might be associated with an unfavorable diagnosis, its immediate effect may be more devastating than the effect of a life event that can be quickly resolved (Miller and Ingham, 1979). In summary, the concept of timing of life events and its effect on depression has received little attention in the literature to date and seems to be an area worthy of further investigation.

Sensate Functions

Figure 4.5 vividly illustrates the increasing probability of significant visual and auditory impairments with advancing age. Almost all elderly people need reading glasses and most need bifocals. As with vision, significant hearing loss, which affects men more often than women, occurs in some 30 percent of all older people. Hearing loss is potentially the most problematic of the perceptual impairments because it can reduce reality testing and lead to marked suspiciousness, even paranoia. Post (1968) described the transient paranoid reaction-syndrome involving older persons living alone, principally women, many of whom have hearing loss, have recently moved, and are devoid of interpersonal contact apart from rent collectors. A National Institute of Mental Health study has shown that there is a marked relationship between hearing loss and depression (National Council on Aging, 1975). In his research, Parker (1969) showed how auditory disability can isolate the person from the rest of society and induce depression.

Other factors such as blindness and loss of tactile response also may be related to depression and isolation. For example, aged persons gradually give up driving as they develop sensory difficulties, especially in sight. They then become more confined to the home and more isolated. Reading, television, hobbies, and activities that have been a source of diversion or

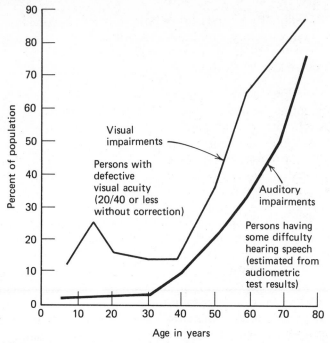

Figure 4.5 Percentage of persons in the United States with visual and auditory impairments, age 6–79 years, 1960–70. (National Center for Health Statistics, *Health United States 1975*, using Health Examination Survey.)

purpose in life are reduced or eliminated. Also, the elderly tend to feel more vulnerable to danger and crime when they are handicapped.

Mistaken or exaggerated stimuli in the environment due to sensory deficits can create as much stress as if they were real. Elderly people thus handicapped are in double jeopardy of negatively distorting reality—at the sensorial and then at the conscious thinking level—thereby doubling their chances for a depressive response.

THOUGHTS

The growing acceptance of the theoretical premise that cognition's mediate response to life events or crises has been referred to as the "cognitive revolution" in psychology (Dember, 1974). It has been strongly and consistently espoused by Aaron Beck, who found support for a cognitive theory of depression from his naturalistic studies, clinical observations, and experimental investigations. Like R. Lazarus (1966), Beck theorized that emotions are responses to cognitions or mental thought processes. In other words, a person's thoughts about a stimulus or stressor determine his emotional reaction to it. Sometimes thoughts or cognitions are distorted by illogical thinking or erroneous perceptions of circumstances. When this happens, non-reality based affective responses like depression or anxiety needlessly occurs.

Cognitive appraisals of stressors include evaluation of their present and future significance upon one's well-being whether the stressors are actual, imagined, or anticipated. When the consciously perceived significance of a stressor includes harm or attack, loss, restraint, or threat, negative emotions result. In contrast, benign and positive cognitive mediation results in positively toned emotions.

Beck termed thought processes that are stable in response to similar types of events "schemata." They develop with experience and time. Some thought schemas, such as those related to aging and age-related losses, may remain latent until activated by circumstances analogous to prior experiences that shaped and embedded negative attitudes, such as an early childhood association with a sickly, crotchety old neighbor. Depending upon the aging person's formative experiences, his or her realization of approaching senescence or physical decline can activate either negative depressogenic views that this stage of life is the end of the line, where one is left standing on the outskirts of life or positive, mood-enhancing views that this is a time of relaxed closure of life that still contains much to experience and enjoy (Lidz, 1968).

Since many of the stressors encountered in old age were never before experienced in life (physical decline, loss of role and status, loss of friends through death), they may stimulate negative, maladaptive depressogenic cognitive responses that previously lay dormant. Also, since the losses characteristically encountered by the elderly are apt to be less amenable to change, prevention, or control than the losses characteristic of earlier developmental stages of life, there is more rational justification for feelings of hopelessness and helplessness.

Finally, if cognitive responses or thought schemas are deeply ingrained and stable, as Davis (1979) has suggested in the case in the elderly, then, in theory at least, this population may be more cognitively prone to depression and more in need of cognitive therapy to correct negatively biased thought patterns related to age-specific events.

In cognitive therapy, the therapist collaborates with the client in identifying and modifying cognitive misconceptions and superstitions in order to correct maladaptive responses (Meichenbaum and Jeirk, 1976). According to Rush and Beck (1978), this process is easier with the mildly depressed, who are able to analyze negative thoughts with some objectivity. As depression worsens, however, it becomes more difficult for the person to evaluate negative interpretations objectively and detect illogic in their own thinking.

Sometimes words alone can trigger negative thoughts: it is words that make reflective and conceptual thinking possible (Lidz, 1968). Even though we think with visual symbols as well as with other sensations and perceptions, words are the switching points, the symbols that we can manipulate in order to shift from one associational trend to another. Word-symbols vary greatly from one person to another, depending upon developmental history, personality, culture, and philosophy of life. The task in therapy is to identify the symbols attached to specific words—to make unconscious symbols conscious, and, by so doing, to gain control over word-symbols that habitually trigger negative meanings and negative affect.

Life review has been extolled by several authors (Butler, 1963; Havinghurst and Glaser, 1972; Tedesseo-Castelnuovo, 1978) for its value in resolving internal conflicts, serving as a buffer against loss and depression and enhancing personal adjustment and ego integrity. According to Erickson (1950), reminiscing is important to the psychological health of the individual in the last stage of life. As the person approaches death, there is an increasing need to examine life experiences and accomplishments in terms of whether life goals have been attained. Undoubtedly, this conscious review process involves the reinterpretation of life events and their significance. In the process, negative perspectives can be changed into positive ones with evidence from the present. As such, life review or reminiscent therapy may simply be another form of cognitive therapy. Whereas cognitive therapy focuses on the cognitive restructuring of *present* events, reminiscent therapy stimulates the same cognitive restructuring of *past* events, in the light of present wisdom and knowledge gained in the intervening years.

Perception of Loss

Loss seems to be a common theme in the distorted and illogical thinking of depressed patients (Beck, 1963). In his long-term study of depressed patients, Beck discovered that depressed patients differed from the nondepressed patients in the way they construed the meaning of experiences, especially those related to loss. They were apt to misinterpret or exaggerate the loss or attach overgeneralized meaning to the loss. Specific thought aberrations included overgeneralization, selective abstraction, arbitrary inferences, and magnification (refer to Chapter 9). Loss experienced by the depressed person may be hypothetical or "pseudo-losses," yet he treats his conjectures as though they were established facts (Beck, 1974).

Schless et al. (1974) concluded from research on neurotic depressive subjects admitted to an in-patient unit that depressed patients view life events as uniformly more stressful. When subjects in that study were asked to rate the stress value of life events listed in the Holmes-Rahe Social Readjustment Scale (Holmes and Rahe, 1967), they not only rated the events as more stressful than nondepressed normal controls, but, even after their depression abated and they were discharged from the hospital, their perception of the stressfulness of the listed events did not change.

The weights they assigned to the events were also independent of the severity of their depression and whether the event had been personally experienced or not. In short, they demonstrated a persistent tendency to perceive stressors in a negative, pessimistic light and, thereby, exaggerate the reality of loss.

J. Becker (1974) proposes that depression should be conceptualized in terms of three types of perceived losses: self-esteem, game, and meaning. The loss of self-esteem goes hand in hand with the loss of hope—hope increases with an increase in self-esteem—and the two are affected by the predisposing internal factor of thoughts and the external factors (which can be facilitative or restrictive) of health, nutrition, finances, mobility or exercise, and social supports.

Game loss in the sense in which Becker uses it is a series of norms or rules for significant action. Game loss is the paramount etiological factor in depression. In the elderly, retirement with its accompanying loss of role could be seen as a "game loss." So too could the experience of being old in a youth-oriented society that offers little guidance in the appropriate behavior and role for the senior citizen, a role that is better defined in traditional culture with a longer history and period of time to develop such roles.

Object loss, according to Becker, is secondary to game loss. The death of a loved one or failing to accomplish a career goal are stressors that can be overcome unless the object loss upsets an entire game by necessitating drastic changes in the way that the game must be played.

Meaning loss refers to a condition of the individual in which he perceives that there are no games worth playing—a loss of meaning or hope. According to Levitt and Lubin (1975), "This apprehension comes to very few," but the elderly at the end of life are more vulnerable to it.

A sense of meaning or purpose in life can be considered as one of man's symbolic possessions (Akiskal and McKinney, 1975). When it is lost, the ego, which is rooted in social reality, may experience a precipitous loss of self-esteem and a profound feeling of hopelessness. Without purpose, there is no motive for going on, for mounting the energy to confront life's stress. The person who throughout his life has found meaning in the pursuit of youth-oriented goals—good looks, material success, status on the job—in old age may find himself devoid of motivators.

Those who choose the pursuit of leisure-time activities as a full-time commitment soon find that perpetual play can confuse them about purpose and value. In time they begin to feel unnecessary to others, and the pursuit of continual pleasure loses its appeal. This play ethic is most often found in age-segregated retirement communities, where it is possible to fill one's social calendar from dawn to dusk. The absence of children and relatives in these communities is also a problem. Without family members close by, it is more difficult to form a sense of being needed in a way that gives purpose to living.

A new existential orientation is necessary in the retirement years. As Aaron Antonovsky (1979) sees it, life worth living requires a sense of coherence, a perception that life is meaningful and manageable. The judgment that life is meaningful and manageable, even when one is bedridden or terminally ill, is a very personal matter to be made only by the person living it. It is an existential question of spiritual and religious dimensions. Belief systems, such as faith in God, fate, or some higher natural order, enable people to create meaning out of life, even out of damaging experiences. Such systems provide answers or explanations for otherwise inexplicable events such as a traumatic accident, death of a loved one, one's own imminent death, and destructive evil such as a Nazi concentration camp. The great philosopher Socrates, anchored in some sense of meaning and purpose, found the motivation to learn how to play the lyre while he awaited death in prison.

Commenting on the special importance of a sense of meaning in old age, Simone De Beauvoir (1972) wrote:

> There is only one solution if old age is not to be an absurd parody of our former life, and that is to go on pursuing ends that give our existence a meaning—devotion to individuals, to groups or to causes, social, political, intellectual or creative work. In spite of the moralists' opinion to the contrary, in old age we should wish still to have passions strong enough to prevent us turning in upon ourselves. One's life has value so long as one attributes value to the life of others, by means of love, friendship, indignation, compassion. When this is so, then there are still valid reasons for activity or speech. People are often advised to "prepare" for old age. But if this merely applies to setting aside money, choosing the place for retirement and laying on hobbies, we shall not be much the better for it when the day comes. It is far better not to think about it too much, but to live a fairly committed, fairly justified life so that one may go on in the same path even when all illusions have vanished and one's zeal for life has died away.

A devotion to some cause or purpose beyond themselves was one constant theme in the lives of people enjoying high well-being who were interviewed by Gail Sheehy for her book *Pathfinders*. But the pursuit of a long life with meaning and purpose is a lifetime pursuit. It is most apt to occur when one's sense of old age is not so grim as to make it not worth the struggle.

Angry Thoughts and Feelings

Freud viewed depression as the inward-turning of the aggressive instinct that for some, was not previously directed at the appropriate object. Hostility is triggered by the loss of an ambivalently loved object. However, this model, which is phrased in metapsychological terms, is not easy to verify empirically. "Even though it is the most widely quoted psychological conceptualization of depression, there is little systematic evidence to substantitate it" (Akiskal and McKinney, 1975).

Research indicates that the redirection of hostility toward outside objects has not been correlated with improvement in depression (Klerman, 1974). It may actually have disastrous consequences (Akiskal and McKinney, 1975). Beck (1974) postulated an alternative explanation of the connection between anger, the direction of its expression and depression:

> I do not believe the cathartic effect of the expression of hostility results in improvement but rather that the mobilization of hostility is effective because it helps to change a person's self-image by giving him a greater sense of control over his environment.

If such is the case, it is assertion skills and control over one's environment that are the critical variables to be manipulated in treating depression. From this perspective, frustrated attempts at controlling one's life and circumstances result in anger and lowered self-esteem.

Ewald Busse, a geriatric psychiatrist at Duke University has proposed that in the elderly anger frequently stems from a loss of self-esteem in the face of lessened ability to obtain basic gratifications and to defend themselves against threats to security (Rosenfeld, 1978) rather than from anger displaced within themselves.

For some people the workplace or children in the family are convenient targets for the venting of displaced anger. As one ages and these targets disappear, so too do the opportunities for catharsis. A generalized infection of angry feelings may result, and when they are projected broadly at people in the environment without apparent cause, the old person may be justifiably seen as crotchety and ill-tempered.

Antecedents of Depressive Thoughts

Thought patterns and specific cognitions vary from one person to another. Factors mentioned in the literature that seem to shape thoughts or perceptions about life events are developmental history, personality characteristics, and culture. A discussion of these factors influencing cognitive interpretation of the meaning of events follows.

DEVELOPMENTAL HISTORY.   In his research, Astrup et al. (1959) concluded that depression in the elderly was often colored by the patient's life experiences and personality traits. In respect to life experiences, Lidz (1968) states that the most frequently aroused emotions in the adult usually depend upon childhood experiences with parents and family. In the case of depression, case histories of depressives reveal early experiences of parental loss or rejection. (McLean, 1976b; Farber, 1968)

In his review of the literature relating orphanhood and adult depression, Beck (1974) reported that approximately 30 percent of severely depressed adults experienced parental loss in childhood. The loss need not be total. Even parental disparagement or ambivalent response to a child can destroy confidence, create feelings of rejection, and predispose one to depression in the future. When parents convey to the child that he is inadequate, he grows up without hope for a favorable outcome from his efforts. He is thereby handicapped in his ability to develop a secure and confident identity and, without a secure identity, he is vulnerable to frustration and despair (Shmagin, 1977).

B. Bressler (1978) has reported that 50 percent of completed suicides and 65 percent of attempted suicides come from broken homes. "Sensitized by unfavorable life circumstances (e.g., early parental loss) or by more insidious conditions over time, individuals are thought to become predisposed to overreact to life circumstances later on" (MacLean, 1976b). When the same or similar losses occur subsequently, the person is apt to make extreme, absolute judgments and view loss as irrevocable or indifference as total rejection.

PERSONALITY CHARACTERISTICS.   People who spend their childhood in setting rigid, perfectionistic goals for themselves are apt to believe that their universe is collapsing when they confront inevitable disappointments later in life (Beck, 1974). Rigidity and perfectionism as a way of life make one depression-prone. In a case history examination of 319 depressed adult psychiatric patients ages 38 to 71, Hamilton and Mann (1954) found that the personality traits of the depressed subjects were consistent with a pattern of superego control: reticence, prudishness, stubbornness (or rigidity), oversensitiveness, penuriousness, and perfectionism. Such high-functioning people tend to take life seriously, to display a lack of imagination and sense of humor, and to have a strong drive for power and control over others (Gordon, 1973). Nevertheless, in commenting upon proposed childhood antecedents of adult depression, MacLean (1976a) has stressed their speculative nature because they depend upon retrospective information that is subject to distortion.

In Freudian terms, people who are more sensitive than others to separation or loss and to depression have been noted to be orally dependent and narcissistic. Obsessive persons, best characterized by their ambivalence and controlled hostility, also appear to be depression-prone (Grauer, 1977).

Stress therapists and cognitive or behavioral theorists note other characteristics of depressed persons, such as behavioral inactivity and deficient communication, socialization, goal-setting, and problem-solving skills (MacLean, 1976a). These skill deficiencies may originate in early childhood learning experiences or may simply be side-effects of depression. The observation that these characteristics are common in depressed patients does not explain causality nor identify which came first, the depression or the characteristics.

Behavioral inactivity is the engagement in fewer pleasant activities and reduced subjective enjoyability of potentially pleasant events. Deficient communication skills usually result in a reduced quantity and range of interaction and/or aversive interaction. Either deficiency deprives the individual of potential sources of positive social reinforcement. When goal-setting skill is deficient, the person is apt to set unrealistic standards and then persist in attempts to attain the goals despite contraindications. The end result of frustrated goal-attainment is a loss of self-esteem and feelings of impotence and hopelessness. Faulty problem-solving skills result in increasing stress and more problems. Discouraged from lack of success, the person gives up, procrastinates, or becomes immobilized. Fortunately, research indicates that all of the aforementioned skills can be operationally defined, measured, and improved through cognitive/behavioral or social skills models of training and therapy (see Chapter 10).

CULTURE.   Different suicide rates in different cultures are not haphazard. Rather, they reflect suicide-producing forces in the culture or the times. In a culture with a high suicide rate, one can expect more unsuccessful suicide attempts, high rates of depression, personalities susceptible to depression, difficulties in living and surviving, weakened support structures and fragmented family ties (Farber, 1968). The values of different cultures are like a divining rod that helps one decide at what point life becomes unlivable.

Cultural traditions combined with religious beliefs shape the value system of a society and tell the people what to think about events. The value systems thus formed profoundly influence the person's attitudes, behaviors, and reactions to life events of which growing old is one. In countries where value systems demanding a meaningful role, respect, and care for the elderly are sufficiently strong to override the cost of providing that care, the elderly enjoy a meaningful and rewarding old age.

Many have proposed that the aged can enjoy a respected place only in primitive societies. This belief presumes that the cultural forces of fragmentation of the family and emphasis on youth/productivity that are pervasive in industrialized societies preclude consideration of the needs of the elderly. Yet, there is a country that has been transformed into an industrial leviathan and not yet abandoned its appreciation and concern for elderly members in the process. The country is Japan.

Religious doctrines in Japan emphasize filial piety as the first expression of veneration for the emperor and, by extension, to all one's ancestors, thus ensuring a remarkable degree of security for the elderly (Hendricks and Hendricks, 1977). After World War II, however, in the wake of rapid industrialization, urbanization, social and geographic mobility, and democratization of the family, many of the traditions regarding the place and treatment of elderly people have changed. Cross-cultural studies show a correlation between these changes and an increase in geriatric depression. However, religious tenets that dictate a creed of respect for one's elders persist to ensure some security for elderly people. These tenets are espoused in the national assembly that continues to enact laws requiring lineal descendants to support their elderly relatives. Consequently, tradition reinforced with legal sanctions supports the extended family with 8 of every 10 elderly living under one roof with children or grandchildren. Since both partners in young couples often work outside the home, grandparents are prized for the necessary role that they play in caring for the child and the house. There are few government programs to support the elderly or attend to their health and social needs. In short, it is religious beliefs primarily that have guaranteed a meaningful role, family involvement, and economic security for the elderly in Japan.

Similarly, in China, the elderly retain a place of respect. *Lao*, which means old, is a term of affection and respect—not derogatory as it is in the West. Like Japan, China is one of the few countries with legal sanctions for sons and daughters to care for their retired parents. If parents are neglected, the children are usually contacted by neighborhood committees, the work units at factories or shops, and the party unit of the Communist party. Visits from these groups usually are sufficient to improve the situation. The government also bolsters the tradition of elderly care as a primary duty through media campaigns. The hero in literature frequently performs heroic deeds or makes great sacrifices to help older people; the young are urged to do the same. As in Japan, two and three generations live in most households in which the elderly play an important role doing household chores, caring for the grandchildren and contributing from their generous pensions to the support of the family. Reporting his observations from a recent trip to China, Paul Green (1983) noted: "In every case we found grandparents delighted with the 'heavenly happiness' of sharing their lives with grandchildren and of living with children who would take care of them as they got older."

In contrast, Senator Frank Moss observes, "It's hell to be old in the U.S." (1979), and Robert Butler echoed the same theme in his book, *Why Survive? Growing Old in America*. In America, unlike China and Japan, the admixture of ethnic groups that have immigrated to the country has resulted in a wide variation of values and practices in caring for the elderly.

In the absence of common religious and cultural traditions, it seems that economic values prevail and new emigrees are enculturated not to moral values of caring for the elderly but to economic goals of social advancement, youth, and productivity. In such a world of tension, of compulsion, of work, and of competition, elderly people are considered a burden. It has been reported that sickly old people are even abandoned by their families in parking lots in New York City, a shocking example of this ethic (*New York Times*, November 1, 1981).

Families, entrusted with the task of enculturating society's children, coming from diverse backgrounds, create their own internal culture or religious orientation. When the economic pressures and values of the larger society conflict with long-held moral precepts about responsibility of the young for the old and vice versa, the family may become a battleground where, in the search for new, creative and mutually satisfying alternatives, new traditions are developed. In the process, each new generation of elderly face a special challenge of defining a role for themselves that is both meaningful and respected and to establish their continuing involvement and value in society. As they become more assertive in carving their place in society and increasing their power over government decision making through political action, their risk for depression and suicide will decrease (Litman, 1981) and their hope for a more rewarding old age will increase.

But perhaps the final resolution of the dilemma regarding the appropriate role of the elderly in society and the extent of the family's responsibility to respect and care for their older members will ultimately be resolved on religious rather than economic bases as is the case in Japan and China. For example, in the apostolic exhortation on the Catholic Family issued by Pope John Paul II, in 1981, he guides Roman Catholic conscience in this regard (Parish Family Digest, 1983). He exhorts that the pastoral activity of the Church must help everyone to discover and make good use of the role of the elderly within the civic and church community and in the family in particular. Specifically, he views the unique and valuable role of the elderly as helping to clarify human values, bridging generation gaps between parents and children and demonstrating the continuity of generations and the interdependence of God's people.

An interesting observation by J. L. Newman (1975) about the treatment of the elderly in diverse cultures and its effect upon the incidence of incontinence is worth reporting here. Newman believes that incontinence may be the result of rejection by society. His theory is based on observations of unexplained incontinence in young, healthy adults who were prisoners of war and who were faced with a feeling of complete rejection by their friends and colleagues. In Eastern countries, e.g., Singapore, incontinence in long-stay wards is quite infrequently seen. Perhaps the different cultural patterns lead to a feeling of less rejection by the family in those oriental cultures. Newman associates incontinence in the elderly with isolation, humiliation, and privation, and feels that an understanding of their needs might reduce the dimensions of the problem.

LOW SELF-ESTEEM AND HOPELESSNESS

According to Beck's (1967) ego-psychological viewpoint, depression-prone individuals tend to expect the worst and to view events negatively whether or not they are inherently so. Incorporated into this negative mind set are usually feelings of loss of control and inability to decrease the threat— that is, helplessness and hopelessness. In fact, Beck asserts that hopelessness and helplessness are the central features of human depression, resulting from a peculiar "cognitive triad" of negative conception of self (low self-esteem), negative interpretations of one's experiences, and a negative view of the future (hopelessness).

Evidence for the existence of the cognitive triad comes from correlational studies conducted by Beck (1974). As he reports:

> We have conducted a series of correlational studies to test these clinical observations. We found significant correlations between the Depression Inventory and measures of pessimism ($r = 0.56$) and negative self-concept ($r = 0.70$). After recovery from depression, the scores on these measures showed substantial decrements, as expected. In a longitudinal study we found that change scores (between the time of admission and discharge) on the measures of pessimism and negative self-concept correlated 0.49 and 0.53, respectively, with the change scores on the Depression Inventory. These findings lent support to the notion that the state of depression is associated with a negative view of the self and the future. The correlation (0.70) between measures of negative view of the future and of negative view of the self supported the concept of the cognitive triad in depression.

Two of the most reliable symptomatic indicators of clinical depression are lowered self-esteem and feelings of hopelessness or helplessness (Masserman, 1970; Minkoff et al., 1973). Drawing from the writings of Bibring, Klerman (1974) concludes that depression may be a response to helplessness and a fall in self-esteem and that helplessness does not occur except when accompanied by a fall in self-esteem. The relationship of these concepts is diagramatically presented in the integrated model of depression presented in Figure 4.3.

Fall in self-esteem, according to Hirshfield (1979), is a hallmark of depression. The depressed person agonizes over losses and regards himself as the "loser." Even before embarking on an undertaking, he expects to be defeated or disappointed. In old age, it is even harder to maintain a sense of self-esteem when the individual returns to a dependency state of earlier life stages. Being dependent in a society that values independence decreases self-esteem.

Suffering from a low estimate of self, the depressed person puts much effort into pleasing others and developing symbiotic relationships (Beck et al., 1977). Generally, theorists agree that people prone to depression depend excessively upon acceptance by other persons for their self-esteem. If others are less accepting of them in old age, due to the loss of youth's beauty or some disfiguring physical handicap (such as a stroke or arthritis), they must either reorient their thinking to develop a new source of self-esteem or they fall into depression, stricken by rejection.

Stereotypes and Self-esteem

Even the well elderly must fight a continual battle to maintain their self-esteem in a society that idolizes youth and fears old age and death. This cult of youth has been perpetuated by both a lack of information and biased information. Commonly, the younger generation in our society lacks information about old age because they have little or no contact with elderly people. With the modern scattering of the extended family across the country, most young people have few opportunities to develop close relationships with senior members of their family. Lack of contact and closeness with their seniors deprives them of an intimate acquaintance with old age and the aging process. If they had that opportunity, they would learn that the majority of those over 65 reside in their own homes, with their spouse, and are essentially well and active—not a depressing picture. Unfortunately, deprived of such first-hand knowledge because their grandparents are either deceased or residing in a distant location or in a cloistered retirement village, the young remain uninformed about aging and depend upon the media to fill in their gaps in knowledge. An analysis of articles from a leading midwestern newspaper concerning aging compared the views of aging projected to the paper's 288,000 readers in 1973 with the views projected in 1963. Content analysis revealed that there had been a significant increase in the number of articles on aging. Nevertheless, the view of aging that the media projected was still outdated, patronizing, and negative (MacDonald, 1973).

Women in our society are especially vulnerable to negative attitudes toward themselves and their own old age. Most women explain failure by finding fault within: it was their own lack of ability, stupidity, carelessness, and worthlessness (Sheehy, 1981). Attributions of basic, irremedial incompetence groom women for a higher incidence of depression than is found in men. The depression that low self-esteem nurtures depletes their abilities and energies to prove otherwise, thereby providing them with evidence that their original belief in their incompetence was well-founded.

The media does its part to accent the incompetence of females, particularly as they age. A study based on 2,741 characters in prime-time network television drama sampled between 1969 and 1971 showed that elderly comprised less than 5 percent of both sexes, about half their share of the real population. Whereas most males in prime-time drama failed because they were evil, females failed because they aged (Hess, 1974). The female characters actually failed more often than they succeeded. Aging in prime-time drama is thus associated with increasing evil, failure, and unhappiness, especially for females.

While media coverage of old age has improved considerably in the years since these studies, biased negative presentations of old age still persist and continue to instruct youth that old age is associated with physical decline, wrinkles, ill-humor, forgetfulness, constipation, and rigid clinging to the past. In the absence of more realistic, real-life models of old age, the young who develop a negative image of the elderly unavoidably project negative, rejecting attitudes toward them. Likewise, modern technological society, which measures success and worth in productivity and job-related status has no yardstick for measuring the value of elderly people, who do not produce and have no jobs. Eisdorfer and Keckich (1980) write:

> If we can look beyond the pathology and the wrinkled lines in the face and see an individual struggling with loneliness, isolation, sensory loss, role attrition, financial concerns, and status loss, then we can begin to see the aged as people like ourselves who happen to be old and subject to the vicissitudes of a nonsupportive environment.

Living in a culture infected with negative prejudices toward gray hair and wrinkles, the elderly are subject to continual discounting and negative feedback that eats away at their self-esteem. Having themselves absorbed the values of the world of work, after retirement they feel different and useless.

When older people who have always measured their worth by their skills, abilities, and/or occupation lose those self-reinforcers, they also lose their sense of worth and depression follows. Melges and Bowlby (1969) observed that most people who later become depressed are highly invested with various personal and interpersonal skills. Such skill-oriented persons are likely to consider themselves at least partly responsible for their fate and would thus tend to blame themselves for failure. If they are highly goal-oriented and inner-directed, believing that they have responsibility and control over what happens to them, they are also more likely to blame themselves for a decreasing number of accomplishments in old age. They are hard, unrelenting, compulsive personal task masters with high standards that they have difficulty adjusting to accommodate to the requirements and abilities of an aging body (Pearson, 1971; Beck et al., 1977).

Hopelessness

In studying the relationship between hopelessness and suicide, M. L. Farber (1968) noted that man is essentially a future-oriented animal. When he views the future without hope, he despairs and suicide pervades his thoughts. Deprived of a future to hope in, he embraces death. Farber proposes that hope is a function of an inverse relationship between competence and threat. Hope $= f$ (competence/threat). Accordingly, as one's sense of competence or self-esteem increases, it overshadows the degree of perceived threat and hope increases.

In a similar vein, P. Lichtenberg (1957) proposed that depression is a manifestation of felt hopelessness regarding the attainment of goals when responsibility for the hopelessness is attributed to one's personal defects. He hypothesized that depression varies in degrees on a continuum according to the amount of hope that the individual perceives in the future. In the mildest form of depression, there is a moderate loss of hope and the success probability may be low for a particular situation. The expectation concerning life in general, however, remains fairly high. As one declines in the continuum of hope, there is an increasing loss of self-esteem until, as illustrated in Figure 4.3, there is no hope for success even in particular situations or by altering one's behavior.

Helplessness

Learned helplessness is a concept introduced by M. Seligman (1975) from his study of the response of animals exposed to electric shock. In his laboratory studies, he found that after repeated exposure to inescapable electric shock, dogs were impaired in their adaptive ability and subsequently made no efforts to avoid shocks that were escapable. Applying these observations to humans, Seligman theorized that when people are repeatedly exposed to uncontrollable outcomes, they come to believe that outcomes are independent of their behavior and, consequently, they reduce their attempt to influence the environment. Fear of inability to control gives rise to depression.

This model has stimulated considerable research on aging in general and on the impact on aged individuals of institutionalization in particular. In his review of aging research using this model, Richard Schulz (1982) noted a common conclusion, that aging is a process characterized by large decreases in the person's ability to control important outcomes due to shrinking financial resources, decreased physical ability, loss of work role, and other causes. With a shrinking sphere of environmental control, withdrawal and high rates of depression result. Exposed to circumstances of extreme helplessness, the mortality rate has been noted to increase in aged institutionalized patients (Grauer, 1977).

To address the pervasive sense of helplessness in depressed elderly, D. Wasylenki (1980) advocated that the therapist take a dominant role in therapy, acting as a powerful, protective, and accepting figure who can help restore feelings of security and confidence. The unproven expectation is that as the patients become convinced of their good standing with the therapist, their self-esteem increases.

SOCIAL SUPPORTS

The significance of social supports and socialization as a major mediating factor in depression has been a constant theme in sociology since Emile

Durkheim's (1858–1917) nineteenth-century work "Suicide." More recently, cognitive or behavioral theorists have identified social skill deficits, isolation and aversive communication as critical variables in the genesis of depression. Since both the quality and quantity of social supports tend to decline precipitously in old age, as a consequence of both personal and societal changes, this part of the depression paradigm has special significance in a geriatric population.

There is virtually universal agreement that the social support available is an important factor in the coping process and may protect a person against the serious consequences following a life event (Miller and Ingham, 1979). Brown and Harris (1978) found that confiding relationships, particularly with spouses or boyfriends, were protective against depression in women. Research by Sarason and colleagues (Sarason et al., 1978; Siegel et al. 1978) indicates that the mere fact of having someone to talk to is to some extent protective, even if one has not made use of this. What still remains unresolved is whether social support is a moderator variable (i.e., protective when a life event is present but not causing symptoms by itself) when there are no life events, or whether lack of social support causes symptoms in its own right.

When Blazer and Williams (1980) compared the 997 depressed elderly people in their community survey with the 850 nondepressed subjects, they found that the major difference in the demographic characteristics between the two groups was that there was a higher incidence of widowed people in the depressed group. Presumably, the loss of a spouse weakens one's support system and, by so doing, increases one's vulnerability for depression. Clearly, the risk for institutionalization is higher in individuals with no family support system: 70 percent of the institutionalized have no family support system. Close positive relationships, on the other hand, appear to facilitate good health and morale even under personal crises. People who can be characterized as having elaborate social networks at their disposal generally live longer than isolates (Berkman, 1977).

In analyzing the characteristics of depressed elderly in the Durham community survey, Blazer and Williams (1980) found that social and economic resources (collectively termed *external mediators* in the depression framework) appeared to be important factors for subjects with symptoms of primary depressive disorder and secondary depressive disorder as well as for those people with medically related depressive symptoms. They also found that these people were more likely to be living alone.

Living arrangements, especially if one is living alone, appears to be an important risk factor in depression and suicide. The Sainsbury (1963) study of suicides in London showed a correlation between suicide and living alone, living in lodgings or boarding houses, and being foreign born. More of the elderly suicides in his study fell into these categories than those of other age groups. B. M. Barraclough (1971) reported that living alone is the social variable with the highest correlation to suicide and, therefore, must represent a significant aspect of the depression and suicide paradigm. While 63 percent of all aged persons live in families, more than 30 percent live alone—most of them women who are widowed (Stotsky, 1972).

Yet, living alone may be an inadequate construct to describe and measure social isolation. For there are many who live alone without experiencing social isolation or depression. The Louis Harris survey (National Council on Aging, 1975) found that 80 percent of the elderly had seen one or more of their children within the previous week. For some, that type of experience may be enough to maintain a sense of caring, belonging, and purpose. And there are others who live alone and like it—valuing their privacy, freedom in decision making, and ability to control the number and type of friendships that they entertain.

Perhaps, then, living alone is but an *indirect* indicator of the quality and intensity of *communication*, the sine qua non of social support. In the absence of communication, people lose the opportunity to learn what effect they are having on others. Because positive self-appraisal is dependent upon the supportive feedback that one receives from others, when it is missing, self-esteem is bound to suffer.

In fact, according to MacLean (1976a), communication is probably the most sensitive measure of depression. Depressed people talk less, more slowly and hesitantly, and with a decreased voice volume. In so doing, they are apt to elicit reactions of advice and support from others. In time, their whining, pessimistic, self-depreciating, complaining, and unheeding response to the advice offered begins to generate anger and resentment from others, who then feel guilty for having those rejecting, unsupportive feelings, and try to compensate by exhibiting ungenuine supportive behaviors. Finally, this internal conflict that people feel around depressed people is so uncomfortable that they avoid association with them; the result for the depressed person thus is more depression (Arkowitz, 1981). Deprived of a social support system, the person finds it harder to weather the storm of life. For communication and, with it, social supports can mediate and balance the forces of stress, in what appears to be an inverse relationship: the stronger the support system, the more stress a person is able to tolerate. Several researchers investigating social correlates of depression have noted that those who lack supportive confiding relationships are at a substantial increased risk for depression (Roy, 1978; Brown and Harris, 1978; Costello, 1982).

In fact, in the Surgeon General's Report on Healthy People and Disease Prevention (1979), it is reported that belonging to a group, access to advice, and the availability of someone to talk to about one's own troubles are psychological protective interacting variables in promoting overall health and resistance to depression.

The personal attachments and affiliations that constitute a support system can include not just family members and friends but pets as well.

Elderly patients can plummet into a severe depression requiring hospital-ization following the death of their sole companion, a dog or a cat. New scientific findings indicate that animals have a very salutory effect on people. "Pets can lower your blood pressure; talking to or petting your dog or cat has a very calming effect on your body" (Surgeon General, 1979)—and mind.

Of course, at times, members of one's support system can exacerbate stress or block coping rather than help. Nevertheless, social support systems can be regarded as an extremely valuable potential coping re-source. In the integrated theory of depression shown in Figure 4.3, support systems have been conceptualized as one of the external factors mediating the psychological coping response to stress.

In earlier times or in agrarian societies, the elderly stayed at home with their children. They were needed to handle chores, watch young children, cook, clean, sew, and earn their keep in dozens of ways; they were an important part of the social structure (Hamalian and Karl, 1976). Now, urbanization and technological change in modern society have increased isolation, loneliness, alienation, and depression (Sobel, 1981). The break-down of the family structure and the increasing mobility of the population has scattered families across the country, leaving elderly people behind in the deteriorating inner city or in small towns adjacent to farming com-munities where farmers retreat when they can no longer handle the laborious task of managing their farms (National Council on Aging, 1975). Others are not left behind: they leave behind family, friends, neighbors—a social support system that may have taken a lifetime to develop. The leavers flee cold climates and boredom to seek the sun and cameraderie of other retirees in senior ghettoes in the Sunbelt. There they are insulated from the outside world that demeans, rejects, and degrades them (Roscow, 1977).

Socialization is the touchstone in the Sunbelt's retirement communities, mobile home courts, or apartment complexes where the elderly congregate. Yet, personal encounters and friendships tend to be superficial ones in these transient, fluctuating communities and, as such, are no substitute for the strong relationships that they left back home. When they do need help, the elderly fail to call upon these new friends. Clients have explained their reluctance to reach out to their neighbors for help by saying that they do not want to burden others, they do not want their neighbors to know their business, they cannot trust them to keep confidences, or they do not want to ask for help for fear that the return expectations for mutual assistance will be more than they can handle.

It takes time and energy to develop meaningful, supportive relationships, and many elderly do not feel that they have the time or energy or, more basically, the desire to invest in relationship building, so they keep to themselves and explain their reticence by saying "I am a very private person." Some of these people lack the skill in developing new friendships because they came from a community where they simply grew up with all their friends, and the social structure (family, schools, churches) took responsibility for building support networks for them. Others have assimilated society's prejudicial attitude toward aging. They reject the aged in their own old age, refuse to associate with senior citizen groups—a convenient meeting ground for network building—for fear that they might become old by association as if it were a communicable disease. The consequence is isolation, lack of a reference group, and caring, attentive, and personalized help when it is needed. When they need them most, families and social supports of many elderly are often nonexistent. In the absence of social support structures for the elderly, social agencies are called upon to fill in the gaps and their personnel are expected to function as surrogate families temporarily and, sometimes, permanently. The consequent pressures upon these agencies, their personnel, and the taxpayers, who support them, are tremendous.

COPING AND ADAPTATION

Coping as defined by Billings et al. (1983) consists of the cognitions and behaviors that serve to appraise the meaning of stressors, to control or reduce stressful life circumstances, and to moderate the affective arousal that often accompanies stress.

According to MacLean (1976a), it is the management strategies for coping and adapting to stress that separates the depressed from the nondepressed population. Klerman (1974) too considers depression to be an adaptational failure rather than a psychological illness. Erickson (1950) used the term *crisis* to refer to developmental stages in which the person undergoes "a decisive encounter with his environment." *Unsuccessful adaptation* at a time of developmental crises, which also occur in old age according to Erickson, can lead to emotional disturbances, which often take the form of depressive reactions (Levin, 1963).

Some older persons who coped quite well throughout most of their lives may succumb to depression in their senior years because the coping mechanisms that they used previously may fail. One such coping mechanism is "keeping busy." While it may have served well earlier in life to siphon off tension from internal conflicts or stressful experiences, it is sometimes not available to an elderly person who is immobilized with a debilitating illness. When such habitual defense mechanisms fail, hospitalized patients revert to an almost childlike, dependent state, feeling hopelessly lost in their search for a way out of their dilemma.

If unsuccessful efforts to adapt begin to characterize large segments of a person's life over a period of at least several weeks, then the person is apt to conclude that he has little control of his life (MacLean, 1976a). Eventually if this pattern continues, one begins to anticipate failure in all

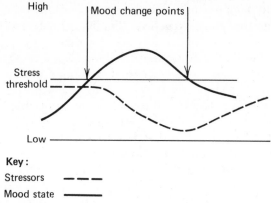

Figure 4.6 Relationship of stress threshold with mood state.

undertakings. In this manner, the vicious cycle of depression is clinched: unsuccessful attempts to cope over a period of time resulting in anticipation of future failure that then generates feelings of low self-esteem and hopelessness leading into depression. This anticipation of failure syndrome is conceptually similar to the cognitive triad of Beck and the learned helplessness hypothesis of Seligman that were explained earlier. MacLean (1976a) states:

> From this point of view an individual who is predisposed to clinical depression (by virtue of an early experience of parental loss, particular child-rearing practices, inadequate coping skills or by virtue of being part of an unsupporting social environment) functions normally over time, rising periodically over the clinical threshold as a function of his inability to cope successively with a particularly large concentration of environmental stressors, before returning to his functional pre-stress baseline.

This concept is illustrated in Figure 4.6.

Depression may result when there is high or low degrees of stress. Levi (1974) has proposed that the relationship between psychosocial stimulation and stress can best be described in a U-shaped curve as shown in Figure 4.7. This model would account for depression found among the elderly in stimulus-sparse environments as discussed in greater detail in Chapter 12.

Stressors that exceed the adaptational threshold may be sudden in occurrence or may be cumulative over time. Small but steady amounts of psychological stress can result from a variety of personal and interpersonal situations that may not be fully appreciated for their stress-producing impact. The search for a single precipitating factor sufficient to cause the depression may be futile or disappointing if it was a minor event that pushed a long-developing stress-accumulating process over the threshold.

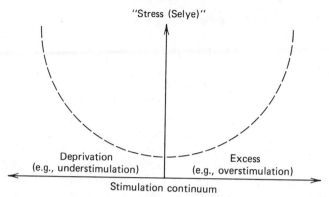

"Stress (Selye)"

Deprivation
(e.g., understimulation)

Excess
(e.g., overstimulation)

Stimulation continuum

Figure 4.7 Relation between physiological stress and level of stimulation. (Levi, L. Psychological stress and disease: A conceptual model. In Gunderson, E. K., and Rahe, R. H., eds., *Life Stress and Illness.* Courtesy of Charles C. Thomas, Publisher, Springfield, Illinois, 1974.)

Yet, if it is true that depression results from inability to cope with and prevent stress, then the logical target of primary and secondary prevention of depression in old age is in the personal preparation for that life stage by developing coping strategies that will reduce the effects of age-specific stressors in one's life.

There is less agreement about the physiological adaptive function of depression. While the "fight or flight" reaction to anxiety-fear has been well traced in the neuroendocrine system following the research of Walter Cannon (1932), the physiological response in depression has only lately been the object of intensive research.

Engel (1962) and Schmale (1970) have postulated that the coping strategies that result in depression involve conservation-withdrawal (akin to repression), denial/internalization (see Figure 4.4) with reduced psychomotor activity, lowered metabolism, and increased parasympathetic activity. In contrast, anxiety reactions elicit fight or flight, acting-out behavior with increased psychomotor activity, increased metabolism, and increased sympathetic activity. These intriguing hypotheses need experimental verification.

Whether the person projects and discharges anxiety into interpersonal situations or instead uses repression and denial and somatic channels to cope with distress (see Figure 4.4) depends upon the ego defense mechanisms or coping strategies employed (Pancheri and Benaissa, 1976).

Management strategies that deviate from the constructive pathways of problem-solving (psychological) and homeostasis (biological) as displayed in Figure 4.4 seem to result in somatic or behavioral disorders.

The formula of variables described in this chapter in the psychological and biological response to a stressor is unique in each person. The sum total of these intervening variables determines how a person will cope with stress. Coping is an act of flexible and resourceful problem-solving.

It occurs when the person seeks out new information, corrects or changes old dysfunctional beliefs about untoward circumstances, and then begins to behave differently and without distress in a very difficult situation.

Those who cope best are more apt to be physically healthy and age more slowly. This was the conclusion of a longitudinal study of 204 men who were students at Harvard in the early 1940s (Valliant, 1978). Psychiatrists evaluated their "adult adjustment" by scoring them on such factors as job success, happiness of their marriages, and number of vacations taken. Of the 59 men who had the best mental health between the ages of 21 and 46, only two became chronically ill or died by age 53. However, of the 48 who had the worst mental health, 18 were seriously sick or dead by that age. It seems that chronic anxiety, depression, and emotional maladjustment, measured in a variety of ways, predicted early aging, defined by irreversible deterioration of health. These data suggest that effective coping and positive mental health is an important part of staying physically healthy.

THE BIOLOGICAL RESPONSE

While knowledge of the neurobiology of human emotions is still in its infancy, research in this area indicates that "the raw stuff of emotion is built into the brain" according to Paul MacLean of the National Institute of Mental Health (quoted by Bigley and Sawhill, *Newsweek*, 1983). "We are on the crest of a neuro-biological revolution," according to another researcher, Bondereff (quoted *ibid*), and therefore, a complete theory of depression must incorporate a description of the biological response.

The amine hypothesis of affective disorders states that depression is associated with a functional deficit of one or more brain neurotransmitter amines at specific central synapses and that, conversely, mania is associated with a functional excess of one or more of these amines (Katz, 1970). The biochemical theory of depression began with the serendiptious finding that reserpine—used in the treatment of hypertension and known to act on neurotransmitters in the brain—had a depressogenic side effect on 15–20 percent of hypertensive patients using the drug. The depressogenic action of reserpine resulted from its ability to deplete the neurotransmitters serotonin and norepinephrine from the brain (Shore and Brodie, 1957). Another associated serendiptious discovery was that monoamine oxidase (MAO) inhibitors such as iproniaizid, when used in the treatment of tubercular patients, produced some mood elevation. This mood elevating action was later discovered to result from the MAO's ability to inhibit the destruction of brain amines, thereby ultimately resulting in elevated brain amine levels. A scarcity of the two neurotransmitters (serotonin and norepinephrine) has been demonstrated in association with depression. In fact, drugs that alleviate depression work by raising the level of these two transmitters.

Neurotransmitters

Neurons are programmed in the language of electricity and chemistry. When an electrical impulse reaches the tip of a neuron's tail, or axon, it fires a chemical called a *neurotransmitter*. This chemical message diffuses across a gap, called a *synapse*, to receptors on the next cell, triggering another electrical impulse that travels down a second axon, until the message reaches millions of neurons.

There are several categories of neurotransmitters. One category is *bioamines*, which are classified by their chemical structure. *Peptides* are another category. The most widely investigated neurotransmitter is nor-epinephrine. It is the transmitter between the presynaptic and postsynaptic nerve ending. The list of neurotransmitters is growing constantly. It includes some hormones that were previously not known to be neurotransmitters. For example, insulin not only controls blood sugar levels in the body but it also carries messages from one part of the body to another. Since 1975, scientists have discovered more than 50 neurotransmitters (Bigley and Sawhill, 1983).

The Neuroendocrine System

The hypothalamus appears to be the neurophysiological mechanism that mediates the psychosocial influences on the sympathoadrenomedulary and the immune system. The chemical that triggers the hypothalamus is thyroid stimulating factor (TSF). The exact means by which psychosocial events are translated into neurological and biochemical events is still to be determined. However, the hypothalamic nerve center at the base of the brain, once triggered, releases its own chemical messengers to the pituitary to which it is connected. As shown in Figure 4.8, corticotropic releasing factor (CRF) stimulates the anterior pituitary to discharge another chemical called adrenocorticotropic hormone (ACTH) into the blood. ACTH then directs the cortex of the adrenal gland to synthesize and secrete glucocorticoids; for example, cortisol.

Depressed patients usually have elevated plasma levels of cortisol. But there is a paradox in regard to depression and levels of cortisone. Naturally occurring hyperfunction of the adrenal cortex, as in Cushing's syndrome, is associated with depressive symptoms, whereas a high level of administered hormone is accompanied by euphoria (Sachar, 1967). Therefore, the mechanism for the production of depressive symptoms in association with high levels of blood cortisol is unclear and still under investigation. Nevertheless, the vegetative symptoms of depression are somatic symptoms that have been traditionally known to be controlled by the action of cortisol on target organs in the body.

The way station for memories and thoughts lies in the limbic system parts, which give rise to emotions (Bigley and Sawhill, 1983). One part,

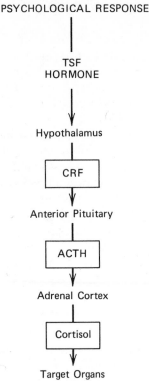

Figure 4.8 Biological (subcortical) response to stress.

the amygdala, seems to process sensations wrapped in an aura of happiness or sadness and index memories together with their associated mood states. For this reason, the remembrance of incidents past is often accompanied by the same emotion that suffused the original experience. Also, memory-retaining neurons in the cortex are like an intricate and sensitive spider's web, reaching out to touch a host of other neurons in the brain's electrical network (Bigley and Sawhill, 1983). That is why a single element in the environment can automatically trigger a memory response that includes a host of thoughts, feelings and sensations. In cognitive-behavioral therapy (refer to chapter 10), the goal is to identify and control automatic thought-memory-feeling response that habitually precipitates sad feelings: to unwrap the feeling-tone aura, examine the memory/thought contents and repackage them in more realistic positive emotions.

Incidentally, norepinephrine, which is usually depleted in depressed patients, seems to act as a "Print it!" command, writing memories in indelible ink (Bigley and Sawhill, 1983). But some memories are so unpleasant that, although they are "printed," they cannot be recalled. Perhaps remembering these things induces such painful feelings that the brain actually prevents their recall.

Research in the age-associated differences in neurophysiological mechanisms has been hampered by the lack of longitudinal studies. However, it appears to be a promising area for future research. To date, studies that have been assembled show adrenal deficiency and increased MAO levels in the elderly. Under basal conditions, it seems to be proved that the cortisol secretion rate is significantly diminished in old age (Blichert-Toft et al., 1980).

There is also a line of research that indicates that social and psychological variables can be manipulated selectively to induce major changes in brain amines. For example, in one experiment, norepinephrine, dopamine, and serotonin levels were most pronounced in mice that had been reared in isolation as compared to group-reared mice. It is this type of research that will eventually define the link between the psychological and biological response to stress in a comprehensive theory of depression. Until then, it is tempting to think of moods packaged in molecules in the body (Blichert-Toft et al., 1980).

DEPRESSION AS A PRECURSOR TO ILLNESS

Depression can predispose a person to physical illnesses in several ways. Depressed diabetic or hypertensive patients may be so disoriented or distracted that they forget to take the medications essential to their health. They are also apt to neglect routine precautions, thereby increasing their risk for accidents. Of broader consequence are the findings of recent studies that there are changes in biological activities related to depression that significantly increase the risk of illness and hospitalization (Schmale, 1958). As a result, depressed people seem more likely to experience a wide range of illnesses than nondepressed people.

The depression to illness link seems to be based in the sympathoadrenomedullary system response to psychosocial stimuli. Lennart Levi (1974) stated that the influence of psychosocial factors on neuroendocrine function, if prolonged or repeated too often, can result in functional disturbances in organs and organ systems. In fact, nearly all physiological variables can be altered by the effects of psychosocial stimuli on brain-glandular (endocrine) function through the common pathway of the hypothalamus. Because the thymus gland, which plays a central role in immune response, relies upon impulses from the hypothalamus in order to initiate immune-system activity, stress-related alterations in thymus gland activity can affect the body's ability to ward off germs and other foreign substances such as cancer cells (Solomon, 1969).

In a recent study, researchers at Mount Sinai Medical Center found a significant decrease in the activity of lymphocytes among 15 men whose wives had died after undergoing treatment for breast cancer (Schleifer et al., 1983). These findings seem to confirm that psychological stress associated with bereavement can weaken the immune system and leave a person vulnerable to disease.

Through its diverse actions on the body, the hypothalamus also has multiple effects on body metabolism. ACTH, which is released by the anterior pituitary under stimulation from the hypothalamus, regulates, among other things the sugar metabolism and the metabolism of minerals, including sodium and water. The thyroid hormones, which are stimulated by ACTH, increase the turnover of carbohydrates, fat, cholesterol, calcium, and magnesium and affect the heart rate and contractibility, total peripheral resistance, secretion of hydrocortisone and growth hormone, and the sensitivity of some tissues to catecholamines (Levi, 1979). The catecholamines are powerful vasoactive agents, with pronounced effects on sugar and fat metabolism. The exact mechanism of these physiological processes and how they vary according to different psychosocial variables has yet to be determined.

Although many studies have already been made in which animals have been exposed to various environmental stimuli, the results are diverse and conflicting due to differing research methods, subjects and control of extraneous influences (Levi, 1979). Many environmental variables such as heat, noise, crowding, and malnutrition may predispose subjects to illness. On the other hand, protective psychosocial interacting variables such as those discussed in the "Psychological Response" section of this chapter can prevent physiological reactions and the diseases for which they may be precursors.

It is these physiological changes that are perfectly normal reactions to stress that may be interpreted by some people as symptoms of disease (as in the case of hypochondriasis). In analyzing this process of psychosomatic onset, Simeons (1961) stated:

> When these once normal and vitally important reactions to fear do reach his conscious awareness, he interprets them as something abnormal and regards them as afflictions. . . . These now largely useless reactions, and their misinterpretation as signs of disease, produce a new—this time conscious—state of alarm: the dread of disease. . . . It is in this way that the vicious cycles which cause psychosomatic disease become established.

Since there is no sharp borderline between normal physiological reactions to stress, hypochondriacal reactions and actual physiological dysfunction leading to disease itself, the definition of where normal ends and disease begins is arbitrary and a function of labeling process. Whereas psychosocial stimuli may produce physiological effects to the point of disease, these stimuli can also influence physiological function to the point of impeding health and the recovery from illness.

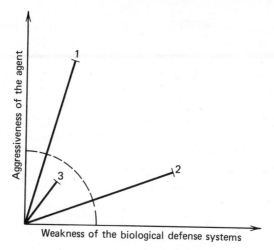

Figure 4.9 The interrelation between aggressiveness of the agent and the biological defense system in the production of a psychosomatic illness. (1) An extremely aggressive agent may lead to illness even when biological defenses are fairly strong. (2) A much weaker agent may result in illness when the defense system is itself weak. (3) A mildly aggressive agent acting against a normally strong defense system does not produce illness. (Pancheri, P., and Benaissa, C. Stress and psychosomatic illness. In Sarason, I. G., and Speilberger, C. D., eds., *Stress and Anxiety*, vol. 5. New York: Hemisphere Publishing Company, 1978.)

Because of this intimate mind-body interdependence, any stress-related illness can be said to be determined by two interacting and independent variables: 1) the type and intensity of the physical pathogenic agent and 2) the resistance of the biological defense systems that are determined by both somatic and psychosocial factors (Pancheri and Benaissa, 1978). In this framework, as illustrated in Figure 4.9, according to the same authors:

> . . . any somatic disease may be regarded as the final outcome of a series of unsuccessful attempts to cope with stress induced by either psychosocial stimuli, physical stimuli, or both.

In conclusion it appears that depression has a multifactorial genesis. Because it is affected by psychological, genetic, developmental, cultural, social and biological factors, it requires holistic assessment and intervention strategies. For the same reason, its prevention and treatment can best be managed by the complementary expertise and research efforts of the multidisciplinary health team.

REFERENCES

Akiskal, H., and McKinney, W. Overview of recent research in depression. *Archives of General Psychology*, 1975, 32:285–304.

Antonovsky, A. *Health, Stress and Coping.* San Francisco: Jossey-Bass, 1979.

Arkowitz, H. Is depression a social disease? Lecture, Psychiatry Grand Rounds, Health Sciences Center, University of Arizona, Tucson, March 11, 1981.

Astrup, C., Fossum, A., and Holmboc, R. A follow-up study of 270 patients with acute affective psychosis. *Acta Psychiatric Neurologica Scandanavica,* 1959, 34, Supp 135.

Barraclough, B.M. Suicide in the elderly. In Ashford Kent (Ed.), *Recent Developments in Psychogeriatrics.* Royal MedicoPsychological Association. *British Journal of Psychiatry,* 1971, Special Pub. No. 6.

Barrett, J.H. *Gerontological Psychology.* Springfield, Ill.: Charles C. Thomas, 1972.

Beck, A.T. Thinking and depression. *Archives of General Psychiatry,* 1963, 9:324–33.

Beck, A.T. *Depression: Clinical, Experimental, and Theoretical Aspects.* New York: Harper & Row, 1967.

Beck, A.T. The development of depression: a cognitive model. In Friedman, R., and Katz, M. (Eds.), *The Psychology of Depression.* Washington, D.C.: Winston, 1974.

Beck, A.T., et al. A new fast therapy for depression. *Psychology Today,* January 1977, 10:94.

Becker, J. *Depression: Theory and Research.* New York: Wiley, 1974.

Berkman, L. Social networks, host resistance and mortality: a follow-up study of Alameda County residents. Unpublished doctoral dissertation, University of California, Berkeley, 1977.

Bigley, C.J., and Sawhill, R. How the brain works. *Newsweek,* February 7, 1983, pp. 40–47.

Billings, A.G., Cronkite, R.C., and Moos, R.H. Social-environmental factors in unipolar depression: comparison of depressed patients and nondepressed controls. *Journal of Abnormal Psychology,* 1983, 92:2:119–33.

Billings, A.G., and Moos, R.H. The role of coping responses and social resources in attenuating the impact of stressful life events. *Journal of Behavioral Medicine,* 1981, 4:139–57.

Billings, A.G., and Moos, R.H. Psychosocial theory and research on depression: an integrative framework and review. *Clinical Psychology Review,* 1982, 2:213–37.

Blazer, D. and Williams, C. Epidemiology of dysphoria and depression in an elderly population. *American Journal of Psychiatry,* April 1980, 137:4:439–44.

Blichert-Toft, M., Lindholm, J., and Kehlet, H. 30 minute ACTH stimulation test as a predictor of hypothalamic-pituitary-adrenocortical function: comparison with metyrapone test. *Acta Medica Scandinavica,* 1980, 207:2:115–17.

Bressler, B. Depression and suicide. *Consultant,* March 1978, 18:123–126.

Brown, G.W., and Harris, J. *Social Origins of Depression: A Study of Psychiatric Disorder in Women.* London: Tavistock, 1978.

Brown, G.W., and Harris, T.O. *Social Origins of Depression: A Study of Psychiatric Disorder in Women.* New York: Free Press, 1978.

Brown, G.W., and Moos, R.H. Social support and functioning among community and clinical groups: a panel model. *Journal of Behavioral Medicine*, 1982, 5:295–311.

Butler, R.N. Life review: an interpretation of reminiscence in the aged. *Psychiatry Journal for the Study of Interpersonal Process*, February 1963, 26:65–76.

Cannon, W.B. *Wisdom of the Body*. New York: W.W. Norton, 1932.

Charatan, F.B. Depression in old age. *New York State Journal of Medicine*, 1975, 75(14):2505–09.

Costello, C.G. Social factors associated with depression: a retrospective community study. *Psychological Medicine*, 1982, 12:329–39.

Costello, C.G., and Wortman, C.B. Depression maintenance and interpersonal control.

Davis, H. The self-schema and subjective organization of personal information in depression. *Cognitive Therapy and Research*, 1979, 3(4):415–25.

De Beauvoir, S. The *Coming of Age*. New York: G.P. Putnam's Sons, 1972.

Dember, W.N. Motivation and the cognitive revolution. *American Psychologist*, 1974, 29:161–68.

Depue, R.A. (Ed.). *The Psychobiology of the Depressive Disorders: Implications for the Effects of Stress*. New York: Academic Press, 1979.

Dohrenwend, B.S., and Dohrenwend, B.J. *Stressful Life Events: Their Nature and Effects*. New York: Wiley, 1974.

Durkheim, E. *Suicide*. Spalding, J.A. (Trans.) New York: Free Press, 1951.

Eisdorfer, C. Stress, Disease and Cognitive Change. In Eisdorfer, C., and Friedel, R. (Eds.), *Cognitive and Emotional Disturbance in the Elderly*. Chicago: New Book Medical Publishers, 1977.

Eisdorfer, C. and Keckich, W. The Normal Psychopathology of Aging. In Cole, J. and Barret, J. (Eds.), *Psychopathology in the Aged*. New York: Raven Press, 1980.

Eliopoulous, C. Chronic care and the elderly: impact on the client, the family and the nurse. *Topics in Clinical Nursing*, April 1981 3:71–83.

Engel, G.L. *Psychological Development in Health and Disease*. Philadelphia: W.B. Saunders, 1962.

Epstein, L.J. Depression in the elderly. *Journal of Gerontology*, 1976, 31:279.

Erickson, E.H. *Childhood and Society*. New York: W.W. Norton, 1950.

Eysenck, H.J. Classification and the problem of diagnosis. In *Handbook of Abnormal Psychology*. Eysenck, H.J. (Ed.), London: Pitman, 1960.

Fahey, C.J. *Annual Report to the President—1981*. Washington, D.C.: Federal Council on Aging, 1981.

Farber, M.L. *Theory of Suicide*. New York: Funk & Wagnalls, 1968.

Farberow, N., and Moriwaki, S. Self-destructive crises in the older person. *Gerontologist*, August 1975, 15:333–37.

Fischer, C.S., and Phillips, S.L. Who is alone? Social characteristics of people with small networks. In Peplau, L., and Perlman, D. (Eds.), *Loneliness: A Source Book of Current Theory, Research and Therapy*. New York: Wiley, 1982.

Gaitz, C.M., and Scott, I. Analysis of letters to "Dear Abby" concerning old age. In Cole, J., and Barret, J. (Eds.), *Psychopathology in the Aged*. New York: Raven Press, 1980.

Goodwin, F.K., and Bunney, W.E., Jr. A psychobiological approach to affective illness. *Psychiatric Annals*, 1973, 3:19.

Gordon, S. The phenomenon of depression in old age. *Gerontologist*, 1973, 13:100–105.

Grauer, H. Depression in the aged: theoretical concepts. *Journal of the American Geriatrics Society*, 1977, 25(10):447–49.

Green, P.S. Growing old in China. *Modern Maturity*. August-September 1983, 26(4):58–59.

Hamalian, L., and Karl, F. *The Fourth World: The Imprisoned, The Poor, The Sick, The Elderly and the Underaged in America*. New York: Dell, 1976.

Hamilton, D.M., and Mann, W.A. The hospital treatment of involutional psychosis. *Proceedings of the American Psychopathological Association's 42nd Meeting*, 1954, pp. 199–209.

Hanson, K. Singing those retirement blues. New York *Daily News*, March 2, 1981, pp 5, 19.

Havinghurst, R., and Glaser, R. An exploratory study of reminiscence. *Journal of Gerontology*, 1972, 27(2):245–53.

Hendricks, J., and Hendricks, C.D. *Aging in Mass Society: Myths and Realities*. Cambridge, Mass.: Winthrop, 1977.

Hess, B.B. Stereotypes of the aged. *Journal of Communications*, 1974, 24:76–85.

Hirshfeld, R.M.A. Treatment of depression in the elderly. *Geriatrics*, 1979, 34(10):51–57.

Holmes, J.H., and Rahe, R.H. The social adjustment rating scale. *Journal of Psychosomatic Research*, 1967, 11:213.

Jarvik, L.F. Aging and depression: some unanswered questions. *Journal of Gerontology*, 1976, 31:324–26.

Katz, M.M. On the classification of depression: normal clinical and ethnocultural variations. In Proceedings of a Symposium, Fieve, R., Ed., *Depression Excerpta Medica*, 1970.

Kempton, M. Learning to wield a cane as a weapon is legacy of old age. *Newsday*, October 6, 1982.

Klerman, G.K. Depression and adaptation. In Friedman, R., and Katz, M. (Eds.), *The Psychology of Depression*. Washington, D.C.: Winston, 1974.

Lazarus, R. *Psychological Stress and the Coping Process*. New York: McGraw-Hill, 1966.

Lerner, M. Sorry, Skinner—it's all in your mind. *Newsday*, September 1, 1982.

Levi, L. Psychosocial stress and disease: A conceptual model. In Gunderson, E.K., and Rahe, R.H. (Eds.) *Life Stress and Illness*. Springfield, Ill.: Charles C. Thomas, 1974.

Levi, L. Psychosocial factors in preventative medicine. *Healthy People*, Background Paper [to the Surgeon General's report], 1979.

Levin, S. Depression in the aged: a study of salient external factors. *Geriatrics*, April 1963, pp. 302–07.

Levitt, E.E., and Lubin, B. *Depression: Concepts, Controversies and Some New Facts*. New York: Springer, 1975.

Lewis, A. "Endogenous" and "exogenous": a useful dichotomy? *Psychological Medicine*, May 1971, 1(3):191–96.

Lichtenberg, P. A definition and analysis of depression. *Archives of Neurology and Psychiatry*, 1957, 77:519–27.

Lidz, T. *The Person*. New York: Basic Books, 1968.

Liem, R., and Liem, J. Social class and mental illness reconsidered: the role of economic stress and social support. *Journal of Health and Social Behavior*, 1978, 19, 139–56.

Lipton, M.A. Age differentiation in depression: biochemical aspects. *Journal of Gerontology*, 1976, 31:293–98.

Litman, R.E. The depressed and suicidal patient. Keynote Address in *The Physician and the Depressed and Suicidal Patient: Proceedings of a Symposium Presented by the University of Arkansas for Medical Sciences*. Nutley, N.J.: Roche Labs, 1981.

Lowenthal, M.G., and Chiriboga, D. Social stress and adaptation: toward a life course perspective. In Eisdorfer, C., and Laraton, M.D. (Eds.), *The Psychology of Adult Development and Aging*. Washington, D.C.: American Psychological Association, 1973.

MacDonald, R. Content analysis of perceptions of aging as represented by the news media. *Gerontologist*, 1973, Part II.

MacLean, P.D. Depression as a specific response to stress. In Sarason, I.G., and Spielberger, C.D. (Eds.), *Stress and Anxiety*, vol. 3. New York: Wiley, 1976a.

MacLean, P.D. Therapeutic decision-making in treatment of depression. In P. Davidson (Ed.), *The Behavioral Management of Anxiety, Depression and Pain*. New York: Brunner/Mazel, 1976b.

Masserman, J.H. *Depressions: Theories and Therapies*. New York: Grune and Stratton, 1970.

Meichenbaum, D., and Jeirk, D.C. The cognitive behavioral management of anxiety, anger and pain. In P. Davidson (Ed.), *The Behavioral Management of Anxiety, Depression and Pain*. New York: Brunner/Mazel, 1976.

Melges, F.T., and Bowlby, J. Types of hopelessness in psychopathological processes. *Archives of General Psychology*, 1969, 20:696–99.

Mendels, J. Electroconvulsive therapy and depression, II: Significance of endogenous and reactive syndromes. *British Journal of Psychiatry*. 1965, 3:682–686.

Meyer, A. A discussion on the classification of the melancholies. *Journal of Nervous and Mental Diseases*, 1905, 32:114.

Miller, M. Suicide after Sixty: The Final Alternative. Monograph copyrighted by Marv Miller, 1978.

Miller, P.M., and Ingham, J.G. Life events to illness link. In Sarason, I.G., and Spielberger, C.D. (Eds.), *Stress and Anxiety*, vol. 6. New York: Wiley, 1979.

Minkoff, K., Bergman, E., Beck, A., et al. Hopelessness, depression, and attempted suicide. *American Journal of Psychiatry*, 1973, 130:455–60.

Moss, F. It's hell to be old in the U.S. *Nursing Dimensions*, Fall 1979, 7:49–51.

Myers, J.K., Lindenthal, J.J., and Pepper, M.P. Life events and psychiatric impairment. *Journal of Nervous and Mental Diseases*, 1971, 152:149–57.

Myers, J.K., Lindenthal, J.J., and Pepper, M.P. Life crises, health status, and role performance. Paper presented at the meeting of the American Psychiatric Association, Boston, May 1968.

National Council on Aging, Inc. *The Myth and Reality of Aging.* A study conducted by NCOA by Louis Harris and Associates, Inc., Washington, D.C.: NCOA, 1975.

Nelson, P.D. Comment in, Gunderson, E.K.E., and Rahe, R.H. (Eds), *Life Stress and Illness.* Springfield, Ill.: Charles C. Thomas, 1974.

Newman, J.L. The prevention of incontinence. In *Eighth International Congress of Gerontology Proceedings*, Washington, D.C., 1975, vol. 2, p. 75.

News Journal of AMA. Grief versus depression in elderly patients. *Journal of the American Medical Association*, 1979, 241(15):1558.

Newsweek. The crisis in Social Security, June 1, 1981 pp. 25–34.

New York Times. Abandoned in parking lot, *New York Times*, November 1, 1981, p. 4.

Neugarten, B. The old and the young in modern societies. In Shanas, E. (Ed.), *Aging in Contemporary Society.* Beverly Hills, Calif.: Sage, 1970.

Pancheri, P., and Benaissa, C. Stress and psychosomatic illness. In Sarason, I.G., and Spielberger, C.D. (Eds.), *Stress and Anxiety*, vol. 5. New York: Halsted Press, 1976.

Parish Family Digest. The Pope speaks. September-October 1983, 38(6):8.

Parker, W. Hearing and age. *Geriatrics*, April 1968, 24:151–52.

Paykel, E.S. Recent life events and clinical depression. In Gunderson, E.K., and Rahe, R.H. (Eds.), *Life Stress and Illness.* Springfield, Ill.: Charles C. Thomas, 1974.

Paykel, E.S. Recent life events in the development of the depressive disorders. In R.A. Depue (Ed.), *The Psychobiology of the Depressive Disorders: Implications for the Effects of Stress.* New York: Academic Press, 1979.

Pearlin, L.I., and Johnson, J. Marital status, life strains and depression. *American Sociological Review*, 1977, 42:704–715.

Pearson, M.M. Solving the diagnostic problems of atypical depression. *Medical Insight*, May 1971, 3:16–21.

Post, F. The factor of aging in affective illness. In Walsh, A., and Oppen, A. (Eds.), Recent Developments in Affective Disorders. *British Journal of Psychiatry*, 1968, Special Pub. No. 2.

Rabushka, A., and Jacobs, B. *Old Folks at Home.* New York: Free Press, 1980.

Rosenfeld, A.H. *New Views on Older Lives*, DHEW Pub. No. (ADM) 78–687. Washington, D.C.: U.S. Government Printing Office, 1978.

Rosow, I. Old people: their friends and neighbors. In Shanas, E. (Ed.), *Family Bureaucracy and the Elderly.* Durham, N.C.: Duke University Press, 1977.

Rush, A., and Beck, A.T. Adults with affective behaviors. In Hersen, M. (Ed.), *Behavior Therapy in the Psychiatric Setting.* Baltimore: Williams and Wilkins, 1978.

Sachar, E.J. Corticosteroids in depressive illness. *Archives of General Psychiatry*, 1967, 17:544–67.

Sainsbury, P. Social and epidemiological aspects of suicide in the aged. In Williams, R.H., Tibbits, C., and Donahue, F. (Eds.), *Process of Aging*, vol. 2. New York: Atherton Press, 1963.

Sarason, I.G., Johnson, James H., and Siegel, J.M. Assessing the impact of life changes: development of the life experiences survey. *Journal of Consulting and Clinical Psychology*, October 1978, 46(5).

Schleifer, S.J., Keller, S.E., Camerino, M. Thornton, J.C., and Stein, N. Suppression of lymphocyte stimulation following bereavement. *Journal of the American Medical Association*, 1983, 250(3).

Schless, A.P., Schwartz, L., and Goetz, C., et al. How depressives view the significance of life events. *British Journal of Psychiatry*, 1974 125:406–410.

Schmale, A.H., Jr. Relationship of separation and depression to disease. *Psychomatic Medicine*, 1958, 20(4):259–77.

Schmale, A.H. The role of depression in health and disease. Paper presented at the American Association for the Advancement of Science meeting, December 1970, Chicago.

Schulz, R. Aging health and theoretical social gerontology: where are we and where should we go. In Eiser, J.R. (Ed.), *Social Psychology and Behavioral Medicine*. New York: Wiley, 1982.

Seligman, M. *Helplessness*. San Francisco: W.H. Freeman, 1975.

Selye, H. *The Stress of Life*, 2nd ed. New York: McGraw-Hill, 1978.

Sheehy, G. *Pathfinders*. New York: William Morrow, 1981.

Shmagin, B.G. The pursuit of unhappiness. *Perspectives in Psychiatric Care*, 1977, 15(2):63–65.

Shore, P.A., and Brodie, B.B. Influence of various drugs on serotonin and norepinephrine in the brain. In Grattini, S. and Ghetti, V. (Eds.), *Psychotropic Drugs*. Amsterdam: Elsevier, 1957.

Siegel, J.M., Johnson, J.H., and Sarason, I.G. *Mood States and the Reporting of Life Change*. Unpublished manuscript. University of Washington, 1978.

Simeons, F.T.W. *Man's Presumptuous Brain*. New York: Dutton, 1961.

Sobel, M. Growing old in Britain. *Aging*, September–October, 1981, 321:8–16.

Solomon, G.F. Emotions, stress, the central nervous system, and immunity. *Annals of the New York Academy of Science*, 1969, 164(2):235–43.

Stotsky, B.A. Social and clinical issues in geriatric psychiatric. *American Journal of Psychiatry*, 1972, 129:117.

Surgeon General. *Healthy People*. U.S. Public Health Service Publication No. 79–55071. Washington, D.C.: U.S. Department of Health, Education and Welfare, 1979.

Sviland, M.A.P. Helping elderly couples to become sexually liberated: psychosocial issues. In LoPiccolo, J., and LoPiccolo, L. (Eds.), *Handbook of Sex Therapy*. New York: Plenum, 1978, 351–60.

Tedesseo-Castelnuovo, P. The mind as a stage; some comments on reminiscence and internal objects. *International Journal of Psychoanalysis*, 1978, 59:19.

Valliant, G.E. Natural history of male psychological health, VI: Correlates of successful marriage and fatherhood. *American Journal of Psychiatry*, June 1978, 135(6):653–59.

Wasylenki, D. Depression in the elderly. *Canadian Medical Journal*, March 8, 1980, 122:525–32.

Weingrad, J. Female scam artists loot the elderly. *New York Post*, October 5, 1982.

Weissmann, M.M., and Myers, J. Affective disorders in a U.S. urban community: the use of Research Diagnostic Criteria in an epidemiological survey. *Archives of General Psychiatry*, 1978, 35:1304–1311.

Westbrook, M.T. Socioeconomic differences in coping with childbearing. *American Journal of Community Psychology*, 1979, 7:397–412.

Wolff, K. *Geriatric Psychiatry*. Springfield, Ill.: Charles C. Thomas, 1963.

Woodruff, D.S. *Can You Live to be 100?* New York: Chatham Square Press, 1977.

Wyler, A.R., Masuda, M., and Holmes, T.H. Magnitude of life events and seriousness of illness. *Psychosomatic Medicine*, 1971, 33:115–22.

Diagnosis

5

Psychological Assessment of Depression in Older Adults

Alfred W. Kaszniak
James Allender

As described in Chapter 2, the psychological assessment of depression in the elderly poses many difficult problems. Some of these problems are created by age-related changes in psychological and physiological functioning, which must be differentiated from specific signs and symptoms of depression. A second source of diagnostic difficulty concerns the need to separate the signs and symptoms of depression from those similar features of other disorders (e.g., organic brain syndromes) for which the elderly are at increased risk. Chapters 2 and 3 reviewed the costs of missed or inappropriate diagnoses. The differential diagnosis of depression in older age poses one of the most difficult task facing clinicians concerned with mental health of the elderly.

The goal of the present chapter is to provide specific guidance in the diagnosis of depression in older age. This goal will be addressed within two major sections. First, the diagnostic criteria for depressive disorders of the Diagnostic and Statistical Manual of Mental Disorders, Third Edition (DSM-III, American Psychiatric Association, 1980) will be presented, with particular attention to special considerations in the application of these criteria to older persons. Second, those most frequently employed assessment instruments (including self-report instruments, behavior rating scales, and individually administered psychological assessment procedures) will be reviewed, with recommendations made concerning those instruments particularly suitable for the assessment of depression in older persons. Chapter 6 will review general issues and specific procedures in the differential diagnosis of depression versus those organic brain syndromes for which the elderly are at particular risk.

DIAGNOSTIC CRITERIA

The DSM-III is the most recent edition of the official diagnostic criteria set forth by the American Psychiatric Association (APA). The first edition of this manual appeared in 1952, and the second edition in 1968. Each edition was designed to be clinically useful while at the same time providing a basis for administrative and research use. Preparation for the development of the DSM-III began in 1974 with an initial draft of the classification schema presented at the Annual Meeting of the APA in May 1975. Discussion of this draft and subsequent revisions occurred at various local, national, and international professional meetings in subsequent years. A series of field trials were conducted from September 1977 to September 1979, with, in all, 12,667 patients (covering a wide age range, from children to older adults) evaluated by approximately 550 different clinicians. A major contribution of these field trials was the opportunity for evaluation of diagnostic reliability by having pairs of clinicians make independent diagnostic judgments of many patients. In general, the DSM-III criteria demonstrate considerably better reliability than the criteria of DSM-II (see Appendix F, APA, 1980). The DSM-III differs from its predecessors in several important dimensions. First, the DSM-III takes a descriptive approach, which is generally atheoretical with regard to etiology. Second, the DSM-III provides specific diagnostic criteria guiding each diagnosis. While these criteria will undoubtedly be revised as new information concerning such variables as clinical course and treatment response becomes available, the present specificity in diagnostic criteria helps to enhance interjudge diagnostic reliability.

Another major departure of the DSM-III is its use of a multiaxial evaluation system. Within this system, an evaluation is made on five axes. Axes I and II include all of the mental disorders, with two classes of mental disorders, personality disorders and specific developmental disorders assigned to Axis II and all other mental disorders assigned to Axis I. Axis III is employed for the classification of physical disorders present. Axis IV ranks the severity of psychosocial stressors and Axis V the highest level of adaptive functioning in the past year. Axes I, II, and III provide the official DSM-III diagnosis, while Axes IV and V are for use in special clinical or research settings. All of the depressive disorders with which this chapter is concerned are classified within Axis I of the DSM-III. Given the limited scope of the present chapter, the focus will be exclusively upon Axis I diagnostic criteria. However, evaluation along all five axes is of considerable value in planning treatment and predicting outcome for any given individual, and careful attention to all of the DSM-III (APA, 1980) is highly recommended.

We have chosen to focus upon the diagnostic criteria of the DSM-III because of its widespread use in North America, as well as some of its virtues. Note, however, that no nosologic system is free of criticism and controversy. The interested reader is directed to Sprock and Blashfield (1983) for a discussion of general and specific issues concerning classification systems. One criticism, particularly relevant to the purposes of the present chapter, is the relative lack of consideration of issues in the diagnosis of older adults. While age of onset is a specific criterion for certain diagnostic categories (e.g., Primary Degenerative Dementia, Senile Onset versus Primary Degenerative Dementia, Presenile Onset), special considerations in application of the diagnostic criteria to older adults are generally not well-specified. In large part, it is the purpose of the next section of the present chapter to alert the reader to these special considerations. As discussed in Chapter 2, depressive disorders appear within the DSM-III in three main sections: 1) Affective Disorders, 2) Adjustment Disorder with Depressed Mood, and 3) Organic Affective Syndrome.

Affective Disorders

The common feature of all syndromes classified as affective disorders within the DSM-III is a *disturbance of mood* (mood here is defined as prolonged and pervasive emotion), generally involving either *depression or elation*, which is not due to any other mental or physical disorder. The class of affective disorders is further subdivided into *Major Affective Disorders*, in which a full affective syndrome is present; *Other Specific Affective Disorders*, in which only a partial affective syndrome is present and is of at least two years duration; and *Atypical Affective Disorders*, a category reserved for those affective disorders not classifiable in either of the two specific classes. The Major Affective Disorders are further subdivided into *Bipolar Disorder* and *Major Depression*, which are distinguished by the presence of a manic episode in the former. Although the first manic episode of Bipolar Disorder typically occurs before age 30 (Loranger and Levine, 1978; APA, 1980, p. 215), it is an important consideration in the evaluation of those older patients suspected of a chronic or recurrent Affective Disorder. Therefore, diagnostic criteria for a manic episode will be briefly reviewed.

Manic Episode

In general, a *manic episode* is characterized by a distinct period during which the predominant mood is either *elevated, irritable, or expansive*, and accompanied by some of the following *associated symptoms*: pressure of speech; flight of ideas; hyperactivity; inflated self-esteem; distractibility; decreased need for sleep; and excessive involvement in activities that have a high potential for painful consequences, a potential not recognized. The specific criteria for diagnosis for a manic episode are provided in Table 5.1.

As described in Table 5.1, the primary criterion is one or more distinct periods with a predominantly elevated, expansive, or irritable mood. The

TABLE 5.1

DSM-III DIAGNOSTIC CRITERIA FOR A MANIC EPISODE

A. One or more distinct periods with a predominantly elevated, expansive, or irritable mood. The elevated or irritable mood must be a prominent part of the illness and relatively persistent, although it may alternate or intermingle with depressive mood.

B. Duration of at least one week (or any duration if hospitalization is necessary), during which, for most of the time, at least three of the following symptoms have persisted (four if the mood is only irritable) and have been present to a significant degree:

(1) increase in activity (either socially, at work, or sexually) or physical restlessness

(2) more talkative than usual or pressure to keep talking

(3) flight of ideas or subjective experience that thoughts are racing

(4) inflated self-esteem (grandiosity, which may be delusional)

(5) decreased need for sleep

(6) distractibility, i.e., attention is too easily drawn to unimportant or irrelevant external stimuli

(7) excessive involvement in activities that have a high potential for painful consequences which is not recognized, e.g., buying sprees, sexual indiscretions, foolish business investments, reckless driving

C. Neither of the following dominates the clinical picture when an affective syndrome is absent (i.e., symptoms in criteria A and B above):

(1) preoccupation with a mood-incongruent delusion or hallucination (see definition below)

(2) bizarre behavior

D. Not superimposed on either Schizophrenia, Schizophreniform Disorder, or a Paranoid Disorder.

E. Not due to any Organic Mental Disorder, such as Substance Intoxication.

(**Note:** A hypomanic episode is a pathological disturbance similar to, but not as severe as, a manic episode.)

Fifth-digit code numbers and criteria for subclassification of manic episode

6— In Remission. This fifth-digit category should be used when in the past the individual met the full criteria for a manic episode but now is essentially free of manic symptoms or has some signs of the disorder but does not meet the full criteria. The differentiation of this diagnosis from no mental disorder requires consideration of the period of time since the last episode, the number of previous episodes, and the need for continued evaluation or prophylactic treatment.

4— With Psychotic Features. This fifth-digit category should be used when there apparently is gross impairment in reality testing, as when there are delusions or hallucinations or grossly bizarre behavior. When possible, specify whether the psychotic features are mood-incongruent. (The non-ICD-9-CM fifth-digit 7 may be used instead to indicate that the psychotic features are mood-incongruent; otherwise, mood-congruence may be assumed.)

Mood-congruent Psychotic Features: Delusions or hallucinations whose content is entirely consistent with the themes of inflated worth, power, knowledge, identity, or special relationship to a deity or famous person; flight of ideas without apparent awareness by the individual that the speech is not understandable.

110

TABLE 5.1   (continued)

Mood-incongruent Psychotic Features: Either (a) or (b):

(a) Delusions or hallucinations whose content does not involve themes of either inflated worth, power, knowledge, identity, or special relationship to a deity or famous person. Included are such symptoms as persecutory delusions, thought insertion, and delusions of being controlled, whose content has no apparent relationship to any of the themes noted above.

(b) Any of the following catatonic symptoms: stupor, mutism, negativism, posturing.

2— Without Psychotic Features. Meets the criteria for manic episode, but no psychotic features are present.

0—   Unspecified.

Source: Reprinted from American Psychiatric Association, *Diagnostic and Statistical Manual of Mental Disorders*, Third Edition, Washington, D.C., APA, 1980.

second major criterion is the episode's duration of at least one week (or any duration if hospitalization is necessary) during which at least three of the listed symptoms (four if the mood is only irritable) have been present and persisted to a significant degree.

Special consideration should be applied in evaluating the presence of some of these features in the elderly patient. First, the category of decreased need for sleep requires evaluation in comparison to age-appropriate expectations. Considerable evidence indicates quantitative diminution in the amount of nighttime sleep with aging, sleep being marked by more frequent and more prolonged awakenings. Thus, evaluation of decreased need for sleep, as part of a possible manic episode, should be based upon comparison to the individual's typical recent sleep pattern, rather than upon comparison to the individual's pattern in earlier life. Again, criteria for a manic episode requires that symptoms such as decreased need for sleep be part of one or more distinct periods with a predominantly elevated, expansive, or irritable mood.

The symptom category "excessive involvement in activities that have a high potential for painful consequences which is not recognized" also needs some special attention. Reckless driving is given as one example in Table 5.1. In the case of an elderly person, a judgment needs to be made as to whether behavior such as reckless driving represents a lack of recognition of potential painful consequences of the act, or limitations posed by sensory, motor, or cognitive deficit.

The application of these criteria to individuals of all ages requires knowing the classification of psychotic features. *Psychotic features* refers to an apparent gross impairment in the ability of the individual to perceive consensually defined reality. Delusions, hallucinations, or markedly bizarre behavior are examples. When such psychotic features are present, they are further subdivided on the basis of whether they are mood congruent or incongruent. *Mood congruence* refers to delusions or hallucinations whose content is consistent with the themes of power, inflated worth, special knowledge or identity, etc. Delusions or hallucinations not so characterized are considered mood incongruent.

Before leaving the discussion of diagnostic criteria for a manic episode, the reader is reminded of the caution that needs to be exercised in applying this diagnosis to the elderly person without a previous history of manic episode. Loranger and Levine (1978) reported data on the age at onset of bipolar affective illness determined for 100 males and 100 females who met the DSM-III criteria for mania. One-third of this sample were hospitalized prior to their twenty-fifth birthday, with at least 20 percent having already shown evidence of illness as adolescents. The peak period of onset was found to be in the early 20s, and onset after age 60 was found to be very rare.

Major Depressive Episode

A *major depressive episode* is characterized by a prominent and persistent *dysphoric mood, usually depression, or a loss of interest or pleasure* in all or almost all usual activities or pastimes. This disturbance is associated with other symptoms, including sleep disturbance, appetite disturbance, change in weight, psychomotor agitation or retardation, feelings of worthlessness or guilt, decreased energy, difficulty concentrating or thinking, and thoughts of death or suicide or suicidal attempts. Table 5.2 presents the specific diagnostic criteria of DSM-III for a major depressive episode.

Special Considerations in Diagnosing Depression in Old Age

Since the DSM-III criteria for major depressive episode were validated in a sample of predominantly younger to middle aged adults (Spitzer et al., 1979), it is conceivable that depression in older individuals manifests differently than depression in younger adults. Results of a study reported by Winokur et al., (1980) suggest that, at least for depressed women, depression with onset in older age is generally comparable to depression with earlier onset. Variables such as premorbid personality characteristics, response to antidepressant drug treatment, relapse during a three-year follow-up period, and the incidence of suicidal thoughts, guilt, psychomotor retardation, and sleep disturbance were found to be comparable between earlier and later onset depressed patients. However, the older onset patients did demonstrate significantly greater weight loss and decrease in sexual drive.

Despite the apparent general comparability of signs and symptoms of depression with onset in younger and older adulthood, special considerations need to be applied when employing the diagnostic criteria to the older individual. First, given the increase risk with older age for a variety

TABLE 5.2

DSM-III DIAGNOSTIC CRITERIA FOR MAJOR DEPRESSIVE EPISODE

A. Dysphoric mood or loss of interest or pleasure in all or almost all usual activities and pastimes. The dysphoric mood is characterized by symptoms such as the following: depressed, sad, blue, hopeless, low, down in the dumps, irritable. The mood disturbance must be prominent and relatively persistent, but not necessarily the most dominant symptom, and does not include momentary shifts from one dysphoric mood to another dysphoric mood, e.g., anxiety to depression to anger, such as are seen in states of acute psychotic turmoil. (For children under six, dysphoric mood may have to be inferred from a persistently sad facial expression.)

B. At least four of the following symptoms have each been present nearly every day for a period of at least two weeks (in children under six, at least three of the first four).

(1) poor appetite or significant weight loss (when not dieting) or increased appetite or significant weight gain (in children under six, consider failure to make expected weight gains)

(2) insomnia or hypersomnia

(3) psychomotor agitation or retardation (but not merely subjective feelings of restlessness or being slowed down) (in children under six, hypoactivity)

(4) loss of interest or pleasure in usual activities, or decrease in sexual drive not limited to a period when delusional or hallucinating (in children under six, signs of apathy)

(5) loss of energy; fatigue

(6) feelings of worthlessness, self-reproach, or excessive or inappropriate guilt (either may be delusional)

(7) complaints or evidence of diminished ability to think or concentrate, such as slowed thinking, or indecisiveness not associated with marked loosening of associations or incoherence

(8) recurrent thoughts of death, suicidal ideation, wishes to be dead, or suicide attempt

C. Neither of the following dominate the clinical picture when an affective syndrome is absent (i.e., symptoms in criteria A and B above):

(1) preoccupation with a mood-incongruent delusion or hallucination (see definition below)

(2) bizarre behavior

D. Not superimposed on either Schizophrenia, Schizophreniform Disorder, or a Paranoid Disorder.

E. Not due to any Organic Mental Disorder or Uncomplicated Bereavement.

Fifth-digit code numbers and criteria for subclassification of major depressive episode
(When psychotic features and Melancholia are present the coding system requires that the clinician record the single most clinically significant characteristic.)

6— In Remission. This fifth-digit category should be used when in the past the individual met the full criteria for a major depressive episode but now is essentially free of depressive symptoms or has some signs of the disorder but does not meet the full criteria.

4— With Psychotic Features. This fifth-digit category should be used when there apparently is gross impairment in reality testing, as when there are delusions or hallucinations, or depressive stupor (the individual is mute and unresponsive). When possible, specify whether the psychotic features are mood-congruent or mood-incongruent. (The non-ICD-9-CM fifth-digit 7 may be used instead to indicate that the psychotic features are mood-incongruent; otherwise, mood-congruence may be assumed.)

113

TABLE 5.2 *(continued)*

Mood-congruent Psychotic Features. Delusions or hallucinations whose content is entirely consistent with the themes of either personal inadequacy, guilt, disease, death, nihilism, or deserved punishment; depressive stupor (the individual is mute and unresponsive).

Mood-incongruent Psychotic Features. Delusions or hallucinations whose content does not involve themes of either personal inadequacy, guilt, disease, death, nihilism, or deserved punishment. Included here are such symptoms as persecutory delusions, thought insertion, thought broadcasting, and delusions of control, whose content has no apparent relationship to any of the themes noted above.

3— With Melancholia. Loss of pleasure in all or almost all activities, lack of reactivity to usually pleasurable stimuli (doesn't feel much better, even temporarily, when something good happens), and at least three of the following:

(a) distinct quality of depressed mood, i.e., the depressed mood is perceived as distinctly different from the kind of feeling experienced following the death of a loved one

(b) the depression is regularly worse in the morning

(c) early morning awakening (at least two hours before usual time of awakening)

(d) marked psychomotor retardation or agitation

(e) significant anorexia or weight loss

(f) excessive or inappropriate guilt

2— Without Melancholia

0— Unspecified

Source: Reprinted from American Psychiatric Association, *Diagnostic and Statistical Manual of Mental Disorders*, Third Edition, Washington, D.C., APA, 1980.

of medical illnesses, and with the possibility of adverse affects of drugs used to treat these illnesses, careful consideration needs to be given to these potential contributors to apparently depressive symptoms. For example, patients with occult carcinoma, particularly carcinoma of the pancreas (Fras et al., 1967) may demonstrate depression-like symptoms, including fatigue, poor appetite and weight loss, and sleep disturbance, before other symptoms that eventually lead to a correct diagnosis. Similarly, patients with cardiac disease frequently complain of sleep disturbance, fatigue, and difficulty with concentration. Depression-like signs and symptoms are also frequently seen as adverse drug effects. These are reviewed in detail within Chapter 7. All these considerations point to the necessity of careful medical as well as psychological evaluation of the older patient suspected of depression.

Evaluation of sleep disturbance in the older patient also requires particular consideration. Fragmented sleep, marked by an increased frequency of awakenings and electroencephalographic (EEG) evidence of a decrease in slow-wave sleep is well documented in depression (Hauri, 1977; Hawkins, 1979). However, healthy older persons, without evidence of depression or other illness, also demonstrate more frequent and longer awakenings and decreased slow-wave sleep in comparison to healthy younger adults (Prinz, 1977; Webb, 1982). Consequently, it may be difficult to determine whether a complaint of sleep disturbance is indicative of depression or merely reflects the older individual's awareness of a change, with increasing age, of sleep quality and pattern. As in a manic episode, it is helpful to inquire carefully about the recency of the perceived change in sleep, as well as its temporal relation to other possible features of a depressive episode.

Age-appropriate expectations also need to be applied to the evaluation of possible psychomotor retardation. A large number of studies reported over the past 100 years has demonstrated behavioral slowing to be perhaps the most significant and ubiquitous change associated with aging (Birren et al., 1980). Hence, evidence of psychomotor slowing inferred from speed of performance on individually administered psychological tests should be based upon comparison to normative data appropriate for the given individual's age. Again, the relative recency of change in speed of behavior, as well as its temporal association with other features can be helpful.

Somewhat different considerations need to be applied to the evaluation of decrease in sexual drive. Cultural stereotype, as well as some older research, has suggested that there is a marked decrease in sexual activity with aging. However, recent investigation (see review by Comfort, 1980) suggests that there is less of an "age change" in sexual activity than has been thought. Lower reported levels of sexual activity in older individuals may represent a mixture of "cohort effects" (a greater number of older individuals always having engaged in a relatively low level of sexual activity), ill health, social pressure, and the lack of an appropriate partner. Hence, one should not necessarily expect that aging will be accompanied by a decrease in sexual response, interest, or activity. However, assessment of sexual drive, when evaluating for the possibility of depression, must take into account the individual's physical health (many diseases result in decreased sexual ability or interest), the availability of a socially acceptable sexual partner, and previous history of sexual behavior.

One area in which older depressed patients may significantly differ from younger patients is in the incidence of hypochondriasis (irrational fear of physical illness), a feature not included within the DSM-III diagnostic criteria for major depressive episode (unless one wishes to consider this as a mood-congruent delusion). As Stenback (1980, pp. 625–626) has pointed out, many authors have been of the opinion that hypochondriacal complaints are the most characteristic feature of depression in older age. In a study of 152 elderly depressed patients consecutively admitted to the Bethlehem Royal Hospital, de Alarcon (1964) found hypochondriasis (defined as a physically unjustified body complaint) present in 64 percent, with no significant difference between the sexes. This is a considerably higher incidence than that found in studies of younger depressed groups (e.g., Stenback and Javala, 1962). Further, Barnes et al., (1981) report that some elderly patients with hypochondriasis who appear depressed to the clinician, and who respond to antidepressant therapy, deny the subjective experience of a depressed mood state. Such patients, given their lack of report of depressed mood, would likely not qualify for a diagnosis of major depressive episode under DSM-III criteria, and would more likely fall under the diagnosis of hypochondriasis, within the general category of Somatoform Disorders (see APA, 1980, pp. 249– 251). This is obviously one area where the diagnostic criteria for major depressive episode, when applied to older individuals, may need revision (see discussion of "Masked Depression" in Chapter 2). Certainly, these considerations indicate the need for careful consideration of possible depression if thorough medical evaluation fails to provide a physiological diagnosis for somatic complaints and concerns.

The possibility of depression must also be seriously considered in older individuals suffering from chronic physical illness. As noted above, differential diagnosis is complicated by various signs and symptoms (e.g., fatigue, poor appetite or weight loss, sleep difficulty) common to both depression and various physical illnesses. Recent research (Okimoto et al., 1982) suggests, at least for medical outpatients, that psychological rather than somatic symptoms may be most discriminating in identifying depression in such patients.

Cyclothymic and Dysthymic Disorder

The DSM-III also contains criteria for other specific affective disorders in addition to Bipolar Disorder and Major Depression. These other specific affective disorders share in common the criteria of illness of at least two years' duration, with either intermittent or sustained mood disturbance and associated symptoms. In addition, these other diagnoses require that a full affective syndrome *not* be present, and that the patient be free of psychotic features.

The essential feature of a *Cyclothymic Disorder* is "a chronic mood disturbance of at least two years' duration, involving numerous periods of depression and hypomania, but not of sufficient severity and duration to meet the criteria for a major depressive or a manic episode (full affective syndrome)" (APA, 1980, p. 218). As can be seen in Table 5.3, the criteria for depressive and hypomanic periods are similar, although representing less severe symptoms, to those of major depressive episode and manic episode, respectively. Further, a lesser number of associated symptoms, in addition to the mood disturbance, are required for making the diagnosis, in comparison to the criteria for major depressive episode or manic episode. Given the similarity of symptom criteria, all of the comments made above concerning special considerations when evaluating older individuals for possible Bipolar Disorder or Major Depression, also apply when considering the possibility of Cyclothymic Disorder. As with Bipolar

TABLE 5.3

DSM-III DIAGNOSTIC CRITERIA FOR CYCLOTHYMIC DISORDER

A. During the past two years, numerous periods during which some symptoms characteristic of both the depressive and the manic syndromes were present, but were not of sufficient severity and duration to meet the criteria for a major depressive or manic episode.

B. The depressive periods and hypomanic periods may be separated by periods of normal mood lasting as long as months at a time, they may be intermixed, or they may alternate.

C. During **depressive** periods there is depressed mood or loss of interest or pleasure in all or almost all, usual activities and pastimes, and at least three of the following:	During **hypomanic** periods there is an elevated, expansive, or irritable mood and at least three of the following:
(1) insomnia or hypersomnia	(1) decreased need for sleep
(2) low energy or chronic fatigue	(2) more energy than usual
(3) feelings of inadequacy	(3) inflated self-esteem
(4) decreased effectiveness or productivity at school, work, or home	(4) increased productivity, often associated with unusual and self-imposed working hours
(5) decreased attention, concentration, or ability to think clearly	(5) sharpened and unusually creative thinking
(6) social withdrawal	(6) uninhibited people-seeking (extreme gregariousness)
(7) loss of interest in or enjoyment of sex	(7) hypersexuality without recognition of possibility of painful consequences
(8) restriction of involvement in pleasurable activities; guilt over past activities	(8) excessive involvement in pleasurable activities with lack of concern for the high potential for painful consequences, e.g., buying sprees, foolish business investments, reckless driving
(9) Feeling slowed down	(9) physical restlessness
(10) less talkative than usual	(10) more talkative than usual
(11) pessimistic attitude toward the future, or brooding about past events	(11) overoptimism or exaggeration of past achievements
(12) tearfulness or crying	(12) inappropriate laughing, joking, punning

D. Absence of psychotic features such as delusions, hallucinations, incoherence, or loosening of associations.

E. Not due to any other mental disorder, such as partial remission of Bipolar Disorder. However, Cyclothymic Disorder may precede Bipolar Disorder.

Source: Reprinted from American Psychiatric Association, *Diagnostic and Statistical Manual of Mental Disorders,* Third Edition, Washington, D.C., APA, 1980.

Disorder, age of onset is usually early in adult life. Therefore, the clinician should be skeptical about applying this diagnosis to an older individual if there is not a clear history, consistent with the diagnosis, going back to early adulthood.

Dysthymic Disorder (or Depressive Neurosis) is "a chronic disturbance of mood involving either depressed mood or loss of interest or pleasure in

TABLE 5.4

DSM-III DIAGNOSTIC CRITERIA FOR DYSTHYMIC DISORDER

A. During the past two years (or one year for children and adolescents) the individual has been bothered most or all of the time by symptoms characteristic of the depressive syndrome but that are not of sufficient severity and duration to meet the criteria for a major depressive episode.

B. The manifestations of the depressive syndrome may be relatively persistent or separated by periods of normal mood lasting a few days to a few weeks, but no more than a few months at a time.

C. During the depressive periods there is either prominent depressed mood (e.g., sad, blue, down in the dumps, low) or marked loss of interest or pleasure in all, or almost all, usual activities and pastimes.

D. During the depressive periods at least three of the following symptoms are present:

(1) insomnia or hypersomnia

(2) low energy level or chronic tiredness

(3) feelings of inadequacy, loss of self-esteem, or self-deprecation

(4) decreased effectiveness or productivity at school, work, or home

(5) decreased attention, concentration, or ability to think clearly

(6) social withdrawal

(7) loss of interest in or enjoyment of pleasurable activities

(8) irritability or excessive anger (in children, expressed toward parents or caretakers)

(9) inability to respond with apparent pleasure to praise or rewards

(10) less active or talkative than usual, or feels slowed down or restless

(11) pessimistic attitude toward the future, brooding about past events, or feeling sorry for self

(12) tearfulness or crying

(13) recurrent thoughts of death or suicide

E. Absence of psychotic features, such as delusions, hallucinations, or incoherence, or loosening of associations.

F. If the disturbance is superimposed on a preexisting mental disorder, such as Obsessive Compulsive Disorder or Alcohol Dependence, the depressed mood, by virtue of its intensity or effect on functioning, can be clearly distinguished from the individual's usual mood.

Source: Reprinted from American Psychiatric Association, *Diagnostic and Statistical Manual of Mental Disorders*, Third Edition, Washington, D.C., APA, 1980.

all, or almost all, usual activities and pastimes, and associated symptoms, but not of sufficient severity and duration to meet the criteria for a major depressive episode (full affective syndrome)" (APA, 1980, pp. 220–21). As shown in Table 5.4, sign and symptom criteria are similar to those for Major Depression, although, again, less severe and requiring a fewer number of symptoms for the diagnosis. Considerations similar to those outlined for Major Depression need to be applied when considering a diagnosis of Dysthymic Disorder in the older patient. For the older person who has never previously demonstrated signs and symptoms sufficient to

TABLE 5.5

DSM-III DIAGNOSTIC CRITERIA FOR ADJUSTMENT DISORDER

A. A maladaptive reaction to an identifiable psychosocial stressor, that occurs within three months of the onset of the stressor.

B. The maladaptive nature of the reaction is indicated by either of the following:

(1) impairment in social or occupational functioning

(2) symptoms that are in excess of a normal and expectable reaction to the stressor

C. The disturbance is not merely one instance of a pattern of overreaction to stress or an exacerbation of one of the mental disorders previously described.

D. It is assumed that the disturbance will eventually remit after the stressor ceases or, if the stressor persists, when a new level of adaptation is achieved.

E. The disturbance does not meet the criteria for any of the specific disorders listed previously or for Uncomplicated Bereavement.

Source: Reprinted from American Psychiatric Association, *Diagnostic and Statistical Manual of Mental Disorders,* Third Edition, Washington, D.C., APA, 1980.

fulfill the criteria for an affective disorder diagnosis, the clinician should be skeptical in applying the diagnosis of Dysthymic Disorder, as age of onset is typically early in adult life. However, a diagnosis of Dysthymic Disorder is appropriate in an older person who has a past history of Major Depression and is in partial remission for a period of at least two years.

Within the category of Affective Disorders, the DSM-III also employs two final diagnostic subcategories, those of Atypical Bipolar Disorder, and Atypical Depression. These categories are reserved for individuals with manic or depressive features, respectively, who cannot be classified as having Bipolar Disorder, Cyclothymic Disorder, Major Depression, Dysthymic Disorder, or Adjustment Disorder with Depressed Mood. Since these are essentially "residual" categories, such diagnoses should only very rarely be used.

Adjustment Disorder

An *Adjustment Disorder*, according to the DSM-III, "is a maladaptive reaction to an identifiable psychosocial stressor, that occurs within three months after the onset of the stressor. The maladaptive nature of the reaction is indicated by either impairment in social or occupational functioning or symptoms that are in excess of a normal and expected reaction to the stressor" (APA, 1980, p. 299). Table 5.5 provides the diagnostic criteria for adjustment disorder. Relevant to the present chapter is the subcategory of *Adjustment Disorder with Depressed Mood*. This diagnosis is employed when the adjustment disorder is characterized by symptoms such as depressed mood, tearfulness, and hopelessness, and where the individual does not fit the criteria for other specific disorders, such as major depression, dysthymic disorder, or uncomplicated bereavement. If the older patient presents with signs and symptoms consistent with Major Depression, for example, this diagnosis should be used, regardless of whether any identifiable psychosocial stressors as apparent precipitants, can be discerned.

Since the older person is at particular risk of loss through bereavement, the major differential diagnostic difficulty is between Adjustment Disorder with Depressed Mood and *Uncomplicated Bereavement*. The latter category is used when a focus of attention or treatment is upon a normal reaction to the death of a loved one. As pointed out in the DSM-III, "a full depressive syndrome frequently is a normal reaction to such a loss, with feelings of depression and such associated symptoms as poor appetite, weight loss, and insomnia. However, morbid preoccupation with worthlessness, prolonged and marked functional impairment, and marked psychomotor retardation are uncommon and suggest that the bereavement is complicated by the development of a major depression" (APA, 1980, p. 333). Also noted in the DSM-III is that, when guilt is present, in uncomplicated bereavement, it is principally focused upon things done or neglected at the time of the death.

The duration of "normal" bereavement has considerable variability among different subcultural groups. In evaluating response to bereavement, the clinician therefore needs to take into account the customs and beliefs of the cultural group to which the individual belongs.

Organic Affective Syndrome

The final area in which depressive signs and symptoms are found within the DSM-III, is that of Organic Mental Disorders, in which a disturbance of mood, secondary to a specific organic factor, might be the principle feature, such as in *Organic Affective Syndrome*, or where depressive features may complicate principally cognitive deficits secondary to organic factors, such as in *Primary Degenerative Dementia* with depression. These diagnoses will be discussed more fully within Chapter 6. In the next section attention is focused upon available procedures for the psychological assessment and quantification of depressive signs and symptoms in the older person.

ASSESSMENT PROCEDURES

The DSM-III provides some guidelines as to how the relevant information and observations are to be obtained with any given patient. In general, however, it presumes that clinicians employing the diagnostic criteria will utilize the skills of their respective disciplines in collecting such data. The purpose of the present section of this chapter is to provide information concerning assessment procedures particularly useful in the diagnosis of depression in the older adult.

Risks to Reliability and Validity in Psychological Assessment of the Elderly

In attempting to evaluate the appropriateness of applying a particular psychological assessment instrument to the older individual, several issues, relevant to psychological research in aging generally, must be addressed. Present space limitations will permit only a highlighting of certain critical points. A more comprehensive discussion of these issues is to be found in recent reviews of methodology in geropsychological research (e.g., Birren and Renner, 1977; Krauss, 1980; Labouvie, 1980; Siegler et al., 1980; Corso, 1981, pp. 201–25; Salthouse, 1982, pp. 19–38).

One particularly salient area of threat to reliability and validity of assessment instruments employed with older persons concerns differences between adult age groups in sensory, motor, and cognitive functioning. As reviewed by Corso (1981, pp. 28–65) visual capability begins to decline during the fourth decade of life, with, by 65 years of age, about half of all people showing a visual acuity of 20/70 or less (five times the proportion of those with a similar index at 45 years of age). Blindness or other serious visual problem affects more than 7 percent of the population between 65 and 74 years of age, and 16 percent of those over the age of 75. Age-associated visual impairment appears to be greater among aging women, as compared to men, and ability to read, watch television, and engage in other visual activities is reduced. Reduced visual capability can itself result in apparent disorientation and behavioral deterioration in older persons (O'Neil and Calhoun, 1975). Changes in the structural proteins of the lens with aging (Harding and Dilley, 1976) results in a variety of types of lens opacity or loss of lens clarity in a large number of older persons (typically grouped under the general term, "cataract"). An obvious implication of these statistics is the need for higher levels of illumination and larger print in questionnaires designed for administration to older persons.

The auditory system is also affected by aging. A well-known phenomenon is presbycusis (another general term that refers to several different types of age-associated changes), in which morphological structure of the inner ear is altered, resulting in decreased auditory acuity, particularly for high frequencies, and hence particularly affecting perception of speech. The association between hearing loss and emotional disturbance, particularly depression, among the elderly has been well documented (e.g., Knapp, 1948; O'Neil and Calhoun, 1975). Thus, as with decreased visual capability, auditory impairment may make a direct contribution to psychological disturbance in the older individual. In addition, attempts to administer self-report questionnaires auditorily (as well as to use interview procedures) may have reliability and validity affected by the patient's auditory ability. Practical implications of auditory problems in the elderly, as well as special considerations in evaluating auditory functioning in the older person are succinctly reviewed by Orchik (1981).

As noted earlier in this chapter, behavioral slowing with age has been one of the most studied areas in all of gerontologic psychology (see Birren et al., 1980). Most self-report instruments are not administered with fixed time limits for either response to individual questions or completion of the entire questionnaire. It is thus unlikely that age-associated behavioral slowing markedly influences reliability and validity of such instruments. However, increasing interest in the application of computers for the administration of self-report instruments will require that response slowing, as well as other age-associated phenomena, be carefully considered in the design of such procedures (e.g., Johnson and White, 1980). Behavioral slowing evaluated in interview or observation-based rating procedures, or through individually administered performance tasks must similarly apply age-appropriate criteria.

It is frequently stated that older individuals tire more rapidly than younger persons. It is often therefore recommended that testing sessions be kept as short as possible (e.g., Piper, 1979). Investigations which have either manipulated or controlled fatigue effects have either failed to demonstrate significant differences (Cunningham et al., 1978; Rust et al., 1979), or have found only slight effects (Furry and Baltes, 1973) upon cognitive test performance of healthy elderly versus younger adults. By inference, it is anticipated that fatigue would have relatively little specific effect upon performance task or self-report instrument responses of healthy older persons. However, acute illness, chronic disease (e.g., chronic cardiac disease), and depression all are associated with the symptom of increased fatigability. Therefore, those employing psychological assessment instruments within clinical settings should try to keep sessions brief, and wherever possible, preferentially select those less lengthy instruments.

Test-taking attitudes and response biases (e.g., tendency to choose socially desirable responses) are particular threats to reliability and validity of self-report inventories (Anastasi, 1982). Elderly persons may be different from younger adults in attitudes relevant to test performance. Various studies (e.g., Botwinick, 1966) have suggested a relationship between adult age and increasing cautiousness. This increased cautiousness among the aged is observed in responses to questions concerned with "life situations" relevant to the elderly, particularly when decisions involve financial matters (Wallach and Kogan, 1961). When provided with a list of risky alternatives, older individuals tend to choose one that involves little risk, unless risk cannot be avoided (Botwinick, 1969). In addition to this apparent cautiousness or reluctance to act when faced with questions concerning relevant life situations, older persons have also been shown to be more cautious in their response to a range of other kinds of tasks. For example, in a task investigating auditory threshold, older persons, more than younger persons, tend to report a sound only when certain about it, and thus will tend to be wrong in saying that a faint sound was not presented when it actually was (Rees and Botwinick, 1971). One practical consequence of this cautiousness would appear to be that traditional hearing tests may overestimate the magnitude of auditory deficit in later life (Botwinick, 1973, p. 115). If increased cautiousness is indeed a pervasive characteristic of aging, this would be expected to introduce a systematic response bias in older individuals' task performance and answers in self-report inventories (see Anastasi, 1982, pp. 520–526). Further, Klassen et al., (1975) have found the degree of social desirability response set to increase with adult age. While procedures are available for the measurement of response bias in sensory, perceptual and memory tasks (Danziger, 1980), as well as for self-report questionnaires (e.g., Edwards, 1957), such procedures have seldomly been applied in clinical assessment instruments otherwise appropriate for the elderly.

Another likely contributor to response bias in self-report instruments employed with the elderly is that of attitudes toward mental health care and psychological difficulty in general. Demographic investigations have clearly established that older persons underutilize mental health care services (Redick and Taube, 1980). Although it is likely that many factors contribute to this underutilization, including economic factors, insufficiency and inappropriateness of mental health services, and negative attitudes and stereotypes of mental health professionals (Gatz et al., 1980), it has also been suggested that older adults are reluctant to consider their life difficulties in psychological terms (Lawton, 1979). (For a more extensive discussion of these issues, see Chapters 2 and 3.)

The preceding discussion, which merely serves to highlight some of the difficulties in the use of all psychological assessment instruments with the elderly, leads to the following conclusion: it cannot be assumed that those assessment instruments that are known to be reliable and valid in application to younger adults will have the same reliability and validity when applied to older individuals. Indeed, Schaie (1978), in his review of the literature concerning external validity (the degree to which a given measure relates to other behavior, particularly in the "real world") of intellectual assessment in adulthood, finds that external validity is not constant either across situations or across different adult age groups. Similarly, self-report instruments that are externally valid when used with younger adults cannot be assumed to have the same validity for older persons. Further limiting measurement validity, is the fact that several psychological assessment instruments contain content that is either irrelevant or inappropriate to older persons (Oberleder, 1967).

Several authors (e.g., McNair, 1979) have questioned whether there is presently sufficient information on the reliability of psychological test responses of elderly, compared to younger adults, to allow informed evaluation of them. Further, it has been pointed out (Kochansky, 1979; McNair, 1979) that there is a relative lack of empirical comparison of the validity of various assessment procedures, thus making it difficult to make educated choices among them. Despite these problems, the clinician or investigator faced with making diagnostic decisions needs some guidance in selecting, from among the large number of available assessment approaches, those that suit his or her particular needs. The following reviews are in the service of such guidance.

Diagnostic Interview-Based Assessment Instruments

"The interview is the cornerstone of psychodiagnosis and has surely been used in diagnosis for thousands of years. It has always been the clinician's personal, subjective effort to gain information and understanding, and it remains the most important tool in clinical assessment and diagnosis" (Wiens and Matarazzo, 1983, p. 313). While it has often been assumed that diagnostic interviewing is an art rather than a science and hence can only be acquired through clinical experience, guidelines are available which can be of considerable help, particularly to the neophyte clinician. Further, there is available a growing body of research concerning interview behavior, and the reliability and validity of interview procedures, which also constitutes an important guide for the clinician (for a review of this literature, see Wiens and Matarazzo, 1983). Despite the availability of guidelines and relevant research, remember that, in developing these skills, there is no substitution for the observation of experienced interviewers and supervised practice in interviewing.

DSM-III Interview Guidance

The DSM-III provides guidance to the interviewer, by employing explicit and specific criteria for each disorder. The interviewer thus knows what information needs to be obtained, in what particular areas. Since duration of symptoms is a specific diagnostic criterion for several of the disorders relevant to the present discussion, the interviewer is directed to a focus upon not only people's current status, but their previous history as well. Particularly useful as an interviewing guide is the DSM-III provision of decision trees for differential diagnosis (APA, 1980, pp. 339–49). Each decision tree provides the clinician with a presenting set of clinical features as a starting point. The clinician can then follow a series of decision rules that provide guidance for the type of questions or other data gathering necessary and enable the efficient pursuit of a diagnosis. Also particularly helpful is the glossary of technical terms provided in Appendix B of the DSM-III (pp.353–368). The examiner is provided with specific definitions, in terms of observable behaviors, for each technical term employed in the DSM-III criteria (e.g., affect, grandiosity, hallucination, mood). By making more explicit the procedure of obtaining relevant data in the making of a diagnosis, as well as the "operational definition" (specification of directly observable features) of terms, the reliability of diagnosis between observers is markedly improved (Spitzer et al., 1979).

Schedule for Affective Disorders and Schizophrenia

Additional guidance in the conducting of structured interviews is also available through application of the Research Diagnostic Criteria (RDC) (Spitzer et al., 1978), and the Schedule for Affective Disorders and Schizophrenia (SADS) (Endicott and Spitzer, 1978). The RDC provides specific inclusion and exclusion criteria for a number of diagnoses, with particular emphasis upon affective disorders. The interrater reliability, a measure of the agreement between different clinicians, when the RDC is applied to adult inpatients with affective disorders, is impressively high (Endicott and Spitzer, 1979). However, the application of the RDC is dependent upon the knowledge and experience of the examiner, since criteria often involve clinical concepts rather than a simple listing of complaints. Another limitation of the RDC is that it is quite complex and time-consuming to administer. The SADS is an interview guide that was developed in conjunction with the RDC, as an attempt to reduce "information variance" (diagnostic and descriptive unreliability that occurs when clinicians have different sources of information about the patient in question) (Spitzer et al., 1975). Use of the SADS ensures coverage of critical areas of possible psychopathology, with part I of the SADS employing items used to describe the features of the current illness at its greatest severity, as well as functioning during the week prior to interview, and part II focusing upon past illness and history. The examiner employing the SADS and the RDC is able to relate findings to diagnostic categories in DSM-III, as many of the diagnostic categories are virtually identical (for detailed comparison, see Williams and Spitzer, 1982).

Use of the SADS and RDC is invaluable to the researcher who wishes to ensure reliable diagnosis. However, the reliability gained through strict inclusion and exclusion criteria results in some patients going undiagnosed within the SADS-RDC criteria. Hence, these procedures may be less useful to the clinician who must always arrive at some diagnosis. However, Dessonville, Gallagher, Thompson, Finnel, and Lewinsohn (1982) have recently demonstrated validity of the SADS interview schedule in the assessment of depression in older persons. They found the SADS to differentiate accurately Major Depression from changes associated with normal aging in healthy elders (including those over 70 years of age). As might be expected from previous discussion within the present chapter, they did find that caution needs to be applied in the interpretation of signs of sleep changes, weight changes, somatic anxiety and phobic tendencies, particularly when diagnosing physically ill older persons. The SADS and RDC are available through the Biometric Research Division of Columbia University.

In addition to the SADS, several other interview-based procedures have been employed in evaluation of depression in older persons. Some of these have been developed specifically for the evaluation of depression;

others are multidimensional and designed for the evaluation of a variety of psychopathologic syndromes. Some have been specifically developed for application with older individuals; others were developed on younger persons and later studied in application to the elderly.

Hamilton Rating Scale for Depression

One of the earliest developed and best known of the interview-based rating scales for depression (originally developed for use with both younger and older depressed patients) is the Hamilton Rating Scale for Depression (HRS-D) (Hamilton, 1960; 1967). The HRS-D is a 17-item inventory of symptoms, rated for severity (on a scale of 0 to 4 for some items and 0 to 2 for others) by an experienced clinician, based upon interview and other data available. While the protocol for the HRS-D does not specifically structure the nature of the interview, guidelines are provided for the specific behavior that is to be considered under each symptom severity rating. The HRS-D includes a range of both psychological symptoms (e.g., depressed mood, guilt, suicidal ideation, difficulties at work, and loss of interest in hobbies and social activities) and physical symptoms (e.g., insomnia, somatic symptoms, hypochondriasis). Hamilton (1960) advises that two raters be used at the same interview, with one conducting the interview and the other asking supplementary questions. A total score for the scale is obtained by summing the numerical ratings for the individual items (multiplying by 2, if only one rater is used, rather than the recommended two).

High interrater reliability has been found for the HRS-D total score. Hamilton (1960), studying 70 adult male depressed patients, reported a correlation coefficient of .90 between the total scores of two raters. Subsequently, Waldron and Bates (1965) found a correlation of .89 between scores obtained by two independent raters of 53 female patients. Examination of the interrelationship of the 17 HRS-D items, via factor analysis of ratings of 152 male and 120 female patients (Hamilton, 1967) indicated four leading factors. The first factor was labeled by Hamilton as a "general factor of depressive illness," and thought to be an over-all measure of the severity of the symptoms. A second factor was a bipolar factor representing "retarded versus agitated depression." Third was another bipolar factor, which contrasted loss of appetite, fatigability, and insomnia against guilt, suicidal ideation, and loss of insight. The fourth was a final bipolar factor with hypochondriasis, weight loss, and loss of insight contrasted against a variety of other symptoms. These factors were generally comparable, particularly the first two, when studied separately for the male and female patients. Mowbray (1972), in a separate study of both in-patients and outpatients with depression, generally confirmed Hamilton's findings concerning the factor structure of the HRS-D, although the bipolarity between agitated and retarded depression did not emerge. Sex differences in factor patterns were also found to be somewhat larger than those observed by Hamilton (1967). While the factor structure thus appears reasonably consistent across different samples of patients which have been studied, no reliability estimates for the factor scores have been reported.

Validity of the HRS-D has been less well-studied. The scale has been reported to be sensitive to the effects of different treatments for depression, such as electroconvulsive therapy (ECT) (e.g., Robin and Harris, 1962) and tricyclic antidepressant pharmacotherapy (e.g., Waldron and Bates, 1965). More recently, Sarteschi et al. (1973) have found the HRS-D able to discriminate between depressed and anxious patients over the age of 60. While this result suggests validity of the HRS-D in the evaluation of depression in older age, the clinician must remain aware that age-specific normative data is not yet available. Hamilton (1967) and Mowbray (1972) have published the means and standard deviations for the 17 HRS-D items, based upon the patients whom they studied (including both younger and older adults). The research of Sarteschi et al. (1973), indicates that age is an important factor to be considered when applying any such data. Sarteschi et al. (1973) found that, in depressive patients over the age of 60, psychotic depressive symptoms were significantly more frequent and severe, and psychomotor retardation or agitation, as well as cognitive difficulty, were significantly more frequent, in comparison to the younger depressives.

An additional caution concerns the use of the HRS-D with medically ill elderly. While good correlation between the HRS-D and a self-report depression measure, the Geriatric Depression Scale (GDS), has been reported for an elderly depressed group (Yesavage et al., 1983), a study of elderly patients with rheumatoid disease (Gallagher et al., 1982) found a somewhat lower correlation between the same two measures. As will be discussed later, in the section concerning self-report measures, the GDS was specifically constructed to minimize physical symptom items. The apparent difference between the HRS-D and the GDS correlations, when studied in depressed versus physically ill patients, may reflect the fact that nine of the seventeen items of the HRS-D concern somatic symptoms. Consistent with this interpretation is the Gallagher et al. (1982) finding that the Zung Depression Rating Scale (which, unlike the GDS, does contain a substantial number of somatic symptom items) had a somewhat higher correlation with the HRS-D than did the GDS in their rheumatoid arthritis patients.

Despite the limitations of the HRS-D in evaluating depression in older adults, it will likely continue to be frequently employed in research, given its history of previous application in treatment-outcome studies. A recent study (Endicott et al., 1981) has demonstrated a procedure for extracting the HRS-D from the SADS, with comparable reliability and validity of the extracted HRS-D score as a substitute for the original HRS-D procedure. Since the SADS, with its specific interview structure, yields quite impressive reliability, extraction of the HRS-D score from the SADS, as recommended by Endicott et al. (1981), would appear to have the advantage of maintaining comparability to previous research employing the HRS-D while also retaining the advantages of the SADS. Maintaining comparability to previous research, through employing the HRS-D abstracted from the SADS would appear to be of particular importance for studies investigating the outcome of therapeutic interventions with depressed elderly, since previous investigation in this area (e.g., Sakalis et al., 1974) has frequently employed the Hamilton scale.

Geriatric Mental Status Interview

The Geriatric Mental Status (GMS) interview is a semistructured interview technique for assessing psychopathology (including depression) in elderly patients, developed by Gurland et al. (1976). The GMS was developed as part of a U.S.-U.K. cross-national project investigating differences between British and American psychiatrists in diagnosis of the elderly. The GMS is administered by a trained interviewer, in a session typically less than one hour, in which between 100 and 200 questions are asked, resulting in ratings on 500 items. The questions of the GMS concern dimensions such as cognitive function, affective state, somatic concerns, and behavioral symptoms which can be rated from the interview. In designing the questions, care was taken to ensure that some of the special considerations necessary when evaluating older patients (detailed earlier in this chapter regarding DSM-III criteria) were included. For example, the examiners were interested in the subjective report of behavioral slowing, since this was thought possibly indicative of a psychiatric disturbance. An item directed at subjective slowing was therefore included. However, in order to differentiate between subjective slowing as an accompaniment of the normal aging process versus that indicative of psychopathology (particularly depression), an additional rating was provided for slowing that had become "worse in the last three months" (Gurland et al., 1976).

Factor analysis of the Geriatric Mental Status interview, based upon data from samples of patients in both the United States and United Kingdom (Gurland et al., 1976), demonstrated 21 factors, one of which was labeled by the investigators as representing depression. Scores for each individual factor are derived for a particular patient by adding the number of positively rated items in a factor. Since scores were standardized on the elderly samples studied in the United States and United Kingdom, normative comparison can be made.

Interrater reliability was evaluated by having a series of recently hospitalized psychiatric patients over the age of 65 interviewed and rated by one of the project psychiatrists, with the remaining project psychiatrists rating the patient by observing the interview. Kappa, an index of agreement which discounts agreements that could have been reached by chance

(Cohen, 1960) was over .70. Items based upon patient self-report and specific tests of memory and orientation provided higher levels of agreement than observation of the patient's spontaneous behavior, expression and speech pattern (Gurland et al., 1976).

It is of interest to note that, when the GMS was employed, no systematic differences were found between American and British psychiatrist raters in their diagnoses (Copeland et al., 1976). Also of importance is the apparent ability of the GMS interview to differentiate patients with organic brain syndromes from those with "functional" psychiatric disorder (Fleiss et al., 1976), a frequently difficult differential diagnosis, as will be discussed in Chapter 6.

Inpatient Multidimensional Psychiatric Scale

The Inpatient Multidimensional Psychiatric Scale (IMPS) (Lorr and Klett, 1966) is another multidimensional rating scale based upon semistructured interview and observation. Ratings on the 75 items of this scale contribute to summary scores for 10 syndromes, which were defined by factor analysis of the original 75 items. While there is not a syndrome scale specifically labeled as depression (due to the fact that the syndrome scales were constructed via factor analysis rather than by keying to diagnostic groups), there are scales with obvious relevance to the diagnosis of depression (e.g., "hostile belligerence," "anxious intropunitiveness," "retardation and apathy"). The IMPS has been employed in a large number of studies of adult psychiatric inpatients, including studies of differential diagnosis and treatment response (see Lorr, 1966, for a summary of this research). Interrater reliability, for several samples of patients studied, ranges from the low .80s to the middle .90s.

Validity demonstrations have included successful discrimination between "open-ward" and "closed-ward" patients, prediction of duration of hospitalization, and general agreement with independent diagnostic categorization. However, the instrument has received relatively little specific attention in application to elderly inpatients. Sarteschi et al. (1973) did report administration of the IMPS to a group of 310 elderly and younger patients, primarily with diagnoses of depression and anxiety disorders. Discriminant function analysis demonstrated the IMPS to differentiate the depressed from other patients. However, similar analysis demonstrated differences between those over and under 60 years of age. Thus, while these results would encourage further development of the IMPS as an assessment instrument for application to older patients, these results also indicate that the norms presently available, which are based on adults of various ages, should not be employed when evaluating the older individual.

Other Multidimensional Interview-Based Rating Scales

While the instruments described in the preceding sections represent the major interview-based rating scales for the specific assessment of psychopathology, with data available regarding application to older individuals, there also exist other multidimensional rating scales, designed for comprehensive assessment of not only psychopathology, but medical, nutritional, economic, and social problems as well. One such instrument is the Comprehensive Assessment and Referral Evaluation (CARE) (Gurland et al., 1977–78). CARE has been shown to record and classify information reliably on the health and social problems of older individuals. It is a semistructured interview guide with an inventory of defined ratings. Because it covers psychiatric, nutritional, medical, economic, and social problems, it appears particularly suitable for use with both already identified patients and nonpatients and may help in determining whether an older individual should be referred to a professional, and to whom (Gurland et al., 1977–78). Because of its multidimensional content, sections of it can be administered by various members of a multidisciplinary team. Should future research support the validity of the CARE instrument, it would appear to have particular promise as a comprehensive assessment tool. However, given the numerous areas assessed by this instrument, depression is not as fully assessed as in some of the other instruments reviewed.

The Older Americans Resources and Services Questionnaire (OARS) (Pfeiffer, 1976), is a multidimensional evaluation technique developed for the Duke University Longitudinal Study of Aging. It is based upon a semistructured interview with ratings of mental and physical health, as well as social and economic resources. Recently, Fillenbaum and Smyer (1981) have demonstrated adequate interrater reliability for the OARS. This feature is important because the various parts of the OARS were specifically designed to be completed by different multidisciplinary team members working independently. Fillenbaum and Smyer (1981) also demonstrated acceptable criterion validity, employing such criteria as an objective economic scale, ratings based on personal interviews by geropsychiatrists, and ratings by physician's associates and physical therapists. As with the CARE, the OARS would thus appear to be very useful in selecting among various referral and service alternatives for the older adult.

The final instrument to be reviewed within this section is the Philadelphia Geriatric Center's Multilevel Assessment Instrument (MAI) (Lawton et al., 1982). This instrument was designed to assess the well-being of older persons in a range of particular areas. Behavioral competence in the domains of activities of daily living, cognition, health, time use, and social interaction is assessed, as well as subjective psychological well-being and perceived environmental quality. Lawton et al. (1982) evaluated the psychometric qualities of these measures by administration of the instrument to 590 older persons from various groups (independent community residents, in-home services clients, and people awaiting admission to an institution). The summary rating scales demonstrated agreement between an interviewer and an independent rater, with either a zero or a one-point discrepancy, in 95 percent of all instances. Intraclass correlations (another reliability index) ranged from .88, for the rating of activities of daily living competence, to a low of .58, for the rating of social interaction. Other measures of reliability (internal consistency and retest reliability), although not impressively high, were found to be acceptable. Validity, assessed by contrasting the different criterion groups (e.g., independently living versus people awaiting admission to an institution), as well as by comparison to clinician and administrator ratings, also generally supported the adequacy of the MAI.

Even though the CARE, the OARS, and the MAI instruments were not specifically designed for the differential diagnosis of depression in the elderly, they are particularly important to consider in the comprehensive evaluation of the older individual. Depression does not present in the older person as an isolated symptom complex, but rather appears within the context of other medical, social, and economic difficulties.

Self-report Instruments

While the interview is the cornerstone of psychological diagnosis, self-report assessment instruments also play an important role. First, such instruments allow for a systematic sampling of symptoms and/or historical information, and ensure that the data obtained are comprehensive and representative. Second, because such instruments can be completed by the patient, without direct participation of the professional, they have the potential for increasing efficiency of the assessment process. Third, there exist explicit standards for the development of such "tests" (see Guion, 1983; Sales, 1983, Appendix D, pp. 689–762), which, when properly applied, result in an instrument with high levels of reliability and validity. Fourth, in addition to the clinical utility of self-report instruments (particularly for purposes of clinical screening and for augmenting the clinical interview), such instruments are important in research, where known properties of reliability, validity, and other psychometric characteristics (see Anastasi, 1982) allow for increased confidence in research results. An important feature of such instruments is the availability of normative data, to which an individual's responses on the instrument can be compared. The examiner thus need not rely entirely upon his or her own personal experience in making judgments concerning the degree to which the patient's symptoms or history diverges from normal expectation. As we have seen in the previous discussion of age-appropriate expectations in applying the DSM-III criteria, and interview-based rating scales, this is a particularly important issue in evaluation of the older patient.

Despite the potential contribution of self-report instruments to assessment, there are also weaknesses and many potential limitations. The most significant weakness is that information is based entirely upon self-report.

Since no direct observation of patient behavior is included within self-report instruments, much that may be important in clinical decision making is omitted. In evaluation of the older patient with severe major depression, self-report instruments may be useless, as it may not be possible to elicit the individual's cooperation in completing the questionnaire. A related weakness is that of susceptibility to bias: patients can easily misrepresent themselves in responding to the questionnaire. Misrepresentation may be motivated by a number of different factors, including the individual's expectation concerning what is the "appropriate" or "socially acceptable" answer, cultural differences in the minimization or exaggeration of complaints, limitations in the individual's ability to comprehend the questions (due to illiteracy for example), attempts to persuade the examiner that one is more seriously ill (e.g., in order to gain admission to hospital), or less seriously ill (e.g., in order to gain discharge from hospital) than is actually the case, and many others. The clinician directly observing the individual during interviewing may be in a position to detect clues to the existence of these sources of bias (e.g., facial expression, body posture, tone of voice). While some available self-report instruments contain specific items designed to detect these sources of bias, instruments available and appropriate for the evaluation of the older individual generally do not.

The weaknesses inherent in self-report instruments argue against any sole reliance upon them in assessment. As stated by Gallagher, Thompson, and Levy (1980, p. 19), "Psychological assessment should not, therefore, simply be equated with procedures of 'psychometric testing,' although standardized tests may be used in the assessment process . . . psychological assessment is better conceptualized as more broadly oriented toward issues of problem solving."

The *potential* limitations of self-report instruments derive primarily from the relative adequacy with which a given instrument meets criteria of reliability, validity, and age-appropriate available norms. Such potential limitations are, as noted, considerably greater for self-report instruments applied to the assessment of older individuals, as compared with application to younger adults.

In the following section, those self-report instruments either specifically designed for use with the elderly, or with known reliability, validity, and appropriate normative data, when applied to the elderly, will be reviewed.

Minnesota Multiphasic Personality Inventory

The Minnesota Multiphasic Personality Inventory (MMPI) is the most widely used self-report assessment instrument by clinical psychologists (Dahlstrom et al., 1972). The MMPI contains four validity scales, helpful in detecting response bias, and 10 clinical scales, one of which is a depression scale. Since the beginning of the development of the MMPI in the late 1930s, an enormous amount of validity research has been compiled (for a brief introductory review, see Butcher and Finn, 1983). In construction of the instrument, items were selected for a certain clinical scale only if they significantly differentiated between a clinical group (e.g., depressed patients) and normal control subjects. Items that failed to differentiate the groups or demonstrated a frequency of response so low in both groups as to provide no information were not included. Unfortunately, the MMPI was developed and validated on primarily younger adults. Research employing the MMPI with older groups suggests that comparison of the older individual to the published norms, based upon younger adults, is inappropriate, and in particular, that the depression scale may be measuring different features in younger and older groups.

Swenson (1961) employed the MMPI with a group of 95 individuals with a mean age of 71.4 years, living within the community. The depression scale was found to be the most elevated scale in 22.6 percent of male profiles and 14.1 percent of female profiles. While this study eliminated those older individuals "with mental disorders intense enough to warrant a psychiatric diagnosis" (Swenson, 1961, p. 302), no other attempt was made to include or eliminate any particular subgroups of older persons. Hence, it could be argued that elevations on the depression scale, in comparison to younger adult norms, reflected physical illness or mental disorder, which might not have come to the attention of a professional. A study reported by Leon et al. (1981), argues against physical illness and undiagnosed depression as being the sole explanations for higher MMPI depression scale scores in the elderly. They report upon a group of 132 individuals who had been repeatedly evaluated in a longitudinal study beginning in 1947, and who were still alive in 1977. At the beginning of the project in 1947, these individuals (all male) had a mean age of 49 years and were physically healthy and emotionally stable. In 1977 the survivors in this longitudinal study had a mean age of 77 years. The depression scale of the MMPI showed a statistically significant increase across the four evaluation points conducted over the 30-year longitudinal study period. While 27 percent of the sample reported death of a close friend over the past year, and 46 percent reported chronic physical illness (typically necessitating the continued care of a physician), at the 1977 evaluation, the presence of chronic disease or the death of a friend did not significantly predict their MMPI depression scores.

Results of a study reported by Harmatz and Shader (1975) suggest that different factors may account for the way in which older versus younger individuals respond to MMPI depression scale items. They collected data on 43 men and 46 women under the age of 35, and compared this to data on 33 men and 43 women over the age of 65 (plus a subsequent group of 40 men over the age of 65), all of whom were healthy volunteers in a psychopharmacologic research study. MMPI Depression Scale items that were answered differently by the young and older samples were seen to fall into two major classes: 1) items involving the acknowledgment of

TABLE 5.6

NEWCASTLE UPON TYNE COMMUNITY AGED MMPI BASIC CLINICAL AND VALIDITY SCALES (MEANS AND STANDARD DEVIATIONS OF MMPI K CORRECTED T SCORES).

	(N = 83) K corrected T Scores		
	M	S.D.	
L	41.3	5.2	**
F	54.8	7.0	**
K	61.5	4.7	**
Hs	73.2	14.2	**
D	67.4	14.5	**
Hy	72.5	10.7	**
Pd	49.6	9.8	
Mf	56.8	11.7	**
Pa	54.5	9.1	**
Pt	58.1	9.5	**
Sc	62.3	10.2	**
Ma	42.3	6.2	**
Si	47.5	6.9	
Standardization sample	Mean 50	Standard Deviation 10 on all scales	

Source: Reprinted with permission from Savage, R., Gaber, L., Britton, P., Bolton, N., and Cooper, A. *Personality and Adjustment in the Aged.* Copyright 1977, Academic Press, Inc., (London) Ltd.

** Difference from standardization significant at $p < 0.01$.

somatic dysfunction or difficulty in performance skills, and 2) items involving demand characteristics of social desirability (see discussion earlier in this chapter concerning sources of response bias in older persons). These results suggest that the MMPI Depression Scale may not be measuring the same construct (i.e., "depression"), in older as compared to younger individuals.

While available research thus argues strongly against the use of the MMPI Depression Scale published norms (derived from younger adults), the possibility remains that norms appropriate to older individuals could be developed, and that the development of such norms might allow for valid assessment of depressive features in older persons. This possibility is suggested by the research of Savage et al. (1977). Reporting on a group of 100 community-dwelling elderly, randomly sampled from persons living in the city of Newcastle upon Tyne in England, they found, similar to other investigators, that this group of aged persons had MMPI depression scale scores (as well as scores on other MMPI scales) significantly greater than that of the standardization sample employed to create the norms for the MMPI (see Table 5.6). However, when this group was separated into psychologically normal individuals versus those having a psychiatric dis-

TABLE 5.7

NEWCASTLE UPON TYNE COMMUNITY AGED MMPI BASIC CLINICAL AND VALIDITY SCALES (MEANS AND STANDARD DEVIATIONS OF MMPI K CORRECTED T SCORES FOR DIAGNOSTIC GROUPS).

| | Diagnosis | | | | |
| | Normal (N = 40) | | Functional (N = 41) | | |
	M	S.D.	M	S.D.	
L			41.8	6.4	
F			56.9	7.6	**
K	61.7	4.3	61.0	4.9	
Hs	64.5	11.1	81.3	13.1	**
D	58.7	8.7	75.8	14.7	**
Hy	66.7	8.6	78.5	9.3	**
Pd	46.5	4.7	54.0	12.4	**
Mf	60.7	11.9	52.4	11.4	**
Pa	51.3	5.6	57.5	10.3	**
Pt	53.3	7.8	62.6	9.1	**
Sc	57.0	7.2	67.5	10.4	**
Ma	41.0	4.9	43.1	7.2	
Si	45.0	4.2	49.9	6.9	**

Source: Reprinted with permission from Savage, R., Gaber, L., Britton, P., Bolton, N., and Cooper, A. *Personality and Adjustment in the Aged*. Copyright 1977, Academic Press, Inc., (London) Ltd.

** Difference significant at p < 0.01.

order ("functional" group), according to the diagnoses of an experienced geropsychiatrist, the MMPI depression scale (as well as other scales) significantly differentiated the groups (see Table 5.7). These results provide some encouragement for the development of age-appropriate norms for the MMPI. However, the reader is cautioned against the application of the Savage et al. (1977) data for any such normative comparison. First, the "normal" group comprised only 40 individuals, a rather small sample for use as a normative referent. Second, there is no insurance that such norms, even if based upon a larger sample, would apply to individuals from other countries and cultures. Further, there is research to suggest (Davis et al., 1973) that even if age-appropriate norms were developed, the MMPI might have less power in discriminating normal from psychiatrically impaired groups for older as compared to younger patients.

A shortened version of the MMPI, the Mini-Mult, (Kincannon, 1968) has also been used with the elderly. Its relative brevity (71 items, as compared to the 550 items of the full MMPI) has encouraged its application in studies of the elderly, particularly in research attempting to determine the epidemiology of depression in older populations (Pfeiffer, 1977; Blazer and Williams, 1980). The Mini-Mult Depression Scale does appear to have some validity in distinguishing healthy elderly from those who are psychiatrically hospitalized, but scores of healthy elders are markedly elevated, in comparison to younger individuals (similar to the findings for the full MMPI), and there are significant sex- and race-related differences in answering (Fillenbaum and Pfeiffer, 1976). Consequently, application of the Mini-Mult should be treated with at least as much caution as the full MMPI, and epidemiologic studies employing this instrument must be interpreted with some skepticism.

Other Multifactorial Personality Inventories

Other multifactorial or "omnibus" personality measures exist, with available data on performance of older individuals. However, most of these, such as the Sixteen Personality Factor Questionnaire (Cattell et al., 1970) have been developed for purposes of measurement of personality dimensions in normal individuals, and have typically not been validated, in application to the elderly, for purposes of assessment of depression or other psychopathological features. (See Costa, 1978 for a brief introductory review.)

Zung Self-rating Depression Scale

Among the single-dimension self-report instruments, the Zung Self-rating Depression Scale (SDS) (Zung, 1965) is one of the most commonly employed. The instrument consists of 20 statements (e.g., "I feel downhearted and blue," "I notice that I am losing weight," "I feel that others would be better off if I were dead," "I get tired for no reason"), each of which the respondent must rate on a 4-point scale, as the item pertains to him or herself (i.e., "a little of the time," "some of the time," "good part of the time," "most of the time"). Zung (1967) administered the SDS to 169 normal subjects, over the age of 65, who were either residents in a retirement home or members of a Golden Age Club. He found this group to score higher on the SDS than a previously studied group of normal individuals under the age of 65, with the older group rating themselves as worst on the predominantly physical symptoms such as sexual enjoyment, decreased appetite, and the presence of diurnal variation (feeling worse in the morning). The least difference, between the older and younger groups, was found on those items which measured mood disturbances. Zung interpreted these findings as indicating a higher incidence of depressive symptoms in older individuals. However, other research has suggested that the somatic items, which appear to account for most of the difference between younger and older normal persons responses, may have different meaning for the old than for the young. The somatic items have been found to not correlate well with either other measures of well-being or the mood disorder items of the SDS (Blumenthal, 1975; Gallagher et al., 1978). One approach to evaluating the reliability of an assessment instrument is to determine its internal consistency, this being the degree to which items of a scale correlate with each other (Nunnally, 1967 pp. 196–198, 210–211). Internal consistency, as measured by coefficient alpha was found to be acceptably high (.86) for a group of 48 "well-functioning senior citizens" (12 males and 36 females) with a mean age of 70.8 (Murkofsky et al., 1978). However, Gallagher et al. (1978) found internal consistency to be unacceptably low, particularly for their group of 107 "old-old" (age 73 to 88) subjects.

Validity of the SDS was demonstrated by Okimoto et al. (1982) in their study of 55 patients, age 60 and older, who were attending a general medical clinic of a Veterans Administration Medical Center. In addition to administering the SDS, these patients were interviewed by a psychiatrist, and 17 (31 percent) were found to meet DSM-III criteria for major depressive disorder. Employing the DSM-III diagnosis as the criterion, the SDS was found to correctly classify 86 percent of the patients (82 percent sensitivity and 87 percent specificity). While such validity estimates are acceptable for a self-report screening instrument, it should be noted that the mean age of the patients studied was 69.4 years. Given the Gallagher et al. (1978) finding of poor reliability in the old-old, the acceptable validity found by Okimoto et al. (1982) might not maintain in application to the old-old.

In summary, research on the SDS indicates that its clinical application requires the use of age-appropriate norms, and that reliability may not be acceptable when the instrument is applied to the old-old. While validity in application to the young-old has been demonstrated, caution should also be employed when using the instrument in assessment of patients with physical illness, given the substantial number of physical symptom items in this scale.

Beck Depression Inventory

Another popular self-report instrument for the assessment of depression is the Beck Depression Inventory (BDI) (Beck et al., 1961). The BDI is a 21-item inventory, assessing depressive symptomatology. While initial report on the development of this inventory (Beck et al., 1961) indicated good reliability, as assessed through internal consistency (split-half reliability coefficient of .93), when applied to younger adult depressed patients, other investigators (e.g., Weckowicz et al., 1967) reported less acceptable reliability with similar samples. Respectable test-retest reliability (.74) has been reported for a three-month test-retest interval, using normal undergraduate students (Miller and Seligman, 1973).

Recently, reliability of the BDI has also been assessed in normal and depressed elderly. Gallagher et al. (1982) administered the BDI to 82 normal and 77 depressed persons (diagnosed by means of the Research Diagnostic Criteria), whose average age was 69.9 and 67.8 years, respectively. The BDI was administered twice to each group, with the intertest interval ranging from 6 to 21 days. Test-retest, split-half, and coefficient alpha reliability estimates were high (.90, .84 and .91, respectively) when both groups were combined. However, as noted by Gallagher et al., these values may have been spuriously high because of the heterogeneous nature of the total sample; therefore the researchers recomputed the reliability estimates for each group separately. For the normal elderly sample, test-retest and split-half reliability were found to be moderately high (.86 and .74, respectively), and coefficient alpha was within the accepted range for a self-report screening instrument (.76). The reliability coefficients for the depressed patients showed slightly less test-retest stability and internal consistency (.79 and .58, respectively), but coefficient alpha remained acceptable (.73). Attempts to improve coefficient alpha in the depressed patient sample by eliminating items that correlated poorly with the total score did not significantly affect it. Gallagher et al. (1982) conclude that the BDI has sufficient internal consistency and stability for use in research and screening applications with older adults.

Other research by Gallagher and colleagues (1983) has recently indicated acceptable validity, with only 16.67 percent misclassification (using a BDI score of 11 or greater as denoting depression) of elderly depressed and nondepressed (by RDC) persons. Although the research reviewed here suggests that the BDI may be preferable, by psychometric criteria to the SDS, one should remain cautious in applying the BDI to older individuals with acute or chronic medical disorders, as 7 of the 21 items refer to symptoms such as fatigue, sleep difficulty, appetite disturbance, weight loss, sexual disinterest, and worry about health.

Center for Epidemiologic Studies Depression Scale

An instrument specifically developed for epidemiologic studies of depression is the Center for Epidemiologic Studies Depression Scale (CES-D) a 20-item self-report symptom rating scale (Weissmann et al., 1977). The scale requires the respondent to rate each of 20 symptom statements on a 4-point scale representing frequency of occurrence (i.e., from "rarely or none of the time" through "most or all of the time"). Although in comparison to the SDS and the BDI, this inventory has a smaller percentage of physical symptom items, information on its specific reliability and validity in application to older adults is not available. Furthermore, for a group of 148 "acutely depressed" younger adults (ages 18 to 65), the CES-D did not correlate highly with an interview and behavior observation rating scale measure of depression (Weissmann et al., 1977). Thus, until further reliability and validity studies with older adults are available, this instrument would not be highly recommended as a self-report measure of depression in the elderly.

Geriatric Depression Scale

Brink and Yesavage and their colleagues (Brink et al., 1982; Yesavage et al., 1983) have reported preliminary validity data on the Geriatric Depression Scale (GDS), a 30-item instrument designed specifically for the assessment of depression in the elderly. Their preliminary research suggests good correlation with an interview and observation rating scale measure of depression (Hamilton Depression Rating Scale) in an elderly sample. The GDS has the advantage of not being heavily loaded with physical symptom items, and of requiring only a "yes" or "no" response to each item, which may have some advantage over the 4-point ratings required on the SDS and the BDI, when applied to older individuals. If continued research supports the reliability and validity of the GDS, it may prove an excellent choice as a self-report measure for assessing depression in the elderly.

Self-concept and Self-esteem Measures

In addition to self-report instruments for the assessment of depressive symptoms, there also exist self-report measures of self-concept and self-esteem, constructs that are relevant to depression. Breytspraak and George (1979) review self-concept and self-esteem instruments that have been used in gerontological research. Two such instruments, the Tennessee Self-Concept Scale (Fitts, 1965) and the Self-Esteem Scale (Rosenberg, 1965) are recommended by Breytspraak and George as having better psychometric development than other available instruments.

Observation-Based Behavior Rating Scales

The interview and self-report instruments reviewed in the preceding section provide the clinician or researcher with a range of tools to assist in the diagnosis and quantification of severity of depression in the older person. However, all of these procedures presume at least some degree of patient cooperation. Such cooperation can generally be anticipated from those individuals whose depression is not so severe as to require hospitalization. The severely depressed patient and some older individuals with chronic neurologic or other physical illness may not be able to provide sufficient cooperation to enable reliable interview or self-report evaluation. In such cases there is a need for reliable and valid assessment procedures that do not depend upon interview or self-report. Observation-based rating scales address this need. Moreover, they provide a means by which behavior relevant to depression can be evaluated in various environmental settings (e.g., hospital or long-term care facility). Observation-based rating scales may thus be particularly important when one wishes to evaluate the generalization of treatment effects beyond the consulting room and into the patient's living environment.

In the following paragraphs those observation-based rating scales developed specifically for use with elderly inpatients will be reviewed. While not exhaustive, this review will focus upon those either best developed or more frequently used scales. Other instruments, either specifically developed for use with the elderly or with possible application to older persons exist. Reference to these additional instruments can be found in the reviews of Salzman et al. colleagues (1972a–c) and of Goga and Hambacher (1977).

In applying the observation-based rating scales reviewed below, or others, caution must be exercised, particularly concerning the assessment of depression. It should be kept in mind that psychometric studies of instruments, such as the Geriatric Mental Status interview, which combine interview and observation-based ratings (Gurland et al., 1976) have found lower interrater reliability for observation, as compared to interview ratings. Further, since all of the observation-based instruments reviewed here are multidimensional, observable signs of depression typically occupy only a small portion of various aspects of behavior rated. The small number of items contributing to the assessment of depressive signs in these scales also contributes to difficulties in attaining retest reliability.

Stockton Geriatric Rating Scale

One of the earliest of rating scales developed specifically for elderly inpatients is the Stockton Geriatric Rating Scale (SGRS) (Meer and Krag, 1964). Both the original version of the scale (Meer and Baker, 1966), as well as a slightly revised version (Plutchik et al., 1970) have demonstrated good interrater reliabilities (in the high .80s) and have been applied to samples of both organically and functionally impaired elderly inpatients. The SGRS contains 33 items, each scored on a 3-point scale, typically by a nurse, nurse aide, or other worker familiar with the patient. Interrater reliabilities do not appear to differ significantly across rater types (e.g., nurse aides, registered nurses, and psychological assistant) (Taylor and Bloom, 1974).

Factor analysis of the Plutchik et al. (1970) revision of this scale (usually referred to as the Geriatric Rating Scale or GRS), finds it to be composed of three factors. The first of these, containing 11 items, appears best described as one of withdrawal or apathy. The second factor, with six items, appears to be characterized by antisocial and disruptive behavior. The third factor, with seven items, contains various items referring to deficits in activities of daily living (e.g., need for assistance in eating, bathing, walking, as well as problems of confusion and incontinence) (Smith et al., 1977).

Validity of the SGRS or the modified GRS has been supported by agreement between the scale scores and clinical evaluation, comparison of scores before and after electroconvulsive treatment, differentiation of elderly patients with organic versus functional disorders, prediction of hospital discharge, and prediction of patient participation in hospital activities (Meer and Baker, 1966; Plutchik et al., 1970; Plutchik and Conte, 1972; Taylor and Bloom, 1974; Dastoor et al., 1975). Various of the studies of the SGRS or the GRS have found hospitalized women to be more impaired than hospitalized men when the total score for this scale is employed. However, the work of Smith et al. (1977) indicated that elderly institutionalized men and women were functioning at the same level in terms of apathy and withdrawal, but women were more impaired than men in activities of daily living and disruptive behavior. These sex differences do not appear to be accounted for on the basis of age or diagnosis differences between the sexes. Given the greater life expectancy of women, as compared to men, these differences may reflect the possibility that the men studied in various of the reported investigations are a more select group than the women (males who survive into older age may be more healthy than comparably aged women). Smith et al., (1977) also suggest the possibility that the sexes may differ in patterns of psychosocial adaptation to institutionalization. Specific empirical support for either of these suggestions is presently lacking.

As a final comment, it should be noted that, while most of the research concerning the SGRS and the GRS has been performed in the United States, the SGRS, as well as a version shortened to almost half the number of items, demonstrate comparable reliability and validity when employed with British hospital populations (Pattie and Gilleard, 1975, 1976, 1978; Gilleard and Pattie, 1977).

Physical and Mental Impairment-of-Function Evaluation

The Physical and Mental Impairment-of-Function Evaluation (PAMIE) (Gurel et al., 1972) is a 77-item observation-based rating scale designed for the assessment of a wide range of behavior in the institutionalized older patient. The 77 items, rated by observation of patient behavior, contribute to scores on 10 factor-analytically derived dimensions: 1) self-care dependent, 2) belligerent/irritable, 3) mentally disorganized, 4) anxious/depressed, 5) bedfast/moribund, 6) behaviorally deteriorated, 7) paranoid, suspicious, 8) withdrawn, apathetic, 9) sensorimotor impaired, and 10) ambulatory. Each item requires the observer (typically a nurse or nurse's aide) to rate patient behavior that had occurred during the week preceding completion of the evaluation. Interrater reliability and validity (employing external criteria including independent measures of physical impairment and death within a one-year follow-up period) have been shown to be acceptable (Gurel et al., 1972). PAMIE factor dimensions have also been reported (in Kaszniak, 1981) to be systematically related to family member reports of patient behavior and family distress, when evaluating chronically ill elderly outpatient participants in a day-care program.

Other Observation-Based Rating Scales

The Sandoz Clinical Assessment–Geriatric (SCAG) (Shader et al., 1974) is an observation-based scale in which ratings are made of 18 symptom areas and an overall global assessment on a 7-point format. It was specifically designed to provide a useful rating instrument for geriatric psychopharmacologic research, and to assist in differentiation between senile dementia and depressive disorders. While ratings are often based upon interviews conducted by a psychiatrist or other trained mental health professional, no structure for such an interview is provided, and the ratings need not be based upon interview alone. Hence, the SCAG is included here among the observation-based assessment instruments.

Shader et al. (1974) examined interrater reliability by having four psychiatrists examine eight subjects (four elderly volunteers and four elderly in-patients) and rate them on the 19 items of the SCAG. The average intraclass correlation coefficient was .75, although several of the items had unacceptably low reliability. Shader et al. (1974) also demonstrated the SCAG to differentiate significantly between elderly volunteers and in-patients. However, their data fail to support good discrimination by the SCAG between depressed and demented inpatients. Thus, although the SCAG may be useful in providing an overall index of severity of psychopathology, its ability to differentiate specific aspects of psychopathology is in question. Further, the interrater reliability on several of the items relevant to the evaluation of depression (e.g., mood depression, irritability, fatigue, appetite) appears unacceptably low, and likely contributes to its lack of validity in differentiating between depressed and other elderly in-patients.

Despite these shortcomings, the SCAG is reviewed here because of its widespread utilization in psychopharmacological research with the elderly. Future attempts to improve the specificity of criteria upon which ratings are to be made might well improve the reliability and validity of the SCAG.

The Nurse's Observation Scale for Inpatient Evaluation (NOSIE) (Honigfeld et al., 1966) is an observation-based rating scale, usually completed by nurses, which is often employed, along with the SCAG, in psychopharmacologic studies. The NOSIE appears to be in need of additional psychometric development and will not be reviewed further here.

Kochansky (1979), in his review of rating scales for assessing psychopathology in the elderly, recommends the Brief Psychiatric Rating Scale (BPRS) (Overall and Gorham, 1962), for the collection of psychopharmacological research data on the elderly. He makes this recommendation primarily on the basis of the brevity of the BPRS and its apparent sensitivity to drug affects. However, the BPRS is also in need of further psychometric development if it is to be applied in the assessment of depression in older individuals.

The final instrument to be reviewed in this section is the London Psychogeriatric Rating Scale (LPRS) (Hersch et al., 1978). While this instrument is basically an extension of the Stockton Geriatric Rating Scale, it contains additional items designed to provide observer ratings of patient cognitive functioning. The LPRS consists of 36 observer-rated items, scored on a 3-point scale, with higher scores reflecting greater degree of disability or functional difficulty. Hersch et al. (1978) studied 55 chronically ill elderly in-patients over an 18-month period, with ratings on the LPRS every third month. Predictive validity was established against criteria of ward placement, outcome (continued hospitalization, discharge, or death) and diagnosis, as well as against the ability of the patient to benefit from particular treatment programs. In addition, a brief prognosis index was developed utilizing the five best discriminating items of the LPRS, which was successful in predicting which patients were most likely to leave the hospital within six months (Hersch et al., 1980). Thus, with the addition of items for evaluation of cognitive functioning, the LPRS may provide a significant improvement over the SGRS.

Individually Administered Performance-Based Measures

Thus far, we have reviewed assessment procedures based upon structured and semistructured interview, self-report inventories, and observation-based rating scales. All of these procedures provide a systematic means of eliciting symptoms (patient complaints) and observing signs (patient behavior). However, it is also often desirable to have reliable and valid assessment of the individual's response ("performance") to specific stimuli.

Systematic observation of behavior in the patient's living environment (i.e., observation-based rating scales) enable assessment of general areas of behavioral competence (e.g., eating, dressing, and ambulatory ability) and general signs of psychopathology (e.g., confusion, socially disruptive behavior, apathy, and motor retardation). The major limitation of such assessment, once reliability and validity of observation can be assumed, is that such general areas of behavior observation do not provide information concerning the specific nature of an individual's behavioral disturbance. For example, the same degree of observed confusion and disorientation can be manifested in different patients for different reasons. One person may be afflicted by depression with impaired arousal, motivation, attention, and concentration. Another individual may be apparently disoriented and confused secondary to a focal brain lesion resulting in a circumscribed memory deficit, with attention and concentration abilities relatively better preserved. A third patient may manifest more general deterioration of a range of cognitive and perceptual functioning, secondary to a degenerative brain disease. Differentiation among these patients is very important— and difficult—as will be discussed further in Chapter 6. Performance-based measures of cognitive functioning may be especially useful in assisting such differentiation.

In addition, even with the patient for whom a confident diagnosis has already been made, it is desirable to have information concerning details of the person's preoccupations, approach to problem-solving and style of response to various stimuli, particularly in planning psychotherapeutic intervention. It is the purpose of this section of the chapter to review the major traditional approaches of the clinical psychologist to such assessment.

Assessment of Intelligence

Intellectual assessment has been a traditional emphasis in the evaluation skills of the clinical psychologist. It is not surprising, therefore, that research on the measurement, characterization of, and factors contributing to intelligence in older age has received more attention than almost any other area of gerontological psychology. This body of research has provided much information of clinical utility, as well as having generated considerable controversy. Even a cursory review of this literature is beyond the scope of the present chapter. However, a firm understanding of the state of our present knowledge in this area, as well as its conceptual and methodological controversies, is critical for the clinician or investigator who wishes to administer and interpret intellectual assessment procedures with older individuals. Therefore, it is strongly recommended that the reader consult recent reviews (e.g., Botwinick, 1977; Willis and Baltes, 1980; Schaie and Giewitz, 1982, pp. 202–39) for an introduction to important data and issues.

Intellectual deterioration has long been part of our cultural stereotype of aging. While both cross-sectional studies (individuals of different ages are compared with one another) and longitudinal studies (a given group of individuals is followed over time) have supported the conclusion that some decline in intellectual ability does occur with normal aging, such decline is less general (not involving as many areas of cognitive functioning), smaller in magnitude, and begins considerably later in adult life than either cultural stereotype or early research in this area would have suggested. This discrepancy between current data and cultural stereotype underscores the need for more than passing familiarity with this literature. As stated by Gallagher et al. (1980), "Knowledge of what to expect in terms of cognitive changes with advancing age is extremely important for clinicians if they are to assess the common presenting problems of the elderly adequately (p. 23)."

Several considerations will have a marked impact upon such expectations. A consideration relevant to the examiner's approach to intellectual assessment with the older test subject is the observation, made by several authors (e.g., Oberleder, 1967; Comfort, 1978), that the older person may be more "threatened" than the younger adult by intelligence testing. The older person, having matured and been educated during a time of less emphasis upon testing and assessment, is less accustomed to such procedures than the younger adult, for whom standardized achievement tests were a ubiquitous aspect of their school experience.

Further, an older person who is experiencing some difficulty in memory or cognitive functioning, or who is apprehensive out of the cultural stereotype of senility and aging, may be fearful of the possible consequences of formal intellectual evaluation (as well as interview-based mental status examinations!). The examiner may, consequently, need to make special efforts to explain the nature and purpose of the assessment and allow the individual sufficient time (including a pretesting practice period in some instances) to become comfortable with the procedures.

All of the considerations concerning special issues in the psychological assessment of older persons detailed earlier in this chapter must also be applied by the examiner assessing intellectual functioning. Increased illumination of visual stimuli, as well as somewhat increased volume and possible repetition of verbal instructions may result from such considerations. Since there is great variability in visual and auditory functioning, as well as expectations and attitudes among older individuals, no strict set of guidelines for the administration of intellectual assessment procedures to the older person would prove adequate. Again, there appears no substitute for familiarity with the geropsychologic literature relevant to this area, as well as supervised practical experience.

In addition to the issues concerning procedures of administration in intelligence testing, current research also markedly influences interpretation of assessment results. The apparent differential decline of intellectual abilities, with those based upon frequently practiced, primarily verbal or "crystallized" (Horn and Cattell, 1967) abilities showing less decline than those requiring rapid speed of response, perceptual integration, and other "fluid" (Horn and Cattell, 1967) abilities, underscores the need for age-appropriate normative data for these differentiable aspects of intelligence.

Research that has simultaneously employed both cross-sectional and longitudinal strategies in the evaluation of intellectual functioning and aging (Schaie and Labouvie-Vief, 1974) has indicated that both cohort (the "generation" to which the individual belongs) and ontogenetic change (change over time in a particular individual's life) make important contributions to intellectual functioning in older adults. Thus, not only must age-specific normative data be available, but such data must also take into consideration the cohort to which the individual belongs. Since the psychological aging (as ontogenetic change) of the cohort of individuals born at the turn of the century may be different from that of individuals born more recently, there is a need for periodic updating of normative data on standard instruments for the assessment of intelligence.

Issues concerning generational versus ontogenetic components of change in adult intelligence also lead to complicated considerations in the construct validity of tests. Tests, as well as individuals, age (see Schaie and Schaie, 1977, p. 695). Hence, tests that were constructed to assess a particular aspect of cognitive functioning for a given cohort in young adulthood could remain valid for that cohort as they age, but might not be valid for successive cohorts. Another way of stating this is that construct validity (the identification of the meaning of a particular hypothetical construct, such as "verbal intelligence," usually through application of factor-analytic approaches) might conceivably be cohort-specific, but ontogenetically invariant. However, other validation criteria, such as predictive validity, could conceivably demonstrate the opposite relationship to cohort and ontogenetic change. For example, the most frequently employed measure of adult intelligence, the Wechsler Adult Intelligence Scale (WAIS) (Wechsler, 1958) has demonstrated predictive validity, for younger adults, against such criteria as educational achievement and occupational status (for comprehensive review, see Matarazzo, 1972). To evaluate the predictive or external validity of this same instrument when applied to the elderly begs the question of what should be considered as appropriate external validators (the older person is usually neither matriculating in an educational institution nor actively participating in a career). This premise, of course, is related to the entire issue of what one is attempting to measure, understand, or predict with intelligence tests administered to the older person. The clinician or investigator needs to consider this question carefully when interpreting the results of intellectual assessment of an older adult. Further, since all age-norms available for presently employed intelligence assessment instruments, such as the WAIS, were developed from cross-sectional studies, and are therefore cohort-specific, Schaie and Schaie (1977) urge the examiner "to substitute the range of birth years for the age range given as of the year the norms were established, to obtain a more accurate reading" (p. 695). They further encourage future test constructors to publish their age-corrected norms in this manner unless data from sequential studies providing estimates of expected changes in norms at given ages are available.

Given the often difficult problem of diagnostically differentiating between symptoms of depression and those of organic brain syndromes resulting in dementia (to be discussed in further detail in Chapter 6), formal intellectual assessment can play a particularly valuable role in the diagnostic process. Such measures have demonstrated sensitivity to the cognitive changes accompanying dementia (see Miller, 1977, for a review of this literature).

In addition, intelligence testing provides an opportunity for the structured observation of behavior relevant to a diagnosis of depression. Behavior, during testing, such as frequent self-critical statements, overconcern with performance, giving up or becoming irritated easily, and expression of apology and guilt may be manifestations of depression. In the WAIS, most of the subtests contributing to the Performance Intelligence Quotient (PIQ) are timed (the individual earns additional points for solving the problem more quickly), whereas most of the subtests contributing to the Verbal Intelligence Quotient (VIQ) are not timed. The psychomotor slowing often seen in depression thus frequently manifests as a PIQ lower than the VIQ. Difficulties with attention and maintaining concentrated effort, also frequent features of depression, may manifest as particularly low scores on those WAIS subtests in which attention and concentration play important roles (e.g., "Digit Span," "Arithmetic," "Digit Symbol").

The appropriate use of formal intelligence assessment thus necessitates going considerably beyond the simple examination of IQ scores. Application of age-appropriate norms, with consideration of cohort versus ontogenetic issues, examination of performance on individual subtests (with particular attention to those cognitive processes most contributory to such subtests), and the careful observation and notation of the individual's behavior and approach to tasks during testing are all of marked importance.

Projective Techniques

Projective techniques also have a long history as part of the assessment armamentarium of the clinical psychologist. Despite heated controversy concerning the appropriateness and utility of such techniques, they continue to be among those most frequently employed instruments in clinical psychological assessment (Klopfer and Taulbee, 1976). Most of this controversy has centered around criticisms concerning inadequate reliability and validity of projective techniques. Empirical attempts to demonstrate reliability and validity have indeed met with relatively little success. However, as pointed out by Kahana (1978, p. 147), these assessment procedures ought not be viewed as "tests," in the formal sense of the term. Projective techniques generally were an outgrowth of psychoanalytic theory, and were thought to portray preconscious or unconscious fantasy, coping, or defense mechanisms and conflicts. Kahana (1978) argues that it is thus difficult to validate data obtained from projective techniques against observed behavior or conscious self-reports. He suggests that analysis of phenomena with presumably similar dimensions, such as dreams, might provide more meaningful validation of projective instruments. Further, he urges that reliability be viewed in more general terms, such as intraindividual similarity of conflicts, coping strategies, and themes, over time or across different tasks.

It is apparent that the controversy concerning projective techniques reflects a broader controversy concerning psychodynamic versus behavioral approaches to understanding human behavior. Whether the clinician or investigator employs projective techniques in the assessment of the older individual will hence more likely reflect one's relative position along this theoretical controversy, rather than considerations based on empirical demonstration of reliability and validity.

Despite the difficulties in employing traditional yardsticks of reliability and validity to projective techniques, they do appear to have some advantages in evaluation of the older person. Kahana (1978) argues that these techniques provide information concerning psychodynamic processes that is critical for intelligent work toward therapeutic change in psychotherapy. This advantage is enhanced by the fact that the examiner must observe the older individual quite closely during administration of the technique, since these procedures are all administered in face-to-face interviews. In their brief review of projective techniques in the psychological assessment of older adults, Gallagher et al. (1980) conclude that

> use of projective techniques may provide a somewhat standardized, ecologically valid avenue for assessing functional status and a useful index of the person's response to unstructured situations. Projective techniques should . . . be considered for inclusion in any comprehensive assessment procedure undertaken with the elderly, particularly when there is little or no opportunity for more natural observation. (p. 29)

Because projective techniques represent clinical assessment procedures heavily dependent upon the background, training, and experience of the examiner, they should not be applied by clinicians or investigators who lack extensive education, as well as supervised practice, in their use. The general review of Klopfer and Taulbee (1976) is recommended for those desiring more information on the current status of projective techniques, and the specific and thorough review by Kahana (1978) is recommended for in-depth coverage of a variety of projective techniques for personality assessment of the older person. The present section will briefly review those major projective techniques most frequently employed in clinical practice, with particular attention to their use in evaluating the elderly.

THE RORSCHACH TEST.   Rorschach's (1942) "Ink-Blot" procedure is probably the best known of all projective instruments. It is also probably the most controversial (cf., Klopfer and Taulbee, 1976). Over the years, several different approaches to administration, scoring and interpretation of the Rorschach have been developed (e.g., Beck et al., 1961; Klopfer and Davidson, 1962; Exner, 1974). Each system is quite complex, and requires considerable time and effort in learning to employ each correctly. Research based upon various of these scoring systems has produced mixed results (see Zubin et al., 1965; Klopfer and Taulbee, 1976), and hence, there is a lack of any consistent evidence of reliability or diagnostic validity for any of the specific systems. However, research has generally indicated diagnostic validity for the Rorschach, based upon clinical impressions by highly experienced examiners (see Zubin et al., 1965, pp. 166–250). This again suggests that the Rorschach, like other projective techniques, is perhaps best conceptualized as an extension of the clinical interview, rather than as a psychometric test procedure.

Studies investigating the Rorschach responses of older individuals (see reviews by Ames et al., 1973; Klopfer, 1974; Kahana, 1978) have shown healthy elderly to perform substantially differently than healthy younger adults. Thus, even the clinician with considerable experience, in administration and interpretation of the Rorschach to younger and middle aged adults, might be prone to diagnostic errors unless age-appropriate expectations are employed. General considerations in the application of any assessment procedure to the older adult, as reviewed earlier in this chapter, also must be applied to evaluation of the Rorschach. Previous research has demonstrated variables such as sensory impairment (Eisdorfer, 1960), intellectual functioning (Eisdorfer, 1963) and "verbosity" (Hayslip, 1981) all to have substantial effects upon the older adult's performance in Rorschach or similar ink-blot testing (e.g., Holtzman et al., 1961).

THEMATIC APPERCEPTION TECHNIQUE AND RELATED PROCEDURES. The Thematic Apperception Test (TAT) (Henry, 1956) is another widely employed projective assessment instrument. The stimuli consist of various drawings, most of which depict individuals in different kinds of interaction. The subject's task is to create a fantasy story, in response to the picture, describing what is happening within the picture, as well as what had happened just before and what will happen just after the scene depicted. As with the Rorschach, many conceptual and methodologic problems are encountered in attempting to evaluate the reliability and validity of the TAT. Zubin et al. (1965, pp. 394–473), in their review of the literature on the TAT available prior to 1965, conclude that, while not generally reliable and valid, the TAT can be scored reliably and interpreted validly under certain specific conditions, for experienced examiners. The TAT has frequently been employed in research with older persons (see review by Kahana, 1978, pp. 153–58), and differences between the responses of healthy older and younger adults have been found. As with the Rorschach, this evidence argues for the need to apply age-appropriate expectations, even for the clinician experienced in using the TAT with younger and middle-aged adults.

One criticism of the TAT has been that its pictures typically depict younger adults, or activities relevant to younger adults. Two different revisions of the TAT exist, which attempt to elicit themes and concerns unique to the aged. The Gerontological Apperception Test (GAT) (Wolk and Wolk, 1971) employs 14 specially designed pictures, each of which depicts an older individual in an age-relevant situation. The Senior Apperception Technique (SAT) (Bellak, 1973, 1975) employs 16 pictures, each showing elderly persons alone or with others in various situations. Research comparing the responses of elderly individuals to these revised techniques versus the traditional TAT cards, has, in general, not demonstrated that these specially designed cards elicit either more detailed or more revealing responses (Fitzgerald et al., 1974; Pasewark et al., 1976; Foote and Kahn, 1979; Stock and Kantner, 1980).

Instruments to Assist in Screening Physical Illness

As described previously in this book (Chapter 2), a number of medical conditions present with signs and symptoms of depression. A recent study of 658 consecutive psychiatric outpatients (Hall et al., 1978) found medical disorders producing psychiatric symptoms in 9.1 percent of these cases, with depression being the single most frequent type of presentation. In the study, those medical conditions considered definitely causative of depressive symptoms included hypothyroidism, pneumonia, infectious viral hepatitis, carcinoma, rheumatoid arthritis, congestive heart failure, and several others. The need for thorough medical evaluation of the older individual presenting signs and symptoms of depression is underscored by the fact that several of these medical disorders are more prevalent in the elderly.

Although there is no substitute for thorough physical examination and medical history, there do exist self-report instruments that have utility in screening for physical illness in the older individual. Some of the instruments appropriate for physical health screening of the elderly have already been discussed under the previous section reviewing multidimensional interview-based observation instruments (e.g., the CARE, the OARS, the MAI).

Other self-report instruments, specifically designed for the evaluation of health status in older persons range from a simple rating of one's own health on a 4-point scale (e.g., Maddox and Douglass, 1973) to more extensive inventories in which type and severity of illness experienced by the individual is questioned (e.g., Rosencranz and Pihlblad, 1970). While validity, against the criterion of physicians' health ratings, has been demonstrated for such self-report measures (e.g., Friedsam and Martin, 1963; Heyman and Jeffers, 1963; Maddox and Douglass, 1973), the clinician or investigator should exercise some caution in the interpretation of such health status self-report measures. Self-perceived health status in the elderly has been shown to be influenced not only by the type and number of symptoms of physical illness, but also by such variables as age, education, race (Cockerham et al., 1983), and participation in paid employment (Soumerai and Avorn, 1983). Such findings emphasize the need to view health status self-report instruments as screening measures to be followed by thorough medical examination.

Another important area in evaluating signs and symptoms of depression in the older person is that of the possible contribution of prescription and nonprescription medications. Pharmacokinetics change with aging (Chapron and Lawson, 1978), with increased risk of drug-induced psychiatric symptoms, particularly when multiple interacting drugs are employed (Hicks et al., 1980). Further, older individuals show considerably greater use, in comparison to younger adults, of over-the-counter medications (Guitman, 1978). These issues are extensively reviewed in Chapter 7.

CONCLUSIONS

As should by now be obvious, no single psychological test, interview procedure, or examination approach can provide an infallible index of depression in older age. The selection of particular assessment approaches will depend upon the background of the examiner, the purpose of the examination (e.g., clinical versus research), the differential diagnoses being considered, the limitations of time and cost involved, as well as the specific technical considerations reviewed within this chapter. It is hoped that this chapter has provided some guidance in the selection of assessment procedures appropriate to the particular examiner's background, purpose, and setting. Accurate diagnosis of depression in older age presents a great challenge. Success in this endeavor can also provide great professional and personal satisfaction.

REFERENCES

American Psychiatric Association. *Diagnostic and Statistical Manual of Mental Disorders, Third Edition.* Washington, D.C.: APA, 1980.

Ames, L.B., Metraux, R., Rodell, J., and Walker R. *Rorschach Responses in Old Age,* rev. ed. New York: Brunner/Mazel, 1973.

Anastasi, A. *Psychological Testing,* 5th ed. New York: Macmillan, 1982.

Barnes, R., Veith, R.C., and Raskind, M.A. Depression in older patients: diagnosis and management. *Western Journal of Medicine,* 1981, 135:463.

Beck, A.T., Ward, C.H., Mendelson, M., Mock, J., and Erbaugh, J. An inventory for measuring depression. *Archives of General Psychiatry,* 1961, 4:53.

Beck, S.J., Beck, A.G., Levitt, E.E., and Molish, H.B. *Rorschach's Test: I. Basic Processes.* New York: Grune & Stratton, 1961.

Bellak, L. *Manual for the Senior Apperception Technique (SAT).* New York: C.P.S., 1973.

Bellak, L. *The TAT, CAT, and the SAT in Clinical Use,* 3rd ed. New York: Grune & Stratton, 1975.

Birren, J.E., and Renner, V.J. Research on the psychology of aging: principles and experimentation. In Birren, J.E., and Schaie, K.W. (Eds.), *Handbook of the Psychology of Aging.* New York: Van Nostrand Reinhold, 1977, pp. 3–38.

Birren, J.E., Woods, A.M., and Williams, M.V. Behavioral slowing with age: causes, organization, and consequences. In Poon, L.W. (Ed.), *Aging in the 1980s: Psychological Issues.* Washington, D.C., American Psychological Association, 1980, pp. 293–308.

Blazer, D., and Williams, C. D. Epidemiology of dysphoria and depression in an elderly population. *American Journal of Psychiatry,* 1980, 137:439.

Blumenthal, M.D. Measuring depressive symptomatology in a general population. *Archives of General Psychiatry,* 1975, 32:971.

Botwinick, J. Cautiousness in advanced age. *Journal of Gerontology*, 1966, 21:347.

Botwinick, J. Disinclination to venture response versus cautiousness in responding: age differences. *Journal of Genetic Psychology*, 1969, 115:55.

Botwinick, J. *Aging and Behavior: A Comprehensive Integration of Research Findings.* New York: Springer, 1973.

Botwinick, J. Intellecultural abilities. In Birren, J.E., and Schaie, K.W. (Eds.), *Handbook of the Psychology of Aging.* New York: Van Nostrand Reinhold, 1977, pp. 580–605.

Breytspraak, L.M., and George, L.K. Measurement of self-concept and self-esteem in older people: state of the art. *Experimental Aging Research*, 1979, 5:137.

Brink, T. L., Yesavage, J.A., Lum, O., Heersema, P.H., Adey, M., and Rose, T.L. Screening tests for geriatric depression. *Clinical Gerontology*, 1982, 10:37.

Butcher, J.N., and Finn, S. Objective personality assessment in clinical settings. In Hersen, M., Kazdin, A.E., and Bellack, A.S. (Eds.), *The Clinical Psychology Handbook.* New York: Pergamon, 1983, pp. 329–44.

Cattell, R.B., Eber, H.W., and Tatsuoka, M.M. *Handbook for the Sixteen Personality Factor Questionnaire.* Champaign, Ill.: Institute for Personality and Ability Testing, 1970.

Chapron, D., and Lawson, I. Drug prescribing and care of the elderly. In Reichel, W. (Ed.), *Clinical Aspects of Aging.* Baltimore: Williams & Wilkins, 1978, pp. 13–32.

Cockerham, W.C., Sharp, K., and Wilcox, J.A. Aging and perceived health status. *Journal of Gerontology*, 1983, 38:349.

Cohen, J. A coefficient of agreement for nominal scales. *Educational and Psychological Measurement*, 1960, 20:37.

Comfort, A. Non-threatening mental testing of the elderly. *Journal of the American Geriatric Society*, 1978, 26:261.

Comfort, A. Sexuality in later life. In Birren, J.E., and Sloan, R.B. (Eds.), *Handbook of Mental Health and Aging.* Englewood Cliffs, N.J.: Prentice-Hall, 1980, pp. 885–92.

Copeland, J., Kelleher, M., Duckworth, G., and Smith A. Reliability of psychiatric assessment in older patients. *International Journal of Aging and Human Development*, 1976, 7:313.

Corso, J.F. *Aging Sensory Systems and Perception.* New York: Praeger, 1981.

Costa, P.T. Objective personality assessment. In Storandt, M., Siegler, I.C., and Elias, M.F. (Eds.), *The Clinical Psychology of Aging*, New York: Plenum, 1978, pp. 119–43.

Cunningham, W.R., Sepkoski, C.M., and Opel, M.R. Fatigue effects on intelligence test performance in the elderly. *Journal of Gerontology*, 1978, 33:541.

Dahlstrom, W.G., Welsh, G.S., and Dahlstrom, L.E. *An MMPI Handbook: Volume I. Clinical Interpretations.* Minneapolis: University of Minnesota Press, 1972.

Danziger, W.L. Measurement of response bias in aging research. In Poon, L.W. (Ed.), *Aging in the 1980s: Psychological Issues.* Washington, D.C., American Psychological Association, 1980, pp. 552–57.

Dastoor, D.P., Norton, S., Boillat, J., Minty, J., Papadopoulou, F., and Muller, H.F. A psychogeriatric assessment program: I. Social functioning and ward behavior. *Journal of the American Geriatric Society*, 1975, 23:465.

Davis, W.E., Mozdzierz, G.F., and Macchitelli, F.J. Loss of discriminative "power" of the MMPI with older psychiatric patients. *Journal of Personality Assessment,* 1973, 37:555.

de Alarcon, R. Hypochondriasis and depression in the aged. *Gerontology Clinics,* 1964, 6:266.

Dessonville, C., Gallagher, D., Thompson, L.W., Finnell, K., and Lewinsohn, P.M. Relation of age and health status of depressive symptoms in normal and depressed older adults. *Essence,* 1982, 5:99.

Edwards, A.L. *The Social Desirability Variable in Personality Assessment and Research.* New York: Dryden, 1957.

Eisdorfer, C. Developmental level and sensory impairment in the aged. *Journal of Projective Techniques,* 1960, 24:129.

Eisdorfer, C. Rorschach performance and intellectual functioning in the aged. *Journal of Gerontology* 1963, 18:358.

Endicott, J., Cohen, J., Nee, J., Fleiss, J., and Sarantakos, S. Hamilton Depression Rating Scale: extracted from regular and change versions of the Schedule for Affective Disorders and Schizophrenia. *Archives of General Psychiatry,* 1981, 38:98.

Endicott, J., and Spitzer, R.L. A diagnostic interview: the Schedule for Affective Disorders and Schizophrenia. *Archives of General Psychiatry,* 1978, 35:837.

Endicott, J. and Spitzer, R.L. Use of the Research Diagnostic Criteria and the Schedule for Affective Disorders and Schizophrenia to study affective disorders. *American Journal of Psychiatry,* 1979, 136:52.

Exner, J.E. Jr. *The Rorschach: A Comprehensive System.* New York: Wiley, 1974.

Fillenbaum, G.G., and Pfeiffer, E. The Mini-Mult: A cautionary note. *Journal of Consulting and Clinical Psychology,* 1976, 44:698.

Fillenbaum, G., and Smyer, M. The development, validity and reliability of the OARS multidimensional functional assessment questionnaire. *Journal of Gerontology,* 1981, 36:428.

Fitts, W. *Manual: Tennessee Self-Concept Scale.* Nashville, Tenn.: Counselor Recordings and Tests, 1965.

Fitzgerald, B.J., Pasewark, R.A., and Fleisher, S. Responses of an aged population on the Gerontological and Thematic Apperception Tests. *Journal of Personality Assessment,* 1974, 38:234.

Fleiss, J., Gurland, B., and Des Roche, P. Distinctions between organic brain syndrome and functional psychiatric disorders: based on the Geriatric Mental State interview. *International Journal of Aging and Human Development,* 1976, 7:323.

Foote, J., and Kahn, M.W. Discriminative effectiveness of the Senior Apperception Test with impaired and nonimpaired elderly persons. *Journal of Personality Assessment,* 1979, 43:360.

Fras, I., Litin, E. M., and Pearson, J.S. Comparison of psychiatric symptoms in carcinoma of the pancreas with those in some other intra-abdominal neoplasms. *American Journal of Psychiatry,* 1967, 123:1553.

Friedsam, H., and Martin, H.A. A comparison of self and physicians' health ratings in an older population. *Journal of Health and Human Behavior,* 1963, 4:179.

Furry, C.A., and Baltes, P.B. The effect of age differences in ability-extraneous performance variables on the assessment of intelligence in children, adults, and the elderly. *Journal of Gerontology*, 1973, 28:73.

Gallagher, D., Breckenridge, J., Steinmetz, J., and Thompson, L. The Beck Depression Inventory and Research Diagnostic Criteria: congruence in an older population. *Journal of Consulting and Clinical Psychology*, 1983, 51:945.

Gallagher, D., McGarvey, W., Zelinski, E.M., and Thompson, L.W. Age and factor structure of the Zung Depression Scale. Paper presented at the 31st Annual Meeting of the Gerontological Society. Dallas, Texas, November 1978.

Gallagher, D., Nies, G., and Thompson, L.W. Reliability of the Beck Depression Inventory with older adults. *Journal of Consulting and Clinical Psychology*, 1982, 50:152.

Gallagher, D., Slife, B., Rose, T., and Okarma, T. Psychological correlates of immunologic disease in older adults. *Clinical Gerontology*, 1982, 1(2):51.

Gallagher, D., Thompson, L.W., and Levy, S.M. Clinical psychological assessment of older adults. In Poon, L.W. (Ed.), *Aging in the 1980s: Psychological Issues*. Washington, D.C.: American Psychological Association, 1980, pp. 19–40.

Gatz, M., Smyer, M.A., and Lawton, M.P. The mental health system and the older adult. In Poon, L.W. (Ed.), *Aging in the 1980s: Psychological Issues*. Washington, D.C.: American Psychological Association, 1980, pp. 5–18.

Gilleard, C.J., and Pattie, A.H. The Stockton Geriatric Rating Scale: a shortened version with British normative data. *British Journal of Psychiatry*, 1977, 131:90.

Goga, J.A., and Hambacher, W.O. Psychologic and behavioral assessment of geriatric patients: a review. *Journal of the American Geriatric Society*, 1977, 25:232.

Guion, R.M. Standards for psychological measurement. In Sales, B.D (Ed.), *The Professional Psychologist's Handbook*. New York: Plenum, 1983, pp. 111–40.

Guitman, D. Patterns of legal drug use by older Americans. *Addictive Disorders*, 1978, 3:337.

Gurel, L., Linn, M., and Linn, B. Physical and Mental Impairment of Function Evaluation in the aged: the PAMIE scale. *Journal of Gerontology*, 1972, 27:83.

Gurland, B.J., Copeland, J., Sharpe, L., and Kelleher, M. The Geriatric Mental Status Interview (GMS). *International Journal of Aging and Human Development*, 1976, 7:303.

Gurland, B.J., Fleiss, J.L., Goldberg, K., Sharpe, L., Copeland, J.R.M., Kelleher, M.J., and Kellet, J.M. A semi-structured clinical interview for the assessment of diagnosis and mental state in the elderly: the Geriatric Mental State Schedule II, a factor analysis. *Psychological Medicine*, 1976, 6:451.

Gurland, B., Kuriansky, J., Sharpe, L., Simon, R., Stiller, P., and Birkett, P. The Comprehensive Assessment and Referral Evaluation (CARE)—rationale, development and reliability. *International Journal of Aging and Human Development*, 1977–78, 8:9.

Hall, R.C.W., Popkin, M.K., Devaul, R.A., Faillace, L.A., and Stickney, S.K. Physical illness presenting as psychiatric disease. *Archives of General Psychiatry*, 1978, 35:1315.

Hamilton, M. A rating scale for depression. *Journal of Neurology, Neurosurgery, and Psychiatry*, 1960, 23:56.

Hamilton, M. Development of a rating scale for primary depressive illness. *British Journal of Social and Clinical Psychology*, 1967, 6:278.

Harding, J.J., and Dilley, K.J. Structural proteins of the mammalian lens: A review with emphasis on changes in development, aging, and cataract. *Experimental Eye Research*, 1976, 22:1.

Harmatz, J.S., and Shader, R.I. Psychopharmacologic investigations in healthy elderly volunteers: MMPI Depression Scale. *Journal of the American Geriatric Society*, 1975, 23:350.

Hauri, P. *The Sleep Disorders*. Kalamazoo, Mich.: Upjohn, 1977.

Hawkins, D.R. Sleep and depression. *Psychiatric Annual*, 1979, 9:391.

Hayslip, B., Jr. Verbosity and projective test performance in the aged. *Journal of Clinical Psychology*, 1981, 37:662.

Henry, W.E. *The Analysis of Fantasy: The Thematic Apperception Technique in the Study of Personality*. New York: Wiley, 1956.

Hersch, E.L., Kral, V.A., and Palmer, R.B. Clinical value of the London Psychogeriatric Rating Scale. *Journal of the American Geriatric Society*, 1978, 26:348.

Hersch, E.L., Merskey, H., and Palmer, R.B. Prediction of discharge from a psychogeriatric unit: development and evaluation of the LPRS prognosis index. *Canadian Journal of Psychiatry*, 1980, 25:234.

Heyman, D., and Jeffers, F. Effect of time lapse on consistency of self-health and medical evaluations of elderly persons. *Journal of Gerontology*, 1963, 18:160.

Hicks, R., Funkenstein, H.H., Dysken, M.W., and Davis, J.M. Geriatric psychopharmacology. In Birren, J.E., and Sloane, R.B. (Eds.); *Handbook of Mental Health and Aging*. Englewood Cliffs, N.J.: Prentice-Hall, 1980, pp. 745–74.

Holtzman, W.H., Thorpe, J.S., Swartz, J.D., and Herron, E.W. *Inkblot Perception and Personality: Holtzman Inkblot Technique*. Austin: University of Texas Press, 1961.

Honigfeld, G., Gillis, R.D., and Klett, C.J. NOSIE-30: A treatment-sensitive ward behavior scale. *Psychological Reports*, 1966, 21:65.

Horn, J.L., and Cattell, R.B. Age differences in fluid and crystallized intelligence. *Acta Psychologica*, 1967, 26:107.

Johnson, D.F., and White, C.B. Effects of training on computerized test performance in the elderly. *Journal of Applied Psychology*, 1980, 65:357.

Kahana, B. The use of projective techniques in personality assessment of the aged. In Storandt, J., Siegler, I.C., and Elias, M.F. (Eds.); *The Clinical Psychology of Aging*. New York: Plenum, 1978, pp. 145–80.

Kaszniak, A.W. Correlates of distress among families of chronically ill elderly. Paper presented at the 89th Annual Meeting of the American Psychological Association, Los Angeles, August 1981.

Kincannon, J.C. Prediction of the standard MMPI scale scores from 71 items: The Mini-Mult. *Journal of Consulting and Clinical Psychology*, 1968, 32:319.

Klassen, D., Homstra, R.K., and Anderson, P.B. Influence of social desirability on symptom and mood reporting in a community survey. *Journal of Consulting and Clinical Psychology*, 1975, 43:448.

Knapp, P.H. Emotional aspects of hearing loss. *Psychosomatic Medicine*, 1948, 10:203.

Klopfer, B., and Davidson, H.H. *The Rorschach Technique: An Introductory Manual.* New York: Harcourt, Brace & World, 1962.

Klopfer, W.G. The Rorschach and old age. *Journal of Personality Assessment,* 1974, 38:420.

Klopfer, W.G., and Taulbee, E.S. Projective tests. *Annual Review of Psychology,* 1976, 27:543.

Kochansky, G.E. Psychiatric rating scales for assessing psychopathology in the elderly: a critical review, in Raskin, A., and Jarvik, L.F. (Eds.); *Psychiatric Symptoms and Cognitive Loss in the Elderly,* Washington, D.C.: Hemisphere, 1979. pp. 125–156.

Krauss, I.K. Between—and within—group comparisons in aging research. In Poon, L.W. (Ed.); *Aging in the 1980s: Psychological Issues.* Washington D.C.: American Psychological Association, 1980, pp. 542–551.

Labouvie, E.W. Identity versus equivalence of psychological measures and constructs. In Poon, L.W. (Ed.); *Aging in the 1980s: Psychological Issues.* Washington, D.C.: American Psychological Association, 1980, pp. 493–502.

Lawton, M.P. Clinical geropsychology: problems and prospects. In *Master Lectures on the Psychology of Aging.* Washington, D.C.: American Psychological Association, 1979. (Originally presented at the meeting of the American Psychological Association, Toronto, August 1978.)

Lawton, M.P., Moss, M., Fulcomer, M., and Kleban, M.H. A research and service oriented multilevel assessment instrument. *Journal of Gerontology,* 1982, 37:91.

Leon, G.R., Kamp, J., Gillum, R., and Gillum, B. Life stress and dimensions of functioning in old age. *Journal of Gerontology,* 1981, 36:66.

Loranger, A.W., and Levine, P.M. Age at onset of bipolar affective illness. *Archives of General Psychiatry,* 1978, 35:1345.

Lorr, M. (Ed.). *Explorations in Typing Psychotics.* London: Pergamon, 1966.

Lorr, M., and Klett, C.J. *Manual: Inpatient Multidimensional Psychiatric Rating Scale, rev. ed.* Palo Alto, Calif.:, Consulting Psychologists Press, 1966.

Maddox, G.L., and Douglass, E.B. Self-assessment of health: a longitudinal study of elderly subjects. *Journal of Health and Social Behavior,* 1973, 14:87.

Matarazzo, J.D *Wechsler's Measurement and Appraisal of Adult Intelligence.* Baltimore: Williams & Wilkins, 1972.

McNair, D.M. Self-rating scales for assessing psychopathology in the elderly. In Raskin, A., and Jarvik, L.F. (Eds.); *Psychiatric Symptoms and Cognitive Loss in the Elderly.* Washington, D.C.: Hemisphere, 1979, pp. 157–168.

Meer, B., and Baker, J.A. The Stockton Geriatric Rating Scale. *Journal of Gerontology,* 1966, 21:392.

Meer, B., and Krag, C. Correlates of disability in a population of hospitalized geriatric patients. *Journal of Gerontology,* 1964, 19:440.

Miller, E. *Abnormal Ageing.* London: Wiley, 1977.

Miller, W.R., and Seligman, M.E.P. Depression and the perceptions of reinforcement. *Journal of Abnormal Psychology,* 1973, 82:62.

Mowbray, R.M. The Hamilton Rating Scale for Depression: a factor analysis. *Psychological Medicine,* 1972, 2:272.

Murkofsky, C., Conte, H.R., Plutchik, R., and Karasu, T.B. Clinical utility of a rapid diagnostic test series for elderly psychiatric outpatients. *Journal of the American Geriatric Society*, 1978, 26:22.

Nunnally, J.C. *Psychometric Theory*. New York: McGraw-Hill, 1967.

Oberleder, M. Adapting current psychological techniques for use in testing the aging. *Gerontologist*, 1967, 7:188.

Okimoto, J.T., Barnes, R.F., Veith, R.C., Raskind, M.A., Inui, T.S., and Carter, W.B. Screening for depression in geriatric medical patients. *American Journal of Psychiatry*, 1982, 139:799.

O'Neil, P.M., and Calhoun, K.S. Sensory deficits and behavioral deterioration in senescence. *Journal of Abnormal Psychology*, 1975, 84:579.

Orchik, D.J. Peripheral auditory problems and the aging process. In Beasley, D.S., and Davis, G.A. (Eds.); *Aging: Communication Processes and Disorders*. New York: Grune & Stratton, 1981, pp. 243–55.

Overall, J.E., and Gorham, D.R. The Brief Psychiatric Rating Scale. *Psychological Reports*, 1962, 10:799.

Pasewark, R.A., Fitzgerald, B.J., Dexter, V., and Cangemi, A. Response of adolescent, middle-aged, and aged females on the Gerontological and Thematic Apperception Tests. *Journal of Personality Assessment*, 1976, 40:588.

Pattie, A.H., and Gilleard, C.J. A brief psychogeriatric assessment schedule: validation against psychiatric diagnosis and discharge from hospital. *British Journal of Psychiatry*, 1975, 127:489.

Pattie, A.H., and Gilleard, C.J. The Clifton Assessment Schedule: further validation of a psychogeriatric assessment schedule. *British Journal of Psychiatry*, 1976, 129:68.

Pattie, A.H., and Gilleard, C.J. The two-year predictive validity of the Clifton Assessment Schedule and the shortened Stockton Geriatric Rating Scale. *British Journal of Psychiatry*, 1978, 133:457.

Pfeiffer, E. *Multidimensional Functional Assessment: The OARS Methodology*. Durham, N.C.: Duke University Center for the Study of Aging and Human Development, 1976.

Piper, M. Practical aspects of psychometric testing in the elderly. *Age and Ageing*, 1979, 8:299.

Plutchik, R., and Conte, H. Change in social and physical functioning of geriatric patients over a one-year period. *Gerontologist*, 1972, 12:181.

Plutchik, R., Conte, H., Lieberman, M., Bakur, M., Grossman, J., and Lehrman, N. Reliability and validity of a scale for assessing the function of geriatric patients. *Journal of the American Geriatric Society*, 1970, 18:491.

Post, F. The relationship to physical health of the affective illnesses in the elderly. In the *Eighth International Congress of Gerontology Proceedings*, Bethesda, Md: Federation of American Societies for Experimental Biology 1:198 1969, vol. 1, p. 198.

Prinz, P.N. Sleep patterns in the healthy aged: relationship with intellectual function. *Journal of Gerontology*, 1977, 32:179.

Redick, R.W., and Taube, C.A. Demography and mental health care of the aged. In Birren, J.E., and Sloane, R.B. (Eds.); *Handbook of Mental Health and Aging*. Englewood Cliffs, N.J.: Prentice-Hall, 1980, pp. 57–71.

Rees, J., and Botwinick, J. Detection and decision factors in auditory behavior of the elderly. *Journal of Gerontology*, 1971, 26:133.

Robin, A.A., and Harris, J.A. A controlled comparison of imipramine and electroplexy. *Journal of Mental Science*, 1962, 108:217.

Rorschach, H. *Psychodiagnostics*. New York: Grune & Stratton, 1942.

Rosenberg, M. *Society and the Adolescent Self-Image*. Princeton, N.J.: Princeton University Press, 1965.

Rosencranz, H.A., and Pihlblad, C.T. Measuring the health of the elderly. *Journal of Gerontology*, 1970, 25:129.

Rust, J.O., Barnard, D., and Oster, G.D. WAIS verbal-performance differences among elderly when controlling for fatigue. *Psychological Reports*, 1979, 44:489.

Sakalis, G., Gershon, S., and Shopsin, B. A trial of Gerovital H-3 in depression during senility. *Current Therapeutic Research* 1974, 16:59.

Sales, B.D. (Ed.) *The Professional Psychologist's Handbook*. New York: Plenum, 1983.

Salthouse, T.A. *Adult Cognition: An Experimental Psychology of Human Aging*. New York: Springer-Verlag, 1982.

Salzman, C., Kochansky, G.E., and Shader, R.I. Rating scales for geriatric psychopharmacology: a review. *Psychopharmacology Bulletin*, 1972a, 8:3.

Salzman, C., Kochansky, G.E., Shader, R.I., and Cronin, D.M. Rating scales for psychotropic drug research with geriatric patients: II. Mood ratings. *Journal of the American Geriatric Society*, 1972b, 20:215.

Salzman, C., Shader, R.I., Kochansky, G.E., and Cronin, D.M. Rating scales for psychotropic drug research with geriatric patients: I. Behavior ratings. *Journal of the American Geriatric Society*, 1972c, 20:209.

Sarteschi, P., Cassano, G.B., Castrogiovanni, P., and Conti, L. The use of rating scales for computer analysis of the affective symptoms in old age. *Comprehensive Psychiatry*, 1973, 14:371.

Savage, R.D., Gaber, L.B., Britton, P.G., Bolton, N., and Cooper, A. *Personality and Adjustment in the Aged*. London: Academic Press, 1977.

Schaie, K.W. External validity in the assessment of intellectual development in adulthood. *Journal of Gerontology*, 1978, 33:695.

Schaie, K.W., and Geiwitz, J. *Adult Development and Aging*. Boston: Little, Brown, 1982.

Schaie, K.W., and Labouvie-Vief, G. Generational versus ontogenetic components of change in adult cognitive behavior: a fourteen-year cross-sequential study. *Developmental Psychology*, 1974, 10:305.

Schaie, K.W., and Schaie, J.P. Clinical assessment and aging. In Birren, J.E., and Schaie, K.W. (Eds.); *Handbook of the Psychology of Aging*. New York: Van Nostrand Reinhold, 1977, pp. 692–723.

Shader, R.I., Harmatz, J.S., and Salzman, C. A new scale for clinical assessment in geriatric populations: Sandoz Clinical Assessment—Geriatric (SCAG). *Journal of the American Geriatric Society*, 1974, 22:107.

Siegler, I.C., Nowlin, J.B., and Blumenthal, J.A. Health and behavior: methodological considerations for adult development and aging. In Poon, L.W. (Ed.); *Aging in the 1980s: Psychological Issues*. Washington, D.C.: American Psychological Association, 1980, pp. 599–612.

Smith, J.M., Bright, B., and McCloskey, J. Factor analytic composition of the Geriatric Rating Scale (GRS). *Journal of Gerontology*, 1977, 32:58.

Soumerai, S.B., and Avorn, J. Perceived health, life satisfaction, and activity in urban elderly: a controlled study of the impact of part-time work. *Journal of Gerontology*, 1983, 38:356.

Spirduzo, W.W. Reaction and movement time as a function of age and physical activity level. *Journal of Gerontology*, 1975, 30:435.

Spitzer, R.L., Endicott, J., and Robins, E. Clinical criteria for diagnosis and DSM III. *American Journal of Psychiatry*, 1975, 132:187.

Spitzer, R.L., Endicott, J., and Robins, E. Research diagnostic criteria rationale and reliability. *Archives of General Psychiatry*, 1978, 35:773.

Spitzer, R.L., Forman, J.B.W., and Nee, J. DSM-III field trials: I. Initial interrater diagnostic reliability. *American Journal of Psychiatry*, 1979, 136:815.

Sprock, J., and Blashfield, R.K. Classification and nosology. In Hersen, M., Kazdin, A.E., and Bellack, A.S. (Eds.); *The Clinical Psychology Handbook*. New York: Pergamon, 1983, pp. 289–307.

Stenback, A. Depression and suicidal behavior in old age. In Birren, J.E., and Sloan, R.B. (Eds.); *Handbook of Mental Health and Aging*. Englewood Cliffs, N.J.: Prentice-Hall, 1980, pp. 616–52.

Stenback, A., and Javala, V. Hypochondria and depression. *Acta Psychiatrica Scandinavica*, 1962, 37 (Suppl. 162):240.

Stock, N.A., Kantner, J.E.: Themes elicited by the Senior Apperception Test in institutionalized older adults. *Journal of Personality Assessment*, 1980, 44:600.

Swenson, W.M. Structured personality testing in the aged: a MMPI study of the gerontic population. *Journal of Clinical Psychology*, 1961, 17:302.

Taylor, H.G., and Bloom, L.M. Cross-validation and methodological extension of the Stockton Geriatric Rating Scale. *Journal of Gerontology*, 1974, 29:190.

Waldron, J., and Bates, T.J.N. The management of depression in hospital: a comparative trial of desipramine and imipramine. *British Journal of Psychiatry*, 1965, 111:511.

Wallach, M.A., and Kogan, N. Aspects of judgment and decision making: inter-relationships and changes with age. *Behavioral Sciences*, 1961, 6:23.

Webb, W.B. Sleep in older persons: sleep structures of 50–60-year-old men and women. *Journal of Gerontology*, 1982, 37:581.

Wechsler, D. *The Measurement and Appraisal of Adult Intelligence*, 4th ed. Baltimore: Williams & Wilkins, 1958.

Wechsler, D. *Wechsler Adult Intelligence Scale—Revised Manual*, New York: The Psychological Corporation, 1981.

Weckowicz, T., Muir, W., and Cropley, A. A factor analysis of the Beck Inventory of Depression. *Journal of Consulting Psychology*, 1967, 31:23.

Weissmann, M.M., Sholomskas, D., Pottenger, M., Prusoff, B.A., and Locke, B.Z. Assessing depressive symptoms in five psychiatric populations: a validation study. *American Journal of Epdemiology*, 1977, 106:203.

Wiens, A.N., and Matarazzo, J.D. Diagnostic interviewing. In Hersen, M., Kazdin, A.E., and Bellack, A.S. (Eds.) *The Clinical Psychology Handbook*. New York: Pergamon, 1983, pp. 309–28.

Williams, J.B.W., and Spitzer, R.L. Research Diagnostic Criteria and DSM-III: an annotated comparison. *Archives of General Psychiatry*, 1982, 39:1283.

Willis, S.L., and Baltes, P.B. Intelligence in adulthood and aging: contemporary issues. In Poon, L.W. (Ed.); *Aging in the 1980s: Psychological Issues.* Washington, D.C.: American Psychological Association, 1980, pp. 260–72.

Winokur, G., Behar, D., and Schlesser, M. Clinical and biological aspects of depression in the elderly. In Cole, J.O., and Barrett, J.E. (Eds.); *Psychopathology in the Aged.* New York: Raven, 1980 pp. 145–53.

Wolk, R.L., and Wolk, R.B. *The Gerontological Apperception Test.* New York: Behavioral Publications, 1971.

Yesavage, J. Self-report scales in assessment of depression. Paper presented at the Talland Memorial Conference on Clinical Memory Assessment in Older Persons, Boston, Mass., October 1983.

Yesavage, J.A., Brink, T.L., Rose, T.L., Lum, O., Huang, V., Adey, M.B., and Leirer, V.O. Development and validation of a geriatric depression rating scale: a preliminary report. *Journal of Psychiatric Research*, 1982–83, 17:37.

Zubin, J., Eron, L.D., and Shumer, F. *An Experimental Approach to Projective Techniques.* New York: Wiley, 1965.

Zung, W.W.K.: A self-rating depression scale. *Archives of General Psychiatry*, 1965, 12:63.

Zung, W.W.K. Depression in the normal aged. *Psychosomatics*, 1967, 8:287.

6

Differentiating Depression from Organic Brain Syndromes in Older Age

Alfred W. Kaszniak
Menachem Sadeh
Lawrence Z. Stern

One of the most difficult problems facing the clinician or investigator is the differentiation of depression from various organic brain syndromes in older age. The American Psychiatric Association's *Diagnostic and Statistical Manual of Mental Disorders, Third Edition* (DSM-III) makes a distinction between *organic brain syndrome*, referring to a group of psychological signs and symptoms without reference to etiology (e.g., Dementia, Delirium) and *organic mental disorder*, which refers to a particular organic brain syndrome in which the etiology is known or presumed (APA, 1980, p. 101). The common feature of all of these disorders is psychological abnormality associated with brain dysfunction. Consequently, diagnosis rests upon both recognition of psychological or behavioral signs and symptoms, as well as demonstration, by means of physical examination, history, or laboratory tests of the presence of a specific organic factor judged to be etiologically related.

The organic brain syndromes categorized by the DSM-III include *Delirium, Dementia, Amnestic Syndrome, Organic Hallucinosis, Organic Delusional Syndrome, Organic Affective Syndrome, Organic Personality Syndrome, Intoxication, Withdrawal,* and a residual category of *Atypical or Mixed Organic Brain Syndrome* (APA, 1980, pp. 103–24). Because there can be a range of etiologies for each of these syndromes, the etiology or pathophysiological process is typically noted on axis III of the DSM-III multiaxial system.

There are two broad categories of *organic mental disorders* classified within the DSM-III. The first includes *Dementia* due to particular neurologic diseases that characteristically appear in older age, and the second contains those *Substance-induced Organic Mental Disorders* (APA, 1980, pp. 124–61). It is beyond scope of the present chapter to review specifics of the diagnostic criteria for all of these disorders. Rather, attention will be focused upon those disorders, more common in older age, which present the greatest difficulty in differentiation from depression.

DEMENTIA IN OLDER AGE

There is general agreement (e.g., Folstein and McHugh, 1978; Roth, 1980) that one of the most difficult yet important diagnostic decisions involves differentiating the signs and symptoms of dementia from those of depression. The DSM-III employs the following criteria for the diagnosis of dementia: 1) a deterioration from a previously acquired level of intellectual ability of sufficient severity to interfere with social or occupational functioning; 2) memory impairment; 3) at least one of the following: a) impairment of abstract thinking, b) impairment in judgement or impulse control and, c) personality change; 4) failure to meet the full criteria for either intoxication or delirium; and 5) either evidence from physical examination, laboratory tests, or history of a specific organic factor judged causally related to the disturbance, or, in the absence of such evidence, the assumption of the existence of an organic factor necessary for the development of the syndrome.

Since the now classic studies of Tomlinson et al. (1968, 1970), several investigators have confirmed that Alzheimer's disease, with its characteristic neuropathology of neuritic plaques, neurofibrillary tangles, and granulovacuolar degeneration, is the cause of the majority of cases of dementia in older age. (For current reviews of this literature, see Roth, 1980; Terry and Davies, 1980; Tomlinson, 1982; Terry and Katzman, 1983.) Across these various neuropathological studies, Alzheimer's disease has been found to account for between somewhat over 50, up to 70 percent of older patients with dementia seen in psychiatric practice. A further 15 to 25 percent are found to have multiple infarctions of the brain, either alone, or in combination with the neuropathology characteristic of Alzheimer's disease. The characteristic neuropathology of Alzheimer's disease has not been seen (at least not to the same extent) in the brains of depressed patients coming to postmortem examination (see Roth, 1980). The course of illness in dementia is also markedly different from that of depression in older age, with, for example, more than three-fourths of patients with dementia found to be dead within two years after admission to hospital, and three-fourths of those with depression found to be still alive (Roth, 1955).

Empirical evidence (see Pfeffer, in press; Roth, 1980) supports the conclusion that dementia of the Alzheimer's type, because of its insidious onset and slow progression, typically does not come to the attention of a professional until several years after the apparent onset of the illness. Once dementia has progressed several years into its course, thorough history-taking (Roth, 1980), careful clinical mental status examination (Folstein and McHugh, 1978), and application of various of the psychological assessment instruments reviewed in Chapter 5 (e.g., Roth and Hopkins, 1953; Trier, 1966; Kendrick and Post, 1967; Fleiss et al., 1976) are successful in differentiating these from the majority of depressed older individuals. However, considerable diagnostic difficulty does occur when dementia is very early in its course, and therefore mild, when the clinician confuses some of the signs and symptoms of dementia with those of depression, or when the older depressed patient presents with significant cognitive deficit.

Difficulty in this differential diagnosis appears to have been particularly common within the United States. Duckworth and Ross (1975) found organic brain syndromes to be diagnosed 50 percent more frequently in New York than in Toronto or London, England. Further, Roth (1959) had noted that the mortality for diagnosed dementias was substantially lower in New York than in England. Both of these observations suggest that diagnoses of disorders more benign than dementia, including depression, have, in the past, frequently been missed by clinicians in the United States.

Difficulties in differentiating dementia from depression in older age appear to be increased by several specific factors. First, as noted previously in this chapter, intellectual functioning does show some, albeit minimal, deterioration with normal aging, blurring the distinction between normal age-changes in intelligence and early indicators of the onset of dementia. Second, cognitive difficulty frequently accompanies depression, particularly for the elderly, and can reach proportions sufficient to be easily confused with that of dementia. Third, signs and symptoms of neurological disorder accompanied by dementia (e.g., Alzheimer's disease, Huntington's disease, Parkinson's disease) have some overlap with those of depression. Fourth, depression can coexist with dementia in these diseases. Finally, there are age-related changes in the brain which are reflected in clinical neurological, neuroradiological, electrophysiological, and neuropharmacological evaluation techniques and can lead to false positive diagnoses of neurologic disorder in the older person. The following paragraphs will review these factors contributing to diagnostic difficulty, with suggestions to assist the clinician or investigator in their resolution.

COGNITIVE FUNCTIONING AND AGING

One source of error in differential diagnosis is the application of inappropriate expectations for cognitive functioning in the elderly. In the preceding chapter, evidence for and issues concerning change in intellectual functioning with aging were discussed. Certainly, as clear from that discussion, the application of normative data based upon younger adults, when employing intellectual evaluation instruments with the elderly, would be inappropriate. Fortunately, the most frequently employed measure of adult intelligence, the Wechsler Adult Intelligence Scale, or WAIS (Wechsler, 1958), is a reliable test instrument, with age-stratified norms. The revised WAIS (WAIS-R) (Wechsler, 1981) improved upon the sampling procedures employed for obtaining older individuals, and provides, therefore, adequate age norms, for seven age groups from 20 through 74 years. Although the WAIS performance appears to reflect validly the cognitive impairment of dementia, there is greater variability among demented, as compared to age-matched healthy elderly, as well as some overlap of the respective score distributions (see Miller, 1977, pp. 33–60). The WAIS and WAIS-R may hence be insufficiently sensitive to mild dementia. Further, with some possible exceptions (e.g., Fuld, 1978), patterns of intellectual deficit, manifest on the WAIS, do not appear specific to any particular dementia etiology.

The presence of memory impairment is one of the DSM-III criteria for the diagnosis of dementia. Neither clinical mental status examination nor the WAIS provide sufficiently sensitive or comprehensive memory evaluation. The most frequently employed instrument for clinical memory assessment is the Wechsler Memory Scale (WMS) (Wechsler, 1945). Some of its psychometric qualities have been criticized (e.g., Erickson, 1978; Erickson and Scott, 1977), but a recent revision of this instrument (Russell, 1975), when correctly scored, demonstrates good interrater reliability (Power et al., 1979). Further, the WMS has been shown to differentiate validly between elderly psychiatric patients with organic brain syndromes and those with depression and other "functional" disorders (Gilleard, 1980).

The WMS, particularly the Russell (1975) revision, would thus appear to provide useful assistance in the evaluation of memory deficit in older persons. But, again, age-appropriate norms must be employed. An ever-increasing body of research demonstrates differences between younger and older adults in both quantitative and qualitative aspects of memory and learning processes (see review by Hartley, et al., 1980). It is thus not surprising that both cross-sectional and longitudinal data show age-related decline in WMS performance (McCarty, et al., 1982). Recently, Haaland et al. (1983) have provided revised WMS norms for ages 65 to over 80. However, the volunteer subjects comprising by their normative sample were better educated than is typical for the general population of these ages. Number of years of formal education has been shown to have a significant effect upon WMS performance, independent of the effects of age, cerebral atrophy (by computerized tomography measurement), and electroencephalographic (EEG) slowing, in older patients suspected of dementia (Kaszniak et al., 1979). Consequently, caution should be employed in using the norms of Haaland et al. unless the patient being evaluated has had nearly the same number of years of formal education as the normative sample. Normative data for older individuals is also available for other memory assessment instruments similar to the WMS, such as the Guild Memory Test (GMT) (Crook et al., 1980). Cautions similar to those noted above should also be applied in using such normative data.

Because, in the earliest stages of dementia, memory may be impaired without significant deficit in measured intelligence, formal evaluation of both intellect and memory are important in the psychological evaluation of the older person suspected of dementia. As dementia progresses, an increasingly large range of cognitive functions are affected with increasing severity. In many patients, progression of dementia results in sufficient impairment that application of instruments such as the WAIS and the WMS is no longer possible (i.e., their level of difficulty exceeds the patient's competence). In such cases, other instruments, with age-appropriate normative data, are available. Several of these are reviewed by Miller (1981).

Depression and Cognitive Deficit

A second factor contributing to difficulties in differential diagnosis is the presence of memory complaint and memory deficit in depression. Research and clinical experience have suggested that older depressed patients frequently complain of memory difficulty, even when objective assessment of memory fails to document deficit in comparison to age-appropriate normative expectation (Kahn et al., 1975). Kahn et al. have speculated that this discrepancy between memory complaint and memory performance in older depressed patients may reflect a general tendency toward pessimistic self-assessment.

In addition to increased memory complaint, research documents the presence of measurable deficit in memory, as well as other cognitive functions, in depression (see reviews by Miller, 1975; McAllister, 1981). Further, it appears that such cognitive deficits are age-associated, with older depressed patients being more likely to manifest such deficits (Donnelly et al., 1980). These deficits have been shown to be reversible, following successful treatment of the depression, with degree of memory improvement being correlated with degree of resolution of depression (e.g., Sternberg and Jarvik, 1976; Stromgren, 1977). Although memory is not the only cognitive function impaired in depression, it has been one of the most consistently documented areas of deficit (see McAllister, 1981).

The presence of reversible cognitive deficit in depression, particularly in the elderly, contributes to problems in the interpretation of formal tests of intellect, memory, and other cognitive assessment instruments. Whitehead (1973), in comparing elderly patients with depression versus those with diffuse brain damage, found the brain-damaged patients to score at generally lower levels on the WAIS than the depressed patients. However, there was no evidence that the patterns of scores were related to diagnosis. Similar subtests of the WAIS were impaired, in comparison to normative expectation, for both groups. Thus, particularly when impairment is quantitatively mild, great caution needs to be exercised in the interpretation of WAIS performance.

Thus, although severity and pattern of measured cognitive deficit will not reliably differentiate depressed from demented patients, recent research on the *qualitative* aspects of memory deficit does provide some assistance. One qualitative dimension, upon which older patients with depression and dementia differ, involves response bias. In general, studies have indicated that elderly depressed patients adopt a more conservative response strategy than older dementia patients (Hilbert et al., 1976; Larner, 1977; Miller and Lewis, 1977). The older depressed patient thus makes fewer false-positive memory errors (identifying an item as having been presented before when it really was not), but also show fewer true-positive (correctly identifying a stimulus as having been presented before) responses. It would thus appear that response bias, rather than true memory disorder, is at fault in the poor memory performance of the elderly depressed patient. Other, more recent research has provided additional evidence in support of this conclusion. Gibson (1981) employed an information-processing analysis (allowing for differential assessment of the theoretically distinct processes of primary and secondary memory) of free recall in a word list learning task. Results suggested that in dementia there is a fundamental breakdown in the process of memory itself, whereas in elderly depressives there is a suppression of normal memory process.

There have been attempts to derive from the studies just described optimal cut-off scores (on a particular memory or learning test) for the differential diagnosis of dementia versus depression in old age (e.g., Larner, 1977). However, further replication and validation would be necessary prior to recommending their general clinical application.

The evidence for response bias in the memory performance of older depressed patients does suggest that qualitative analysis of memory and other cognitive abilities would be of clinical utility. The present authors, as well as others (e.g., Wells, 1979) have noted that the older depressed patients manifesting apparent cognitive deficit frequently give "don't know" answers in intelligence or memory assessment (conservative response bias), whereas dementia patients show fewer such responses and typically make several "near miss" errors or manifest obvious guessing.

A second qualitative aspect of memory performance in depressed patients, which may be helpful in differentiating them from patients with dementia, involves the hypothetical cognitive processes of arousal, attention, concentration, and motivation. Recent research by Weingartner and colleagues (Weingartner et al., 1981; Weingartner, 1983) has indicated that depressed patients experience their greatest difficulty in memory tasks that require elaborate or "effortful" (Hasher and Zacks, 1979) organization and processing of material to be remembered. In contrast, dementia patients appear to have difficulty in all memory tasks, including those in which "automatic" (Hasher and Zacks, 1979) memory encoding is presumed to be involved (Weingartner, 1983). Further, Weingartner finds that degree of memory difficulty in "effortful" processing memory tasks is correlated with Hamilton Depression Rating Scale and Beck Depression Inventory scores. The memory performance of depressed patients was also found to correlate with ability to sustain effort in squeezing a hand dynamometer (presumably indexing effort and fatigability). Weingartner et al. (1981) have speculated that disruption of arousal and activation in depression may thus contribute to apparent memory difficulty. This may also explain the clinical observation (e.g., Wells, 1979) that elderly depressed patients, with apparent cognitive dysfunction, frequently demonstrate little effort to perform even simple cognitive tasks, appear to "give up" easily, and frequently show marked variability in performance on tasks of presumably similar difficulty. These qualitative features of memory performance are of clinical utility in differentiating depression from dementia (the dementia patient typically appears to struggle to perform tasks and demonstrates relatively consistent poor performance on tasks of similar difficulty).

The appearance of marked cognitive deficit, in the absence of evidence of neurologic or other medical etiology, has often been labeled *pseudodementia*, a term first introduced by Kiloh (1961). Kiloh's original description was of 10 patients with functional psychiatric disorders, who manifested features such as impairment of orientation, memory, intellect, and judgement, which are typically associated with dementia. Kiloh (1961) emphasized depressive illness in the etiology of pseudodementia, and others have employed the term almost exclusively in reference to depressed patients (e.g., Post, 1975). However, the appearance of pseudodementia can also occur in various other disorders, including hysterical syndromes and schizophrenia (Kiloh, 1961; Wells, 1979; Bienenfeld and Hartford, 1982; Maletta et al., 1982).

The clinical problem of pseudodementia has attracted considerable recent attention from the psychiatric community, resulting in the publication of many case studies, observations on small series of patients, and systematic studies. For more details, the reader is referred to several recent reviews of this literature (Post, 1975; Wells, 1979; Janowsky, 1982; McAllister, 1983). From these reviews one can abstract several useful clinical features which assist in differentiating depressive pseudodementia from dementia. Most authors (e.g., Wells, 1979; Roth, 1980; Janowsky, 1982) emphasize the marked importance of careful history-taking in this differential diagnostic process. Typically, progressive cerebral degenerative disorders, such as dementia of the Alzheimer type, begin insidiously with a history extending back for several years. In contrast, depressive pseudodementia often presents with symptoms of short duration (no more than a few weeks to a month) before medical help is sought, and there is apparent rapid progression of symptoms after onset. A history of previous psychiatric dysfunction is also much more common in pseudodementia than in true dementia.

Careful interview concerning presenting symptoms is also helpful. While the dementia patient, at least at middle to later stages of the disorder, typically complains very little of memory deficit or other cognitive deficit, the depressive pseudodementia patient will complain considerably of these difficulties, often with elaborate detail and examples, emphasizing disability and highlighting failures. The dementia patient's complaints are typically more vague, with efforts to conceal disability, and evidence of pride in even trivial accomplishments. The dementia patient may hence appear relatively unconcerned about his or her illness, while the depressive pseudodementia patient usually communicates a strong sense of distress. The dementia patient's behavior is typically consistent with the clinically observed severity of cognitive dysfunction (e.g., the patient with apparent memory deficit is observed getting lost on the way to his or her hospital room). The depressive pseudodementia patient will often demonstrate incongruities between behavior and apparent severity of cognitive deficit. Other differentiating features, best observed during the course of formal intellectual or memory assessment, have already been reviewed.

These observations underscore the necessity for careful history-taking, behavior observation, and comprehensive evaluation of affective and cognitive features. Greater diagnostic accuracy has been demonstrated for such multidimensional, as compared to unidimensional assessment approaches (Gurland et al. 1982; Gurland and Toner, 1983).

Depression and Depression-like Symptoms in Neurologic Disorders

The final contributor to differential diagnostic difficulty is the presence of depression and depression-like symptoms in a variety of neurologic disorders which are more frequent in the elderly. It is beyond the scope of the present chapter to discuss these disorders in any detail. However, critical features, particularly those contributing most to differential diagnostic difficulty, will be highlighted, with recommendations, wherever possible, to assist in diagnosis.

Depression in Primary Degenerative Dementia

Several authors (e.g., Demuth and Rand, 1980; Miller, 1980; McAllister and Price, 1982; Reifler et al., 1982) have recently drawn attention to the occurrence of coexisting depression and cognitive deficit in primary degenerative dementia (the term used by the DSM-III to refer to dementia of the Alzheimer type and related, e.g., Pick's, disorders). Older references to this coexistence (e.g., English, 1942) also can be found. The importance of diagnosing coexisting depression in primary degenerative dementia is emphasized by the occurrence of suicide and suicide attempt in these patients (Post, 1962), as well as indirect self-destructive behavior, which may serve as an alternative form of suicide (Nelson and Farberow, 1980). Efforts at differential diagnosis are further encouraged by case reports of depression in primary degenerative dementia responding to treatment, such as electroconvulsive therapy (Demuth and Rand, 1980). Whereas some authors (Busse, 1975; Pfeiffer, 1977) have suggested that depressive symptoms are most common in the early stages of dementia, others (e.g., Demuth and Rand, 1980) have observed depression in patients with severe dementia. Similarly, in studies of larger series of patients, some (Reifler et al., 1982) have found the rate of coexisting depression to decrease significantly with greater severity of cognitive impairment, whereas others (Kaszniak et al., 1981) fail to find any significant relationship between severity of depressive symptoms and severity of cognitive impairment. At present it would appear most prudent to conclude that depressive symptoms can occur at any point in the course of dementia.

To date, relatively little systematic research has been focused upon the nature of depression in primary degenerative dementia. The available research does suggest that different approaches to the assessment of depression may yield quite different results. Miller (1980) administered the Hamilton Depression Rating Scale and the Beck Depression Inventory, among other measures, to groups of normal, depressed, and "organic brain syndrome" elderly patients. On the Hamilton, an interview-based rating scale, all three groups were differentiated, with the normal group showing the lowest score, the depressed group the highest score, and the "organic" group an intermediate score. However, on the Beck, a self-report instrument, both depressed and "organic" groups scored significantly higher than the normal group, but were not significantly distinguishable from each other. While one might question the validity of a self-report instrument when administered to dementia patients (for whom difficulties in language comprehension and decreased insight are common), it should also be pointed out that instruments such as the Hamilton and the Beck focus upon different aspects of depressive symptoms.

An attempt to examine the pattern of depressive symptoms in elderly patients with dementia of the Alzheimer type (Kaszniak et al., 1981), by contrasting dementia and normal control subjects on the various items of the Hamilton, suggested that features such as depressed mood, slowing of thought and action, suspiciousness and loss of insight may be more frequent than "vegetative" manifestations (e.g., sleep disturbance, appetite loss, constipation). However, sampling issues (the dementia patients were selected to be relatively early in the course of dementia, and without a previous history of depression or other psychiatric disorder) and consideration of the fact that individual item reliability is considerably less than total score reliability for the Hamilton, requires that such results be interpreted with considerable caution. Recent research (Breen et al., 1984) also indicates that neither level nor pattern of intellectual (WAIS) or memory (WMS) test performance is accurate in differentiating dementia patients with and without coexisting depression.

A final difficulty in attempting to assess coexistent depression in dementia is generated by the similarity of certain features of dementia and depression. For example, the dementia patient may be careless in cleanliness and personal grooming, suggesting the possibility of depression-related apathy. Decreased variability of facial expression in dementia may be interpreted as the loss of interest or pleasure seen in depression. Tendency toward such interpretation may be increased by the desire of the clinician to find a treatable disorder, such as depression (Morstyn et al., 1982).

Depression in Parkinson's Disease

Symptoms of depression have long been known to be associated with Parkinson's disease. Patrick and Levy (1922) found affective symptoms of varying severity to be common in a group of 146 Parkinson's patients, while Jackson et al. (1923) drew attention to the appearance of affective symptoms often months or years before the development of typical Parkinsonian signs. Other psychological disturbances, such as personality change, confusion, memory dysfunction, agitation, and anxiety have been described in clinical accounts of Parkinson's disease (Schwab and England, 1958). The use of formal assessment procedures for depression such as the Hamilton Depression Rating Scale has supported these clinical impressions of the association of depression with Parkinson's disease, with prevalence estimates ranging from 20 to 90 percent (see review by Mayeux, 1982). Such estimates likely vary not only because of differences in the composition of the research samples, but also because of difficulties in the assessment of depression in Parkinson's disease.

Bradykinesia (slowness of movement) contributes to difficulties in diagnosis of depression. Parkinsonian patients have delayed initiation of movements, general poverty of motor activity, and reduced facial gestures, difficult to differentiate from the psychomotor slowing and constricted emotional expression of depression. In addition to bradykinesia, there is bradyphrenia (slowness of thought), with both this feature and movement slowing appearing to be more common in older Parkinson's disease patients (Wilson et al., 1980). Thus, the relatively immobile, slowly responsive patient with a masklike expression may easily be thought to be apathetic or depressed, whereas the patient's subjective mood may not be markedly altered. This emphasizes the necessity of evaluating psychological symptoms as well as physical signs in the diagnosis of depression in Parkinson's disease. Additional help may be provided by observing the patient while on levodopa therapy. Usually with such treatment, the bradykinesia improves, and even patients with severe long-standing disease may experience periods of relatively good mobility.

The etiology of depression in Parkinson's disease is not well understood. The occurrence of depression prior to motor signs would suggest a DSM-III diagnosis of *Organic Affective Syndrome* (APA, 1980, pp. 117–18), indicating that the depression is thought due to the specific organic condition of Parkinson's disease. However, some patients appear to develop depressive symptoms during the first year after the onset of motor signs (see Mayeux, 1982) and may well be depressed as a reaction to the disabling nature of their disease. In the latter case, a diagnosis of Major Depressive Episode (providing that the diagnostic criteria are met) might be more appropriate.

Early reports had suggested some improvement of depressive symptoms with levodopa therapy (e.g., Barbeau, 1969; Yahr et al., 1969). However, later studies, typically employing more objective measurement, showed little or no mood improvement, although the motor signs of the disease did respond to the drug (Marsh and Markham, 1973; Brown et al., 1978). The apparent improvement of depressive symptoms reported in earlier studies may have been due to some lessening of the "reactive" component of depression, thought to be in response to the motor disability. Tricyclic antidepressants, particularly those with minimal central anticholinergic activity, appear to be helpful in treating depression associated with Parkinson's disease, and have been used simultaneously with levodopa treatment (see Mayeux, 1982).

Another feature contributing to problems in the diagnosis of depression in Parkinson's disease, is the presence of cognitive impairment in a substantial number of patients. Memory and visual-perceptual skills have been among those most frequently reported as impaired, and studies employing careful psychometric assessment of cognitive deficit have documented its association with older age, longer duration of illness, bradykinesia, and severity of functional disability in Parkinson's disease (see review by Mayeux, 1982). Cognitive impairment may greatly limit the extent to which self-report of depressive symptoms can be relied upon in evaluation.

Depression in Huntington's Disease

Huntington's disease (HD) is a chronic, progressive, degenerative neurologic disorder that is inherited as an autosomal dominant trait. The onset of HD most often occurs during middle adulthood, with average life expectancy, once a diagnosis has been made, of approximately 15 years (although with great individual variability). Consequently HD, although not typically thought of as a disease of old age, does affect older persons. Huntington (1872), in his original description declared insanity, with a tendency to suicide, as a major feature of this hereditary disease.

Other manifestations of HD include progressive involuntary movement disorder (typically chorea but occasionally akinesia and rigidity), as well as progressive dementia (Butters et al., 1979). Psychiatric manifestations of the disease include personality changes, schizophrenia-like syndromes, paranoid delusions, and affective disorders, with some authors (e.g., McHugh and Folstein, 1975; Folstein et al., 1979) believing depression to be the most prominent manifestation. In a recent study of 30 HD patients, carefully employing DSM-III diagnostic criteria, Caine and Shoulson (1983) fround 24 of the patients to demonstrate substantial behavioral abnormality, including affective and schizophrenic syndromes, personality changes, and disorders that could not be classified adequately. However, Caine and Shoulson (1983) found no correlation between the severity of dementia and the psychopathology in their group of HD patients. They also found antidepressant pharmacotherapy to benefit the somatic signs of their patients' affective disorders without altering their dysphoric mood.

Given the apparent onset of HD in middle age, most elderly HD patients will demonstrate signs, or history, of involuntary movement disorder. However, depression and attempted suicide may occur many years prior to the onset of involuntary movements in HD. Reactive depression, perhaps based on the knowledge of the hereditary nature and prognosis of the disease, may also occur (see Pearson, 1973).

Diagnosis of Depression in Other Neurologic Disorders

While primary degenerative dementia, Parkinson's disease, and Huntington's disease certainly do not exhaust the list of neurologic disorders in which depression can present in the elderly, these three syndromes do serve to illustrate some of the differential diagnostic problems. Hypothyroidism, neurosyphilis, infectious disease (either primarily affecting the central nervous system or having secondary affect upon central nervous system functioning) and carcinoma are among a number of other disorders that can present with problems in the differential diagnosis of depression (see Hall et al., 1978). In addition to the careful psychological evaluation of depressive signs and symptoms in such patients, thorough neurological evaluation plays an obviously important role. Within the following paragraphs, issues concerning neurological evaluation of the elderly will be briefly addressed.

AGING AND THE BRAIN

Critchley (1956) drew attention to the problems of interpretation of neurological signs and symptoms in the elderly. Like psychological signs and symptoms, age-related changes in the central nervous system frequently require a different interpretation of neurological examination findings in older versus younger individuals. Despite a growing body of literature concerning age-related changes in the nervous system (see Katzman and Terry, 1983), the neurobiology of aging is still in a descriptive stage, and we are far from comprehending the nature of most of the processes involved.

The major morphological and physiological changes that characterize aging in the brain are decreased size, loss of neurons in selected areas of the brain, reduction of dendritic arborization, decreased enzymatic activity involved in neurotransmitter synthesis, loss of receptors, and accumulation of intracellular deposits. However, it is generally unclear how these changes are correlated with functional changes associated with aging (cf., Terry, 1978). Further, the etiology of age-related alterations in brain structure and function remains an enigma. Even the most familiar pathological process accompanying aging, neuronal loss, remains a puzzle for the histologist. Neurons appear to die without signs of neuronophagia, inflammation, or significant intracellular changes, and seem to disappear without a trace, leaving no clue as to the mechanism of their death (see Katzman and Terry, 1983). It is unclear whether age-related neuronal loss is a genetically programmed expression, an accidental process, an "autoimmune" reaction, a response to environmental toxins, or the result of some toxic effect of accumulated waste materials.

In addition to primary changes within the central nervous system, in the elderly the brain is obviously affected by hormonal, immunological, cardiovascular, and other systemic changes that can influence brain function. Such factors require careful consideration when interpreting results of the neurologic examination in the older person.

The Neurological Examination in Older Age

The general principles of neurological evaluation, including thorough history-taking and the procedures of the examination, are applicable to the elderly. Special considerations include the need to consider history-taking from other sources of information, such as relatives or friends, when sensory or cognitive deficit limits the reliability of history-taking from the older patients. Evaluation of the contribution of various systemic disease processes, as well as previous and present medications (see Chapter 7) also complicate neurological evaluation.

Some of the alterations in the aging nervous system may not be evident in the formal neurological examination yet may cause functional difficulties. Thus, as in the neurological examination of the younger child, the clinician must concentrate on functional observations as well as the results of bedside examination. Furthermore, critical to the accurate interpretation of the neurological examination of the older person is an understanding of what should be considered "normal" for a given individual's age. The following paragraphs discuss changes that one should expect on neurological examination of the elderly but otherwise healthy patient.

Mental Status

Various issues concerning the evaluation of cognitive and effective functioning in older age have already been discussed previously in this chapter. Given subtle changes in intellect and memory which appear to accompany normal aging, the clinician would appear to be well advised to rely upon formal mental status examination procedures for which there is available age-appropriate normative data. Several of those best-developed of such procedures have been reviewed in detail elsewhere (e.g., Kaszniak, in press).

Motor Function

The effect of age upon motor function is perhaps the most readily observed of all features in the neurologic examination, and appears to be the result of changes in the central and peripheral nervous system, as well as within muscle. The posture becomes somewhat flexed and rigid, resembling the Parkinsonian posture (Teravainen and Calne, 1983). The gait is often marked by small steps, flexed extremities with reduced arm movements, and slight forward flexion of the body (Murray et al., 1969). Parkinson's disease can be excluded by the absence of typical rigidity, bradykinesia, and resting tremor. Minor extrapyramidal signs in older persons, including mild rigidity and poverty of movement, should not, alone, lead to the incorrect diagnosis of Parkinson's disease. Critchley (1956) had suggested that these age-related changes are actually features of mild extrapyramidal disorder, and indeed, cell loss accompanying aging often selectively affects the striatum and substantia nigra (Corsellis, 1976). Also suggesting similarity of pathophysiological process in normal brain aging and Parkinson's disease is the observation that in the residual cells of the basal ganglia, there is a marked loss of activity of tyrosine hydroxylase, the rate-limiting enzyme of dopamine synthesis (McGeer et al., 1977).

Muscle strength has been found to be reduced by 20 to 45 percent in the sixth to eighth decades of life, compared to that of the third decade (Potvin et al., 1980). The most affected muscles are the leg flexors; grip strength is relatively better preserved. This is commonly accompanied by some muscle wasting. This atrophy affects the entire masculature but is especially observed in the small muscles of the hands and in association with deformed arthritic joints (Critchley, 1956). Fasciculations are usually not observed and, if present, should be considered abnormal. The histological correlates of reduced muscle strength with aging include muscle fiber loss, reduction of fiber size and type grouping, and appear to be the result of myopathic as well as denervation and reinnervation processes.

The examination of muscle tone often reveals mild rigidity, sometimes only during activation of the contralateral limb (Cooper's sign). This may be another feature of the extrapyramidal dysfunction previously discussed. It should be noted, however, that tone is also frequently increased in association with joint disease.

Reflexes

The absence of ankle reflexes in the elderly is a common neurological finding, reported by many of the early writers concerned with the neurology of aging (e.g., Critchley, 1931; Howell, 1949). Ankle-jerk reflexes appear to be elicitable in 99 percent of all patients when reinforcement maneuvers are used (Ellenberg, 1960), but in older patients Carter (1979) reported inability to obtain ankle jerks in 31 percent, even with vigorous reinforcement techniques.

Knee jerk and upper limb reflexes usually persist; infrequently they may be absent (Prakash and Stern, 1973). The abdominal reflexes may be difficult to obtain in middle life, with increasing loss with age.

Critchley (1956) discussed the difficulty in interpreting plantar responses in old age. He found clear-cut flexor plantar responses to be not common, but a true extensor response to be quite exceptional, although occasionally seen. Klawans, and colleagues (1971) also reported the rare occurrence of extensor plantar responses in otherwise neurologically normal older persons. This may be a sign of subclinical disorder, such as cervical spondylosis with subclinical myelopathy. However, the observance of a Babinski sign in the older individual should call for a thorough investigation to rule out occult neurological disease.

In the examination of an older patient, the clinician will often try to elicit so-called primitive or release reflexes, such as the palmomental and snout reflexes. Although such reflexes have traditionally been related to bilateral cortical disease, great caution needs to be exercised in interpreting their presence in the older individual. In fact, a palmomental reflex can be elicited in all normal people with a strong enough stimulus, and a snout reflex appears to be present in half of healthy older individuals (Koller et al., 1982). Koller et al. (1982) failed to find any correlation between the presence of primitive reflexes and apparent cerebral atrophy (by CT scan) or results of psychometric evaluation of cognitive functioning. It would appear then, that these primitive reflexes are of relatively little clinical value in the neurological assessment of older individuals.

Sensory Function

The decrease of vibration sense with age has been recognized for many years (e.g., Critchley, 1931) and confirmed by numerous studies (Prakash and Stern, 1973; Potvin et al., 1980). Reduction of vibration sense is most frequently noticed in the toes and ankles, less frequently in the upper parts of the lower extremities, and only rarely in the upper extremities (Klawans et al., 1971). Loss of position sense follows the same pattern as vibration sense, but is less frequent. Since loss of vibration and position sensation is positively correlated with loss of ankle reflexes, it is most likely due to similar mechanisms, as discussed.

Other somatosensory modalities, such as light touch, two-point discrimination, temperature and pain, also demonstrate some age-related changes (see Corso, 1981, pp. 175–200). However, these modalities are typically found to be intact on clinical neurologic examination.

The Cranial Nerves

Although not always clinically examined, it is important to know that olfactory function is reduced in the elderly. Prakash and Stern (1973) found that only one-third of the people they studied (age range of 69 to 94 years) had intact sense of smell.

Critchley (1931, 1956) noted that, with advancing age, pupils tend to become myotonic with sluggish reaction to light and accommodation. This clinical observation was confirmed by later studies (Prakash and Stern, 1973; Carter, 1979). Pupillography shows a decrease with age of velocity and degree of constriction, as well as pupillary size (e.g., Kummick, 1959). These changes have been related to structural changes in the pupillary sphincter muscle by some observers (e.g., Critchley, 1956).

Critchley (1931, 1956) also observed that upward gaze and convergence are often impaired in the elderly. This has become widely accepted among neurologists and is considered normal. Sharpe and Sylvester (1978) have also reported subclinical dysfunction with age of smooth pursuit movements in the horizontal plane.

As discussed in the previous chapter, significant impairment of visual acuity occurs frequently in older individuals. In addition to the contribution of cataracts, already discussed, another major cause is senile macular degeneration, a term used for various incurable degenerative processes in the posterior pole of the aged eye. It should be remembered that other disorders which impair visual acuity in the elderly, including cataracts and glaucoma, are potentially treatable (Wright and Hendkind, 1983).

Auditory perceptual difficulties accompanying aging, such as presbycusis, have also been discussed within the previous chapter. As already noted, auditory functioning may be difficult to assess in the older individual and may itself contribute to behavioral changes and apparent cognitive impairment. Early recognition of hearing impairment is important, not only as a possible expression of occult disease, but also because of the possibility of restoration by use of an appropriate hearing aid. The mechanism of presbycusis appears to involve both the peripheral auditory system, including loss of hair cells and cochlear neurons, and the central auditory system (Baker, 1981).

Tremor

Trembling hands are popularly considered as one of the signs of older age. So-called senile tremor may also involve the head, trunk, legs, and voice. It is apparently an exaggeration of physiological tremor and thus similar to essential or familial tremor. The main importance of recognizing senile tremor is to distinguish it from Parkinsonian tremor. The former is typically a rapid, fine sustention and intention tremor, while the latter is a slow, coarse, alternating resting tremor (Fahn, 1972).

Autonomic Function

Impairment of autonomic function is common in old age. The most significant alterations occur in cardiovascular, thermoregulatory, and secretory functions. Caird et al. (1973) described a drop of 20 millimeters of mercury or more in systolic blood pressure with postural change in 30 percent of a group of subjects 75 years of age or older. Other cardiovascular reflexes, such as heart rate and blood pressure responses to Valsalva maneuver and tachycardia during tilting, are diminished in the elderly. (Gross, 1979). Such change in autonomic function in the elderly explains the increased frequency of orthostatic hypotension with advanced age. The common use of drugs with possible hypotensive effect such as antihypertensives, levodopa, phenothiazines, diuretics, and tricyclic antidepressants, contributes to the prevalence of this disorder.

Old age is also associated with impairment of thermoregulatory function. Rectal temperature declines in older men and the difference between rectal and skin temperature increases with age (Fox et al., 1973). During exposure to cold, older people may fail to maintain their core temperature, which continues to fall throughout cold exposure. A high proportion of older persons have low resting peripheral blood flow and fail to respond to cold by peripheral vasoconstriction (Collins et al., 1977). During exposures to a hot environment, core temperature rises significantly with age, and finger blood flow has been found to be reduced (Fennel and Moore, 1973). Sweating occurs in only about half of the elderly exposed to heat (Fox et al., 1973). Decreased thermoregulatory function with age contributes to the increased risk of two potentially fatal conditions, accidental hypothermia and heat stroke.

LABORATORY PROCEDURES IN NEUROLOGICAL EVALUATION

In addition to history-taking and physical examination, laboratory procedures play an important role in neurological evaluation particularly for older persons. As with other diagnostic procedures, knowledge about age-related changes in relevant anatomy and physiology is important for appropriate interpretation. Some of the most relevant (for purposes of differential diagnosis of depression and organic brain syndromes in older age) neurophysiologic, neuroradiologic, and neuropharmacologic procedures will be discussed in the following paragraphs.

Electroencephalography (EEG) and Evoked Responses

The alpha frequency in the EEG has been shown to slow with increasing adult age. In middle life, the alpha rhythm is found to be at approximately 10 cycles per second (Hz). It decreases to approximately 9.5 Hz at age 70, 9 Hz at age 80, and 8.5 Hz after age 90 (Drechsler, 1978; Hughes and Cayaffa, 1977). The cause for this slowing is not known. Moreover, while this age-effect is generally true for any large population studied, individual subjects may have no change in EEG frequency with aging, and these alterations appear to have little clinical importance. Not infrequently, slow, irregular, theta activity may be recorded from one or both temporal regions (Busse et al., 1956). This does not necessarily indicate any underlying disorder, and in the absence of other evidence of central nervous system disease, should be considered a normal variant.

More diffuse distribution of theta activity, or slowing into the delta range is typically indicative of cerebral disease. While systemic disease and drug effects can produce such slowing, in their absence, diffuse EEG slowing is most frequently seen in primary degenerative dementia in older age (Muller and Schwartz, 1978). Further, the degree of EEG slowing has been shown to be correlated with the degree of cognitive impairment in primary degenerative dementia (e.g., Johannesson et al., 1979; Kaszniak et al., 1979), and is somewhat predictive of mortality (Kaszniak et al., 1978). Despite the utility of examination of the EEG frequency in differential diagnosis, it must be remembered that patients in the early stages of primary degenerative dementia may not demonstrate any significant EEG slowing. More recent innovations in the analysis of EEG frequency data, such as examination of topographic measures of EEG coherence (e.g., O'Connor et al., 1979) may prove to be useful diagnostic aids, if adequate age-appropriate normative data can be developed.

Evoked-reponse studies have revealed that adult aging has only minimal effect on the early components of the evoked potential (EP), whereas later components have shown significantly increased latencies in older age groups. Generally, similar changes have been found in studies of visual evoked responses (Celesia and Daly, 1977), auditory evoked responses (Goodin et al., 1978), and somatosensory evoked responses (Desmedt and Cheron, 1980). Given these age-related changes in evoked responses, as well as considerable individual variability, it is not surprising that attempts to employ evoked response studies in differentiating dementia from other disorders (including depression) in older age have produced mixed results (e.g., Levy et al., 1971; Hendrickson et al., 1979; Squires et al., 1980; Pfefferbaum, 1983). Pending further research and the availability of adequate age-appropriate normative data, evoked response studies should not be relied upon in attempting to differentiate depression from dementia in older age.

Computerized Tomographic (CT) Scanning

CT scanning, allowing for the visualization of intracranial anatomy, can have particular value in the neurological evaluation of the older person, given its sensitivity to various focal structural lesions of the brain. However, its diagnostic utility in helping to differentiate depression from primary degenerative dementia in older persons remains highly questionable (see Fox et al., 1979).

Even without formal measurement, visual inspection readily reveals ventricular enlargement with advancing adult age. Various measurement procedures have revealed that, by the eighth decade, there is an increase of approximately 15 percent in ventricular size (e.g., Barron et al., 1976; Yamaura et al., 1980). Increased width of cortical sulci, though more difficult to assess, has also been demonstrated to be age-associated (Jacoby et al., 1980). Although, as a group, patients with primary degenerative dementia demonstrate ventricular and sulcal enlargement, in comparison to a normal age-matched group, there is considerable overlap (e.g., Wilson et al., 1982). Not infrequently, the CT scan of a markedly demented patient shows only minimal ventricular and sulcal enlargement. Thus, despite some degree of correlation between degree of cognitive deficit and CT scan measures of ventricular and sulcal enlargement in primary degenerative dementia (e.g., Kaszniak et al., 1979), such measures do not appear to be presently reliable for either diagnostic or prognostic purposes (Kaszniak et al., 1978). Bird (1982) provided a comprehensive recent review of the literature in this area.

New approaches to the analysis of CT scan data, such as those based upon tissue density measures (e.g., Naeser et al., 1980) have been suggested by some to hold diagnostic promise (see Bird, 1982). However, reported failures to find CT scan density measure differences between demented and healthy older persons (e.g., Wilson et al., 1982) argues against any immediate clinical application of such measures.

Other Laboratory Procedures

Although not developed to the point of present clinical application, there are newer radiologic techniques that may eventually prove to be of assistance in differentiating depression from organic brain syndromes in older age. Measurement of cerebral blood flow, using inhalation of radioactively labeled xenon (e.g., Gustafson et al., 1981) is one such procedure.

Another such procedure, which has generated considerable recent interest, is that of positron emission tomography (PET) (Frackowiak, et al., 1981; Benson, 1982). This procedure allows visualization of tomographic measures of regional cerebral metabolism, which have been shown to be sensitive to brain activity during various perceptual and cognitive processes (e.g., Mazziotta et al., 1982). Some of the excitement concerning possible clinical applications of this procedure derives from recent observations that PET measures of cerebral metabolism do not appear to change with normal aging, but are quite sensitive to the presence of dementia of the Alzheimer type (de Leon et al., 1983; Friedland et al., 1983). PET scanning equipment is at present available at very few medical centers and remains plagued by many technical difficulties in its use and interpretation.

Finally, mention must be of possible future diagnostic application of nuclear magnetic resonance (NMR) imaging (James et al., 1981). This procedure has been shown to provide extremely detailed visualization of intracranial structures, is sensitive to the molecular composition of tissue, and may have fewer practical limitations than PET scanning.

Recently, interest has focused upon the possible use of "pharmacological challenge," such as the dexamethasone suppression test, in the diagnosis of depression in older age. Chapter 7 reviews this procedure, and available research literature concerning it. It should be noted that results of its application in attempts to differentiate dementia from depressive pseudodementia have been mixed (e.g., McAllister et al., 1982; Spar and Gerner, 1982), arguing against its reliability in this diagnostic application.

Finally, note should be made of the importance of routine laboratory procedures (e.g., blood counts, blood urea nitrogen, T_4, serum protein electrophoresis, electrocardiogram, etc.) to rule out other possible (and often treatable) causes of apparent dementia (see Kaszniak et al., 1979).

NEUROPSYCHOLOGICAL ASSESSMENT

Neuropsychological assessment is a term collectively applied to a wide range of cognitive and affective measures with known relationship to brain structure and function (see Filskov and Boll, 1981; Heilman and Valenstein, 1979; Lezak, 1983). Given the highly specialized nature of this field, it is beyond the scope of the present chapter to review its specifics. Recent reviews (e.g., Albert, 1981; Klisz, 1978; Price et al., 1980) have provided detailed evaluation of the application of neuropsychological assessment procedures with the elderly. Much of the discussion earlier in this chapter of issues in the assessment of intelligence and memory with older persons apply equally to neuropsychological assessment procedures. Age-appropriate norms have not yet been adequately developed for most of the more frequently employed neuropsychological assessment procedures. However, there has been, in recent years, a dramatic increase in the amount of research focusing upon neuropsychological assessment of older persons, and much has been learned, through application of such procedures, about the nature of cognitive deterioration in dementia (see Kaszniak, in press). Neuropsychological assessment, performed by a competent clinical neuropsychologist who is familiar with this literature, can contribute substantially to the diagnostic process (see Fuld, 1978).

Even with the increasingly better development of neuropsychological assessment procedures, with improved age-appropriate normative data, the clinician must not neglect the critical importance of careful clinical observation and history taking. History of the onset and course of illness may be one of the most critical variables for the diagnosis of various disorders, such as multi-infarct dementia, in older age (Hachinski et al., 1975; Rosen et al., 1980).

REFERENCES

Albert, M.S. Geriatric neuropsychology. *Journal of Consulting and Clinical Psychology*, 1981, 49:835.

American Psychiatric Association. *Diagnostic and Statistical Manual of Mental Disorders, Third Edition*. Washington, D.C., APA, 1980.

Baker, R.H. The neuroaudiologic evaluation of the geriatric patient. In Slasle, W.R. (Ed), *Geriatric Neurology: Selected Topics*. New York, Futura, 1981, pp. 131–72.

Barbeau, A. L-dopa therapy in Parkinson's disease: a critical review of nine years' experience. *Canadian Medical Association Journal*, 1969, 101:791.

Barron, S.A., Jacobs, L., and Kinnel, W.R. Changes in the size of normal lateral ventricles during aging determined by computed tomography. *Neurology*, 1976, 26:1011.

Benson, D.F. The use of positron emission scanning techniques in the diagnosis of Alzheimer's disease. In Corkin, S., Davis, K.L., Growdon, J.H., Usdin, E., and Wurtman, R.L. (Eds.), *Aging. Volume 19: Alzheimer's Disease: A Report of Progress*. New York, Raven, 1982, pp. 79–82.

Bienenfeld, D., and Hartford, J.T. Pseudodementia in an elderly woman with schizophrenia. *American Journal of Psychiatry*, 1982, 139:114.

Bird, J.M. Computerized tomography, atrophy and dementia: a review. *Progress in Neurobiology*, 1982, 19:115.

Breen, A.R., Larson, E.B., Reifler, B.V., Vitaliano, P.P., and Lawrence, G.L. Cognitive performance and functional competence in coexisting dementia and depression. *Journal of the American Geriatric Society*, 1984, 32:132.

Brown, E., Brown, G.M., Kofman, O., and Ovarrington, B. Sexual function and affect in Parkinsonian men treated with L-dopa. *American Journal of Psychiatry*, 1978, 135:1552.

Busse, E.W. Aging and psychiatric diseases of late life. In Arieti, S. (Ed.), *American Handbook of Psychiatry*, 2nd ed. *Volume IV: Organic Disorders and Psychosomatic Medicine*. New York, Basic Books, 1975, pp. 67–89.

Busse, E.W., Barnes, R.H., Friedman, E.L., and Kelty, E.J. Psychological functioning of aged individuals with normal and abnormal electroencephalograms. I: A study of non-hospitalized community volunteers. *Journal of Nervous and Mental Diseases*, 1956, 124:135.

Butters, N., Albert, M.S., and Sax, D. Investigations of the memory disorders of patients with Huntington's disease. In Chase, T.N., Wexler, N.S., and Barbeau, A. (Eds.), *Advances in Neurology. Volume 23: Huntington's Disease*. New York, Raven, 1979, pp. 203–13.

Caine, E.D., and Shoulson, I. Psychiatric syndromes in Huntington's disease. *American Journal of Psychiatry*, 1983, 140:728.

Caird, F.I., Andrews, G.R., and Kennedy, R.D. Effect of posture on blood pressure in the elderly. *British Heart Journal*, 1973, 35:527.

Caird, F.I. Examination of the nervous system. In Caird, F.I. (Ed.), *Neurological Disorders in the Elderly*. Bristol, England: Wright, 1982, pp. 44–51.

Carter, A.B. The neurologic aspects of aging. In Rossman, I. (Ed.), *Clinical Geriatrics*, 2nd ed., Philadelphia: Lippincott, 1979, pp. 292–94.

Celesia, G.G., and Daly, R.F. Effects of aging on visual evoked responses. *Archives of Neurology*, 1977, 34:403.

Collins, K.J., Dore, C., Exton-Smith, A.N., Fox, R.H., MacDonald, I.C., Woodward, P.M. Accidental hypothermia and impaired homeostasis in the elderly. *British Medical Journal*, 1977, 1:353.

Corsellis, J.A.N. Ageing and dementias. In Balckwood, W., and Corsellis, J.A.N. (Eds.), *Greenfield's Neuropathology*. London, Edward Arnold, 1976, pp. 796–848.

Corso, J.F. *Aging Sensory Systems and Perception*. New York, Praeger, 1981.

Critchley, M. The neurology of old age. *Lancet*, 1931, 1:1119.

Critchley, M. Neurological changes in the aged. *Journal of Chronic Diseases*, 1956, 3:459.

Crook, T., Gilbert, J.G., and Ferris, S. Operationalizing memory impairment for elderly persons: the Guild Memory Test. *Psychological Reports*, 1980, 47:1315.

de Leon, M.J., Ferris, S.H., George, A.E., Christman, D.R., Fowler, J.S., Gentes, C., Reisberg, B., Gee, B., Emmerich, M., Yonekura, Y., Brodie, J., Kircheff, I.I., and Wolfe, A.P. Positron emission tomographic studies of aging and Alzheimer disease. *American Journal of Neuroradiology*, 1983, 4:568.

Demuth, G.W., and Rand, B.S. Atypical major depression in a patient with severe primary degenerative dementia. *American Journal of Psychiatry*, 1980, 137:1609.

Desmedt, J.E., and Cheron, G. Somatosensory evoked potentials to finger stimulation in healthy octogenarians and in young adults: wave forms, scalp topography and transit times of parietal and frontal components. *Electroencephalography and Clinical Neurophysiology*, 1980, 50:404.

Donnelly, E.F., Waldman, I.N., Murphy, D.L., Wyatt, R.J., and Goodwin, F.K. Primary affective disorder: thought disorder in depression. *Journal of Abnormal Psychology*, 1980, 89:315.

Drechsler, F. Quantitative analysis of neurophysiological processes of the aging CNS. *Journal of Neurology.* 1978, 218:197.

Duckworth, G.S., and Ross, H. Diagnostic differences in psychogeriatric patients in Toronto, New York and London, England. *Canadian Medical Association Journal,* 1975, 112:847.

Ellenberg, M. The deep reflexes in old age. *Journal of the American Medical Association,* 1960, 174:463.

English, W.H. Alzheimer's disease: its incidence and recognition. *Psychiatric Quarterly,* 1942, 16:91.

Erickson, R.C. Problems in the clinical assessment of memory. *Experimental Aging Research,* 1978, 4:255.

Erickson, R.C., and Scott, M.L. Clinical memory testing: a review. *Psychological Bulletin,* 1977, 84:1130.

Fahn, S. Differential diagnosis of tremors. *Medical Clinics of North America,* 1972, 56:1363.

Fennel, W.H., and Moore, R.E. Responses of aged men to passive heating. *Journal of Physiology,* (London), 1973, 231:118.

Filskov, S.B., and Boll, T.J. (Eds.), *Handbook of Clinical Neuropsychology.* New York: Wiley, 1981.

Fleiss, J., Gurland, B., and Des Roche, P. Distinctions between organic brain syndrome and functional psychiatric disorders: based on the Geriatric Mental State interview. *International Journal of Aging and Human Development,* 1976, 7:323.

Folstein, S.E., Folstein, M.F., and McHugh, P.R. Psychiatric syndromes in Huntington's disease. In Chase, T.N., Wexler, N.S., and Barbeau, A. (Eds.), *Advances in Neurology. Volume 23: Huntington's Disease.* New York: Raven, 1979, pp. 281–89.

Folstein, M.F., and McHugh, P.R. Dementia syndrome of depression. In Katzman, R., Terry, R.D., and Bick, K.L. (Eds.), *Aging. Volume 7: Alzheimer's Disease: Senile Dementia and Related Disorders.* New York: Raven, 1978, pp. 87–93.

Fox, R.H., Even-Paz, Z., Woodward, P.M., and Jack, J.W. A study of temperature regulation in Yemenite and Kurdish Jews in Israel. *Philosophical Transactions of Royal Society of London,* 1973, 266:149.

Fox, J.H., Kaszniak, A.W., and Huckman, M. Computerized tomographic scanning not very helpful in dementia. *New England Journal of Medicine,* 1979, 300:437.

Fox, R.H., Woodward, P.M., Exton-Smith, A.N., Green, M.F., Donnison, D.V., and Wicks, M.H. Body temperature in the elderly: a national study of physiological, social, and environmental conditions. *British Medical Journal,* 1973, 1:200.

Frackowiak, R.S., Possilli, C., Legg, N.J., DuBoulay, G.H., Marshall, J., Lenzi, G.L., and Jones, T. Regional cerebral oxygen supply and utilization in dementia: a clinical and physiological study with oxygen-15 and positron tomography. *Brain,* 1981, 104:753.

Friedland, R.P., Budinger, T.F., Ganz, E., Yano, Y., Mathis, C.A., Koss, B., Ober, B.A., Huesman, R.H., and Derenzo, S.E. Regional cerebral metabolis alterations in dementia of the Alzheimer type: Positron emission tomography with [^{18}F] fluorodeoxy-glucose. *Journal of Computer Assisted Tomography,* 1983, 7:590.

Fuld, P.A. Psychological testing in the differential diagnosis of the dementias. In Katzman, R., Terry, R.D., and Bick, K.L. (Eds.), *Aging. Volume 7: Alzheimer's Disease: Senile Dementia and Related Disorders*. New York, Raven, 1978, pp. 185–93.

Gibson, A.J. A further analysis of memory loss in dementia and depression in the elderly. *British Journal of Clinical Psychology*, 1981, 20:179.

Gilleard, C.J. Wechsler memory scale performance of elderly psychiatric patients. *Journal of Clinical Psychology*, 1980, 36:958.

Goodin, D.S., Squires, K.C., Henderson, B.H., and Starr, A. Age related variations in evoked potentials to auditory stimuli in normal human subjects. *Electroencephalography and Clinical Neurophysiology*, 1978, 44:447.

Gross, M. Circulatory reflexes in cerebral ischaemia involving different vascular territories. *Clinical Sciences*, 1970, 38:491.

Gurland, B., Golden, R., and Challop, J. Unidimensional and multidimensional approaches to the differentiation of depression and dementia in the elderly. In Corkin, S., Davis, K.L. Usdin, E., and Wurtman, R.L. (Eds.), *Aging. Volume 19: Alzheimer's Disease: A Report of Progress*. New York, Raven, 1982, pp. 119–25.

Gurland, B., and Toner, J. Differentiating dementia from nondementing conditions. In Mayeux, R., and Rosen, W.G. (Eds.), *The Dementias*. New York: Raven, 1983, pp. 1–17.

Gustafson, L., Risberg, J., and Silfverskjold, P. Cerebral blood flow in dementia and depression. *Lancet*, 1981, 31:275.

Haaland, K.Y., Linn, R.T., Hunt, W.C., and Goodwin, J.S. A normative study of Russell's variant of the Wechsler Memory Scale in a healthy elderly population. *Journal of Consulting and Clinical Psychology*, 1983, 51:878.

Hachinski, V.C., Iliff, L.D., Du Boulay, G.H., McAllister, V.L., Marshall, J., Russell, R.W., and Symon, L. Cerebral blood flow in dementia. *Archives of Neurology*, 1975, 32:632.

Hall, R.C.W., Popkin, M.K., Devaul, R.A., Faillace, L.A., and Stickney, S.K. Physical illness presenting as psychiatric disease. *Archives of General Psychiatry*, 1978, 35:1315.

Hartley, J.T., Harker, J.O., and Walsh, D.A. Contemporary issues and new directions in adult development of learning and memory. In Poon, L.W. (Ed.). *Aging in the 1980s: Psychological Issues*. Washington, D.C.: American Psychological Association, 1980, pp. 239–52.

Hasher, L., and Zacks, R.T. Automatic and effortful processes in memory. *Journal of Experimental Psychology: General*, 1979, 108:356.

Heilman, K.M., and Valenstein, E. (Eds.). *Clinical Neuropsychology*. New York: Oxford University Press, 1979.

Hendrickson, E., Raymond, L., and Post, F. Averaged evoked responses in relation to cognitive and affective state of elderly psychiatric patients. *British Journal of Psychiatry*, 1979, 134:494.

Hilbert, N.M., Niederehe, G., and Kahn, R.L. Accuracy and speed of memory in depressed and organic aged. *Educational Gerontology*, 1976, 1:131.

Howell, T.H. Senile deterioration of the central nervous system. *British Medical Journal*, 1949, 1:56.

Hughes, J.R., and Cayaffa, J.J. The EEG in patients at different ages without organic cerebral disease. *Electroencephalography and Clinical Neurophysiology*, 1977, 42:776.

Huntington, G. On chorea. *Medical and Surgical Reports*, 1972, 26:317.

Jackson, J.A., Free, G.B.M., and Pike, H.V. The psychic manifestation in paralysis agitans. *Archives of Neurology and Psychiatry*, 1923, 10:680.

Jacoby, R. Dementia, depression and the CT scan. *Psychological Medicine*, 1981, 11:673.

Jacoby, R.J., Levy, R., and Dawson, J.M. Computed tomography in the elderly. I: The normal population. *British Journal of Psychiatry*, 1980, 136:249.

James, A.E., Partain, C.L., Holland, G.N., Gore, J.C., Rollo, F.D., Harms, S.E., and Price, R.R. Nuclear magnetic resonance imaging: the current state. *American Journal of Radiology* 1981, 138:201.

Janowsky, D.S. Pseudodementia in the elderly: differential diagnosis and treatment. *Journal of Clinical Psychiatry*, 1982, 43:19.

Johannesson, G., Hagberg, B., Gustafson, L., and Ingvar, D.H. EEG and cognitive impairment in presenile dementia. *Acta Neurologica Scandinavica*, 1979, 59:225.

Kahn, R.L., Zarit, S.H., Hilbert, N.M., and Niederehe, G. Memory complaint and impairment in the aged. *Archives of General Psychiatry*, 1975, 32:1569.

Kaszniak, A.W. The neuropsychology of dementia. In Grant, I., and Adams, K. (Eds.), *Neuropsychological Assessment of Neuropsychiatric Disorders*. New York: Oxford University Press, 1985.

Kaszniak, A.W., Fox, J.H., Gandell, D.L., Garron, D.C., Huckman, M.S., and Ramsey, R.G. Predictors of mortality in presenile and senile dementia. *Annals of Neurology*, 1978, 3:246.

Kaszniak, A.W., Garron, D.C., Fox, J.H., Bergin, D., and Huckman, M.S. Cerebral atrophy, EEG slowing, age, education, and cognitive functioning in suspected dementia. *Neurology*, 1979, 29:1273.

Kaszniak, A.W., Wilson, R.S., Lazarus, L., Lessor, J., and Fox, J.H. Memory and depression in dementia. Paper presented at the Ninth Annual Meeting of the International Neuropsychological Society, Atlanta, Ga., February 1981.

Katzman, R., and Terry, R. Normal aging of the nervous system. In Katzman, R., and Terry, R. (Eds.), *The Neurology of Aging*. Philadelphia: F.A. Davis, 1983, pp. 15–50.

Kendrick, D.C., and Post, F. Differences in cognitive status between healthy, psychiatrically ill, and diffusely brain-damaged elderly subjects. *British Journal of Psychiatry*, 1967, 113:75.

Kiloh, L.G. Pseudo-dementia. *Acta Psychiatrica Scandinavica*, 1961, 37:336.

Kini, M.M., Leibowitz, H.M., Colton, T., Nickerson, R.J., Ganley, J., and Dawber, T.R. Prevalence of senile cataracts, diabetic retinopathy, senile macular degeneration, and open angle glaucoma in the Framingham Eye Study. *American Journal of Ophthalmology*, 1978, 85:28.

Klawans, H.L., Tufo, H.M., Ostfeld, A.M., Shekelle, R.B., and Kilbridge, J.A. Neurologic examination in an elderly population. *Diseases of the Nervous System*, 1971, 32:274.

Klisz, D. Neuropsychological evaluation in older persons. In Storandt, M., Siegler, I.C., and Elias, M.F. (Eds.), *The Clinical Psychology of Aging*. New York: Plenum, 1978, pp. 71–96.

Koller, W.C., Glatt, S., Wilson, R.S., and Fox, J.H. Primitive reflexes and cognitive function in the elderly. *Annals of Neurology*, 1982, 12:302.

Kummick, L.S. Pupillary psychosensory restitution and aging. *Journal of the Optical Society of America*, 1959, 44:735.

Larner, S. Encoding in senile dementia and elderly depressives: a preliminary study. *British Journal of the Social and Clinical Psychology*, 1977, 16:379.

Levy, R., Isaacs, A., and Behrman, J. Neurophysiological correlates of senile dementia. II: The somatosensory evoked response. *Psychological Medicine*, 1971, 1:159.

Lezak, M.D. *Neuropsychological Assessment*, 2nd. ed. New York: Oxford University Press, 1983.

Maletta, G.J., Pirozzolo, F.J., Thompson, G., and Mortimer, J.A. Organic mental disorders in a geriatric outpatient population. *American Journal of Psychiatry*, 1982, 139:521.

Marsh, G.G., and Markham, C.H. Does levodopa alter depression and psychopathology in Parkinsonism patients? *Journal of Neurology, Neurosurgery, and Psychiatry*, 1973, 36:925.

Mayeux, R. Depression and dementia in Parkinson's disease. In Marsden, C.D., and Fahn, S. (Eds.), *Movement Disorders*. London: Butterworth, 1982, pp. 75–95.

Mazziotta, J.C., Phelps, M.E., Carson, R.E., and Kuhl, D.E. Tomographic mapping of human cerebral metabolism: auditory stimulation. *Neurology*, 1982, 32:921.

McAllister, T.W. Cognitive functioning in the affective disorders. *Comprehensive Psychiatry*, 1981, 22:572.

McAllister, T.W. Overview: pseudodementia. *American Journal of Psychiatry*, 1983, 140:528.

McAllister, T.W., Ferrell, R.B., Price, T.R., and Neville, M.B. The dexamethasone suppression test in two patients with severe depressive pseudodementia. *American Journal of Psychiatry*, 1982, 139:479.

McAllister, T.W., and Price, T.R.P. Severe depressive pseudodementia with and without dementia. *American Journal of Psychiatry*, 1982, 139:626.

McCarty, S.M., Siegler, I.C., and Logue, P.E. Cross-sectional and longitudinal patterns of three Wechsler Memory Scale subtests. *Journal of Gerontology*, 1982, 37:169.

McGeer, P.L., McGeer, E.G., and Susuki, J.S. Aging and extrapyramidal function. *Archives of Neurology*, 1977, 34:33.

McHugh, P.R., and Folstein, M.F. Psychiatric syndromes of Huntington's chorea: a clinical and phenomenologic study. In Benson, D.F., and Blumer, D. (Eds.), *Psychiatric Aspects of Neurological Diseases*. New York: Grune & Stratton, 1975, 267–286.

Miller, E. *Abnormal Ageing*. London: Wiley, 1977.

Miller, E. The differential psychological evaluation. In Miller, N.E., and Cohen, G.D. (Eds.), *Clinical Aspects of Alzheimer's Disease and Senile Dementia*. New York, Raven, 1981, pp. 121–38.

Miller, E., and Lewis, P. Recognition memory in elderly patients with depression and dementia: a signal detection analysis. *Journal of Abnormal Psychology*, 1977, 86:84.

Miller, N.E. The measurement of mood in senile brain disease: examiner ratings and self-reports. In Cole, J.O., and Barrett, J.E. (Eds.), *Psychopathology in the Aged*. New York: Raven Press, 1980, pp. 97–122.

Miller, W.R. Psychological deficit in depression. *Psychological Bulletin*, 1975, 82:238.

Morstyn, R., Hachanadel, G., Kaplan, E., and Gutheil, T.G. Depression vs. pseudodepression in dementia. *Journal of Clinical Psychiatry*, 1982, 43:197.

Muller, H.F., and Schwartz, G. Electroencephalograms and autopsy findings in geropsychiatry. *Journal of Gerontology*, 1978, 33:504.

Murray, M.P., Kory, R.C., and Clarkson, B.H. Walking patterns in healthy old men. *Journal of Gerontology*, 1969, 24:164.

Naeser, M.A., Gebhardt, C., and Levine, H.L. Decreased computerized tomography numbers in patients with presenile dementia: detection in patients with otherwise normal scans. *Archives of Neurology*, 1980, 37:401.

Nelson, F.L., and Farberow, N.L. Indirect self-destructive behavior in the elderly nursing home patient. *Journal of Gerontology*, 1980, 35:949.

O'Connor, K.P., Shaw, J.C., and Ongley, C.O. The EEG and differential diagnosis is psychogeriatrics. *British Journal of Psychiatry*, 1979, 135:156.

Patrick, H.T., and Levy, D.M. Parkinson disease: a clinical study of one hundred and forty-six cases. *Archives of Neurology and Psychiatry*, 1922, 7:711.

Pearson, J.S. Behavioral aspects of Huntington's chorea. In Barbeau, A., Chase, T.M., and Paulson, G.W. (Eds.), *Advances in Neurology. Volume I: Huntington's Chorea*. New York: Raven, 1973, pp. 701–12.

Pfeffer, R.I. Degenerative neurologic disease: Alzheimer's disease, senile dementia of the Alzheimer's type, and related disorders. In Holland, D. (Ed.), *Textbook of Public Health*. New York: Oxford University Press, 1984.

Pfefferbaum, A. Event-related potentials in the diagnosis of dementia. Paper presented at the Talland Memorial Conference on Clinical Memory Assessment of Older Adults, Boston, October 1983.

Pfefferbaum, A., Ford, J.M., Wenegrat, B., Tinklenberg, J.R., and Kapell, B.S. Electrophysiological approaches to the study of aging and dementia. In Corkin, S., et al. (Eds.), *Aging. Volume 19: Alzheimer's Disease: A Report of Progress*. New York: Raven, 1982, pp. 83–91.

Pfeiffer, E. Psychopathology and social pathology. In Birren, J.E., and Schaie, K.W. (Eds.), *Handbook of the Psychology of Aging*. New York: Van Nostrand-Reinhold, 1977, pp. 650–71.

Post, F. *The Significance of Affective Symptoms in Old Age*. London: Oxford University Press, 1962.

Post, F. Dementia, depression, and pseudodementia. In Benson, D.F., and Blumer, D. (Eds.), *Psychiatric Aspects of Neurologic Disease*. New York: Grune & Stratton, 1975, pp. 99–120.

Potvin, A.R., Syndulko, T., Tourtellotte, W.W., Lemmon, J.A., and Potvin, J.H. Human neurologic function and the aging process. *Journal of the Geriatric Society.*, 1980, 28:1.

Power, D.G., Logue, P.E., McCarty, S.M., Rosenstiel, A.K., and Ziesat, H.A. Inter-rater reliability of the Russell Revision of the Wechsler Memory Scale: an attempt to clarify some ambiguities in scoring. *Journal of Clinical Neuropsychology.*, 1979, 1:343.

Prakash, C., and Stern, G. Neurological signs in the elderly. *Age and Ageing*, 1973, 2:24.

Price, L.J., Fein, G., and Feinberg, I. Neuropsychological assessment of cognitive function in the elderly. In Poon, L.W. (Ed.), *Aging in the 1980s: Psychological Issues*. Washington, D.C.: American Psychological Association, 1980, pp. 78–85.

Reifler, B.V., Larson, E., and Hanley, R. Coexistence of cognitive impairment and depression in geriatric outpatients. *American Journal of Psychiatry*, 1982, 139:623.

Rosen, W.G., Terry, R.D., Fuld, P.A., Katzman, R., and Peck, A. Pathological verification of ischemic score in differentiation of dementias. *Annals of Neurology*, 1980, 7:486.

Roth, M. The natural history of mental disorders arising in the senium. *Journal of Mental Science*, 1955, 101:281.

Roth, M. Mental health problems of aging and the aged. *Bulletin of the World Health Organization*, 1959, 21:257.

Roth, M. Senile dementia and its borderlands. In Cole, J.O., and Barrett, J.E. (Eds.), *Psychopathology in the Aged*. New York: Raven, 1980, pp. 205–32.

Roth, M., and Hopkins, B. Psychological test performance in patients over 60. I: Senile psychosis and the affective disorders of old age. *Journal of Mental Science*, 1953, 99:439.

Russell, E.W. A multiple-scoring method for the assessment of complex memory functions. *Journal of Consulting and Clinical Psychology*, 1975, 43:800.

Schwab, R.S., and England, A.C. Parkinson's disease. *Journal of Chronic Diseases*, 1958, 8:488.

Sharpe, J.A., and Sylvester, T.O. Effect of aging on horizontal smooth pursuit. *Investigations in Ophthalmology and Visual Science*, 1978, 17:465.

Spar, J.E., and Gerner, R.H. Does the dexamethasone suppression test distinguish dementia from depression? *American Journal of Psychiatry*, 1982, 139:238.

Squires, K.C., Chippendale, T.J., Wrege, K.S., Goodin, D.S., and Starr, A. Electrophysiological assessment of mental function in aging and dementia. In Poon, L.W. (Ed.), *Aging in the 1980s: Psychological Issues*. Washington, D.C.: American Psychological Association, 1980, pp. 125–134.

Sternberg, D.E., and Jarvik, M.E. Memory function in depression. *Archives of General Psychiatry*, 1976, 33:219.

Stromgren, L.S. The influence of depression on memory. *Acta Psychiatrica Scandinavica*, 1977, 56:109.

Teravainen, H., and Calne, D.B. Motor system in normal aging and Parkinson's disease. In Katzman, R., and Terry, R. (Eds.), *The Neurology of Aging*. Philadelphia: F.A. Davis, 1983, pp. 85–110.

Terry, R. Senile dementia. *Federation Proceedings*, 1978, 37:2837.

Terry, R.D., and Davies, B. Dementia of the Alzheimer type. *Annual Review of Neurosciences*, 1980, 3:77.

Terry, R., and Katzman, R. Senile dementia of the Alzheimer type: defining a disease. In Katzman, R., and Terry, R. (Eds.), *The Neurology of Aging*. Philadelphia: F.A. Davis, 1983, pp. 51–84.

Tomlinson, B.E. Plaques, tangles and Alzheimer's disease. *Psychological Medicine*, 1982, 12:449.

Tomlinson, B.E., Blessed, G., and Roth, M. Observations on the brain in non-demented old people. *Journal of Neurological Science*, 1968, 7:331.

Tomlinson, B.E., Blessed, G., and Roth, M. Observations on the brains of demented old people. *Journal of Neurological Science*, 1970, 11:205.

Trier, T.R. Characteristics of mentally ill aged: a comparison of patients with psychogenic disorders and patients with organic brain syndromes. *Journal of Gerontology*, 1966, 21:354.

Wechsler, D. A standardized memory scale for clinical use. *Journal of Psychology*, 1945 19:87.

Weingartner, H. Forms of memory impairment: toward the development of a biologic model of cognitive function. Paper presented at the Talland Memorial Conference on Clinical Memory Assessment of Older Adults, Boston, October 1983.

Weingartner, H., Cohen, R.M., Murphy, D.L., Martello, J., and Gerdt, C. Cognitive processes in depression. *Archives of General Psychiatry*, 1981, 38:42.

Wells, C.E. Pseudodementia. *American Journal of Psychiatry*, 1979, 136:895.

Wells, C.E. Pseudodementia and the recognition of organicity. In Benson, D.F., and Blumer, D. (Eds.), *Psychiatric Aspects of Neurologic Disease, Volume II*. New York: Grune and Stratton, 1982, pp. 167–78.

Whitehead, A. The pattern of WAIS performance in elderly psychiatric patients. *British Journal of the Social and Clinical Psychology*, 1973, 12:435.

Wilson, R.S., Fox, J.H., Huckman, M.S., Bacon, L.D., and Lobick, J.J. Computed tomography in dementia. *Neurology*, 1982, 32:1054.

Wilson, R.S., Kaszniak, A.W., Klawans, H.L., and Garron, D.C. High speed memory scanning in Parkinsonism. *Cortex*, 1980, 16:67.

Wright, B.E., and Hendkind, P. Aging changes and the eye. In Katzman, R., and Terry, R. (Eds.), *The Neurology of Aging*. Philadelphia: F.A. Davis, 1983, pp. 149–65.

Yahr, M.D., Duvoisin, R.C., Schear, M.J., Barrett, R.E., and Hoehn, M.M. Treatment of Parkinsonism with levodopa. *Archives of Neurology*, 1969, 21:343.

Yamaura, H., Ito, M., Kubota, K., and Matsuzawa, T. Brain atrophy during aging: a quantitative study with computed tomography. *Journal of Gerontology*, 1980, 35:492.

Intervention

7

Drug Treatment

James E. Spar

Depressive disorders in the elderly are generally responsive to a wide range of therapeutic approaches; some depressed older patients, however, appear to be resistant to treatment unless appropriate psychoactive medications are added to the therapeutic regimen. As older patients are particularly susceptible to side-effects and adverse reactions from drugs, it is important to distinguish patients who are likely to gain from drug treatment from those who are not. Although there are no absolute clinical criteria upon which to base such a decision, a review of the general psychiatric literature provides some useful guidelines.

DRUG TREATMENT GUIDELINES

Patients who exhibit the following cluster of neurovegetative symptoms are more likely to respond to tricyclic antidepressants than those who do not have these somatic symptoms (Bielski and Fridel, 1976): sleep disturbance (particularly early morning awakening); appetite disturbance (particularly if weight loss is present); loss of libido; diurnal (occurring twice in one day) variation of mood (especially if mood is worse in the morning and improves toward evening); constipation; and anhedonia, or inability to experience pleasure from normally pleasurable activities. These symptoms are usually accompanied by psychomotor retardation (slowed behavior) or agitation (purposelessly driven motor behavior) and mood disturbance that is pervasive, persistent, and clearly distinguishable from "normal" depression of mood (i.e., transient "everyday life" depression).

A somewhat different cluster of symptoms, including increased sleep and appetite, high levels of anxiety, and hypochondriasis has been shown in some studies to be preferentially responsive to a different class of antidepressant medication, the monoamine oxidase inhibitors (Robinson et al., 1978). For both syndromes, the presence of hallucinations or delusions can complicate treatment with tricyclic or monoamine oxidase inhibiting medications, and often requires the addition of antipsychotic medications to the antidepressant regimen, or, in the most refractory cases, a switch to electroconvulsive therapy (ECT). Finally, the depressive phase of manic-depressive illness (officially, bipolar affective illness) may respond to lithium carbonate treatment alone or may require the addition of an antidepressant.

The preceding remarks are derived from the literature on adults, but may not, in the long run, turn out to be completely applicable to the elderly. At least three other syndromes that may be conceptualized as "variants" of the depressive syndromes described above also occur in elderly patients and are responsive to tricyclic and monoamine oxidase inhibiting agents or ECT. These syndromes are:

1. Multiple somatic complaints. Physical symptoms such as nausea, headache, abdominal pain, constipation, joint pain, tiredness, and dizziness appear in chronic intermittent clusters that are resistant to usually effective medical intervention. The syndrome is distinguished from hypochondriasis and somatization disorder by its late onset and the presence of neurovegetative features associated with depressive illness.
2. Paranoid psychosis. Many of the neurovegetative features of depressive illness are present, but mood disturbance per se may be absent or overshadowed by persecutory delusions, with or without accompanying hallucinations.
3. Pseudodementia. Features of dementia that are usually associated with organic brain disease are present but are reversible with successful treatment of the underlying depressive illness. Again, neurovegetative features are often present. Pseudodementia is a particularly important syndrome in that, when it is not recognized, appropriate treatment may be withheld and the patient may be inappropriately referred for chronic institutionalization.

THE CONCEPT OF ENDOGENOUS DEPRESSION

Why are depressed patients with neurovegetative symptoms more responsive to antidepressant medications than others? The most widely held view is that neurovegetative signs and symptoms reflect *endogenous* depression—depression that occurs because of a biochemical abnormality in the central nervous system of the afflicted individual. Until recently, endogenous depression was believed to arise "from within," independent of life events, unlike the "reactive" depression that commonly follows stressful or painful life events (for example, the death of a spouse, being fired from an important job, or a major illness). However, this distinction has given way to the common clinical observation that, in fact, endogenous depression often occurs following such life events, and that depression without

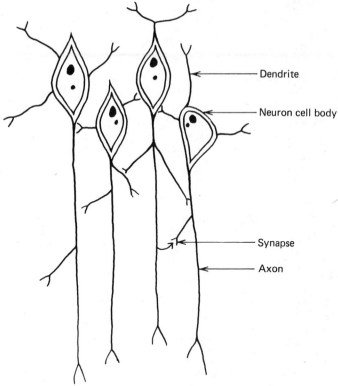

Figure 7.1 Schematic illustration of anatomical organization of neurons in the brain.

endogenous features can occur spontaneously in the absence of traumatic life events, as if "arising from within." The next section reviews current thinking regarding the biochemical abnormalities associated with endogenous depression.

The Biochemical Basis of Mood Regulation

Contemporary theories of mood regulation are primarily concerned with the neurochemistry of synaptic transmission. The relevant concepts may be reviewed with the aid of a few basic propositions and a few schematic illustrations. The central nervous system (the brain and spinal cord) is composed of several billion nerve cells, or neurons, embedded in a gelatinous mass of supporting cells composed mainly of water and fat (Figure 7.1). Each neuron has up to several thousand branches (axons and dendrites), which fan out into the gelatinous mass and come very close to the branches and bodies of other neurons. However, none of these axons, dendrites, or cell bodies makes direct physical contact with

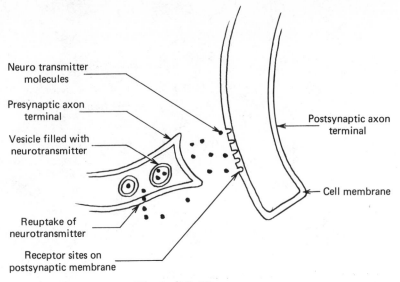

Figure 7.2 The synapse.

the others. Each neuron is therefore physically separate from every other neuron but must communicate with other neurons in order for perception, mood, thought, or behavior to occur. This communication crosses the small spaces between cells and cell branches via a unit called the *synapse* (Figure 7.2). Although nervous impulses are communicated *along* neurons via a wave of electric current, communication *between* neurons occurs only via chemicals (neurotransmitters) that the "sending" (presynaptic) neuron secretes into the synaptic space. Following release from the presynaptic cell, neurotransmitter molecules diffuse across the synaptic space and temporarily bind to specific receptor molecules on the "receiving" (post-synaptic) neuron, initiating a chain of chemical events in the postsynaptic neuron that results in the propogation of the electrical impulse.

Assuming that "mood" is produced by the activity of some group of neurons in the brain, a way to regulate mood would be to regulate the communication between these neurons. How might this regulation be accomplished? To answer this question it will be helpful to review some steps that are known to be involved in synaptic transmission. First, the presynaptic neuron must manufacture the appropriate neurotransmitter. The neurons must absorb the necessary ingredients from the bloodstream and synthesize them into the finished product via a series of intracellular chemical reactions that are dependent upon catalytic enzymes also synthesized by the neuron. Following synthesis, the neurotransmitter is stored within the cell inside membranous capsules, or vesicles. When the electrical impulse reaches the area of the synapse, these vesicles move to the presynaptic cell membrane surface, merge with the cell membrane, and release their neurotransmitter into the synaptic space. The neurotransmitter then diffuses across to the postsynaptic receptor, temporarily attaches, and then is released and degraded by enzymes present in the synaptic space. The neurotransmitter molecules that escape degradation, or in some cases the products of that degradation, are then reabsorbed by the presynaptic neuron. Once inside the presynaptic neuron, they may be further degraded by other enzymes, may be resynthesized into new neurotransmitters, or, if undegraded transmitter is reabsorbed, recapsulized for subsequent re-release. Even in this simplified version of the process, there are several steps where regulation could occur: The rate of absorption of neurotransmitter components; the rate of synthesis of neurotransmitter; the rate of synthesis of catalytic enzymes; the number of vesicles released per impulse; the rate of degradation of neurotransmitter; the rate of re-uptake of neurotransmitter or its components; and the number and sensitivity of postsynaptic receptors could all affect the net amount of neurotransmission per unit time. Although it is not known which of these steps are normally regulated in the functioning brain, it is known that certain pharmacologic agents influence some of these steps and, in so doing, appear to influence mood when administered to experimental subjects, animal or human.

How then do these processes relate to the psychiatric treatment of mood disorders? Consider the following account of mood-generation. The brain receives and integrates information (neuronal impulses) from the senses, checks it against stored information (memory), and assigns it an interpretation, modifies it with other information gathered from internal sensors that monitor body chemistry and position, and routes the final product into several neuronal pathways that ultimately impinge upon neurons that control internal computational and gross motor behavior. The organism's subjective experience of this neuronal activity is "mood." In this very simple scheme, the mood experienced by the individual is a product of perception and interpretation of external and internal events embodied in neurobiochemical processes in the brain. Intervention to influence mood could occur as either external perceived events (psychotherapy) or internal biochemical processes (pharmacotherapy). The following sections of this chapter will be concerned specifically with the latter variety of intervention; the rest of this book is concerned with the former.

How Antidepressant Drugs Work

Almost all of the antidepressant medications in present use are believed to influence mood by directly or indirectly influencing the rate of synthesis, release, re-uptake, degradation, or receptor-site binding of the monoamine neurotransmitters norepinephrine, serotonin, and dopamine, which are believed to be involved in mood-regulating pathways in the brain. The direction of this influence is in all instances toward *increasing* the relative availability of neurotransmitter to the postsynaptic receptor. *Tricyclic antidepressants* block the re-uptake of neurotransmitter by the presynaptic neuron; the *monoamine oxidase inhibitors* retard degradation of neurotransmitter by inactivating the degrading enzyme monoamine oxidase; and the *psychostimulants* stimulate more rapid release of neurotransmitter, and, to some extent, directly stimulate postsynaptic receptors.

Knowledge of these mechanisms of drug action has contributed to several related hypotheses about brain biochemistry in depressive illness. These hypotheses, which can be collectively termed "monoamine deficiency hypotheses," assert that endogenous depression is caused by, or at least associated with, *reduced* neurotransmission (by norepinephrine and/or serotonin) in mood-regulating pathways in the central nervous system. These hypotheses were predominant in biological psychiatry from the mid-1960s until the late 1970s, at which time several challenging lines of observation emerged. These included: 1) Although the effects of tricyclic antidepressants or monoamine oxidase inhibitors on neurotransmitters are known to occur within hours of their administration, most depressed patients treated with these agents experience little or no relief of depression immediately. In fact, most patients require two to three weeks of daily drug ingestion before maximum improvement occurs, even when maximum drug dosage is attained in a week or less. Moreover, this delay cannot be accounted for by the amount of time required to build up a proper level of the drug in the bloodstream, as it is known that maximum levels can be reached in about five days or less. 2) Certain experimental agents, such as iprindole and fluoxitine, do not appear to affect norepinephrine or serotonin, but do appear to be effective antidepressants. 3) Changes in *receptor sites* occur in brain tissue of experimental animals that are administered antidepressant agents, but only if the agents are administered for a week or more. Specifically, the brains of rats that have been administered antidepressant drugs daily for several weeks have reduced density of beta-adrenergic (norepinephrine) receptors compared to untreated rats. This phenomenon, known as "down-regulation," has been observed in response to a range of agents known to be effective for depression, including tricyclic antidepressants, monoamine oxidase inhibitors, and electroconvulsive therapy (Charney et al., 1981). These observations suggest that, following acute administration of antidepressants, neurotransmission is *increased*, resulting in little or no change in symptomatology. Then, after several weeks of overstimulation, postsynaptic receptors down-regulate, resulting in a *reduction* of neurotransmission. Depressed neurotransmission reduces information flow in the brain and, with it, the symptoms of depression.

While definitive interpretation of these and other observations concerning receptors remains to be articulated, it seems certain that the postsynaptic receptor is a promising site for future study and will probably turn out to be of major importance in theories of the action of antidepressant medications.

Antidepressant drugs also affect the brain in other ways. Most interfere with neuronal transmission that takes place via the neurotransmitter acetylcholine and with the action of histamine, a brain substance that may also be neurotransmitter. Although it is possible that antidepressant properties are related to these effects as well, a comprehensive theory based upon these effects has not yet emerged.

DRUGS THAT CAUSE DEPRESSION

If some drugs can influence neurotransmission so as to alleviate depression, may not other drugs work in the opposite way and *produce* depression? The answer to this question is, not surprisingly, affirmative, and it is in fact well documented that chronic ingestion of drugs that reduce the synaptic availability of norepinephrine, such as reserpine and propanolol, is associated with depression. However, many other drugs, with mechanisms of action not clearly related to norepinephrine or serotonin, have also been associated with depression. Table 7.1 lists these agents, most of which can have several types of association with mood disturbance:

1. After chronic ingestion (several weeks of daily or near daily ingestion at normal dosages), the patient may develop a full neurovegetative depressive syndrome that *does not remit* when the drug is stopped. This pattern, which seems to occur more often in people with a family or personal history of depressive illness, can be conceptualized as *drug-induced* depression.
2. During chronic ingestion, a depressive syndrome of minor or major proportion, as above, may occur that *improves or remits entirely* when the offending agent is discontinued. This reaction is labeled as *drug-dependent* depression.
3. A depressive syndrome of minor to major proportions may follow the discontinuation of a chronically ingested medication. This is a particularly important syndrome in people who abuse psychostimulant medications such as amphetamine and cocaine. This pattern is known as *drug-withdrawal* depression.
4. Finally, and perhaps most common, is occurrence of lethargy, tiredness, irritability, and/or sleep disturbance in association with chronic medication ingestion. However, in this pattern, an actual *mood* disturbance (i.e., pervasive and prominent depression) may not be present. This pattern may be thought of as *drug-simulated depression.*

These four types of drug-related mood-disturbance may occur in any person in various combinations at various times. A drug regimen that was

TABLE 7.1

DRUGS THAT CAN CAUSE DEPRESSION

Analgesics
All narcotic analgesics, including synthetics; e.g., codeine, morphine, meperidine (Demerol), pentazocine (Talwin)
ibuprofen (Motrin)
indomethacin (Indocin)
naproxen (Naprosyn)
zompirac sodium (Zomax)

Anti-Anxiety Agents (Minor Tranquilizers)
All benzodiazapines; e.g., diazepam (Valium), chlordiazepoxide (Librium), lorazepam (Ativan), oxazepam (Serax)
meprobamate (Miltown)
alcohol

Antihypertensive Agents
alpha-methyl dopa (Aldomet)
clonidine (Catapres)
guanethidine (Ismelin)
propanalol (Inderal)
reserpine (various trade names)

Antipsychotic Agents (Major Tranquilizers)
All, including chlorpromazine (Thorazine), haloperidol (Haldol), thiothixine (Navane), fluphenazine (Prolixin), thioridazine (Mellaril), molindone (Moban)

Cancer Chemotherapeutic Agents

L-asparaginase	DTIC
vincristine	actinomycin D
procarbazine	nitrogen mustard
hexamethylenamine	Ftorafur
o,p–DDD	cis-platinum
tamoxifen	

Sedative—Hypnotics
benzodiazapine hypnotics; e.g., flurazepam (Dalmane), triazolam (Halcyon), temazepam (Restoril)
barbiturate hypnotics
    phenobarbital (various trade names)
    pentobarbital (Nembutal)
    secobarbital (Seconal)
    amybarbital (Amytal)
other hypnotics
    methyprylon (Noludar)
    ethchlorvynol (Placidyl)
    glutethimide (Doriden)
    methaquaalone (Quaalude)

Miscellaneous
cimitidine (Tagamet)
oral contraceptives
steroids; e.g., dexamethasone (Decadron), prednisone

tolerated well until last week may this week, for poorly understood reasons, produce depression. Accordingly, the physician should take a very careful drug history from all depressed patients. If the patient is regularly taking any of the agents listed in Table 7.1 the physician should, if possible, reduce the dosage or consider replacement with alternatives *before* initiating specific treatment for depression. Unfortunately, many of the listed agents are useful and appropriate for specific conditions and for specific patients and cannot always be replaced.

DRUGS THAT ALLEVIATE DEPRESSION

The major categories of agents that alleviate depression include 1) tricyclic antidepressants, 2) monoamine oxidase inhibitors, 3) psychostimulants, 4) lithium, and 5) the "second-generation" antidepressants. There are also other psychoactive agents that are *not* specific antidepressants but are sometimes useful as adjuncts to specific antidepressant treatment. These include minor tranquilizers, major tranquilizers, and sedative-hypnotics. The following section will review the basic clinical pharmacology of these agents and will discuss, where appropriate, special considerations that pertain when these agents are prescribed for elderly patients.

Tricyclic Antidepressants

These agents have been the mainstay of pharmacologic treatment for depression since their introduction in the mid-1950s. Although they are all structurally similar, there are some differences in their antidepressant potency and their profile of side-effects. Table 7.2 lists the tricyclics presently available in the United States. One subcategorization of the tricyclic antidepressants is based upon their relative potency in blocking presynaptic neuronal re-uptake of serotonin and norepinephrine. In general, the *tertiary* tricyclics, such as amitriptyline, imipramine, and doxepin, are effective in blocking serotonin and norepinephrine re-uptake, while the *secondary* tricyclics, including desipramine and nortriptyline, only block the re-uptake of norepinephrine.* This distinction may be important, as there is some evidence for the occurrence of biochemical subtypes of depression that are differentially responsive to the effects of tertiary and secondary tricyclics (Maas, 1975). However, since research in this area is not yet conclusive, currently, the choice of one tricyclic over another is usually based upon the pattern of side effects rather than efficacy.

---

* Tertiary and secondary refer to the number of methyl groups that are attached to the terminal carbon atom in the side chain of the antidepressants molecule. Molecules with three methyl groups are called tertiary antidepressants, and those with two methyl groups are called secondary antidepressants.

TABLE 7.2
ANTIDEPRESSANTS AVAILABLE IN UNITED STATES

Trade Name	Generic Name	Relative Potency	
		Anticholinergic	Sedative
Tricyclic Antidepressants			
Aventyl	nortriptyline	Low	Low
Elavil	amitriptyline	High	High
Norpramine	desipramine	Low	Low
Sinequan	doxepin	High	High
Surmontil	trimipramine	Medium	Medium
Tofranil	imipramine	Medium	Medium
Vivactyl	protriptyline	Low	Low
Monoamine Oxidase Inhibitors			
Marplan	isocarboxazid	Low	Low
Nardil	phenelzine	Low	Low
Parnate	tranylcypromine	Low	Low
Psychostimulants			
Benzedrine	amphetamine	Low	Low
None	cocaine hydrochloride	Low	Low
Dexedrine	dextroamphetamine	Low	Low
Desoxyn	methamphetamine	Low	Low
Ritalin	methylphenidate	Low	Low
Metrazol	pentylenetetrazol	Low	Low
Cylert	sodium pemoline	Low	Low
Second-generation Antidepressants			
Asendin	amoxapine	Low	Low
Ludiomil	maprotiline	Low	Low
Sernyl	trazodone	Low	High

All of the tricyclic antidepressants can produce, in varying degrees, the following side-effects: sedation, postural hypotension (a drop in blood pressure when arising from a lying or sitting position that may be accompanied by dizziness or lightheadedness), and *anticholinergic symptoms* (symptoms that result from the blockade of postsynaptic receptor binding of acetylcholine) including dry mouth, blurry vision, constipation, difficulty urinating, increased heart rate, worsening of certain types of glaucoma, and mental confusion, the latter particularly in patients with Alzheimer's type dementia. In addition, some tricyclics can slow the rate of electrical conduction of the heart. Therefore, pretreatment screening electrocardiograms are recommended for elderly patients, especially those who have pre-existing heart disease. Those patients experiencing Alzheimer's disease, urinary retention, constipation, or postural hypotension are also at relatively higher risk and should be followed very closely when treated with these agents.

The appropriate *dosage* varies among tricyclics and among individuals; in general, the higher the dose, the greater the likelihood of a favorable response, with the practical dosage limit usually determined by the patient's tolerance of side-effects. Dosages should be gradually increased (i.e., raised by 25 mg every two to five days as tolerated) until clinical response occurs or the highest *comfortable* dosage is attained. The average dosage required by elderly patients is between 125 and 150 mg per day, for most tricyclics. Dosages required with doxepin may be somewhat higher, and of protriptyline significantly lower. Tricyclics may be administered in divided doses or at bedtime in a single dose. The peak response to tricyclic antidepressant medications may require three to four weeks *at maximum dosage* to develop; as it may require one to two weeks to reach maximum dosage, the depressed older individual should anticipate that maximum relief may be six or more weeks away from the onset of therapy. Table 7.2 presents the relative cholinergic and sedative side-effect potency of the tricyclics.

Monoamine Oxidase Inhibitors

These agents are effective antidepressants that work by inhibiting the activity of the enzyme monoamine oxidase, an enzyme responsible for the degradation of serotonin and norepinephrine. Those available in the United States are listed in Table 7.2. There are no clinically important subtypes.

Monoamine oxidase inhibitors (MAOIs) do not impair cardiac conduction, but they can cause postural hypotension and may have weak anticholinergic effects. Their most important side-effect is potentiation of the effects of stimulant-type drugs, ingestion of which by people taking MAOIs can produce dangerous elevations of blood pressure. Even certain foods rich in the amino acid tyramine, which is a precursor for (ingredient in the synthesis of) norepinephrine and dopamine, can cause hypertensive crisis in people taking monoamine oxidase inhibitors. Consequently, absolute avoidance of certain medications and a measure of dietary control is required to safely prescribe these agents. Table 7.3 lists some of the stimulant-type drugs and tyramine-containing foods that must be avoided by patients taking MAOI's. Otherwise, patient management is similar to that recommended for the tricyclics; dosages are gradually increased until maximum comfortable dosage is reached, with response anticipated in the same three to four-week range. As mentioned earlier, there is some evidence that people with atypical neurovegetative depression, with hypersomnia rather than insomnia, weight gain rather than weight loss, and high levels of anxiety and hypochondriasis, may be preferentially responsive to these agents. Of course, elderly patients who cannot be relied upon to follow the medical and dietary restrictions should not be treated with these agents.

TABLE 7.3

DRUGS AND FOODS THAT CAN CAUSE HYPERTENSIVE CRISIS IN PATIENTS
TAKING MONOAMINE OXIDASE INHIBITORS

Category Drugs	Comments
Anti-Parkinson Agents	
L-dopa (Larodopa, Sinemet)	
amantadine (Symmetrel)	
Bronchodilators	
epinephrine (Adrenalin, various trade names)	
isoproterenol (Isuprel, other trade names)	
metaproterenol (Alupent)	
terbutaline (Brethine)	
Decongestants	All found alone and in combination in
pseudoephedrine	various cold and allergy remedies, including
phenylephrine	nasal sprays and drops, syrups, pills,
Neo-Synephrine	capsules.
ephedrine	
phenethylamine	
phenylpropanolamine	
Psychostimulants (all, see Table 7.2)	
diethylpropion hydrochloride (Tenuate)	
Foods	These foods are high in tyramine and should
	be avoided in every case. Individual
Aged cheese	medical consultation should be sought
Aged wine	about other restrictions of foods that contain
Pickled foods	tyramine in lesser amounts.

Psychostimulants

This category of medication includes the amphetamines, cocaine, penty-
lenetetrazol, and methylphenidate, all of which are capable of producing
transient elevation of mood in normal individuals as well as depressives.
Because of this property, which is not shared by the other agents considered
in this chapter, these agents have all been associated with illegitimate use
and abuse, and have consequently been relatively neglected by mainstream
clinical psychopharmacologic researchers in the past several decades.
Psychostimulants are known to curb appetite and interfere with sleep and
can cause increased heart rate and blood pressure. Paranoid reactions,
including psychosis, have been observed following chronic high-dose
ingestion. Of the available psychostimulants, methylphenidate appears to
produce the fewest of these side-effects and is safest for elderly patients.
Although comparative trials (most of which were conducted in the late
1950s and early 1960s) have shown methylphenidate to be generally
inferior to tricyclic antidepressants for long-term treatment of depression,
the relative intolerance of some older patients for the side-effects of first-

line agents (i.e., tricyclic antidepressant, MAOIs), has focused more attention on the psychostimulants, and several authors have proposed a significant, if limited role for these agents in depressed geriatric patients (Katon and Raskind, 1980). Approximately two-thirds of depressed elderly patients sustain transient mood elevation from a single test dose of methylphenidate, and an unknown (but apparently small) proportion of these "acute responders" to methylphenidate will continue to respond if treatment is continued for weeks or months. Dosages of up to 45 mg a day, in divided doses timed to avoid interfering with meals or bedtime, are well tolerated and produce little to no cardiovascular side-effects.

Lithium Salts

Lithium is unique among the agents considered herein in that it is not a large, complex organic molecule but a simple salt, found in abundance in nature; mined, not manufactured. Its mode of action at the biochemical level is still not well understood, nor is its range of usefulness, although it is believed to be primarily effective in preventing the mood swings in bipolar affective (manic-depressive) illness, and secondarily as an acute treatment for mania or hypomania. Some studies suggest that it may also be effective for acute treatment or prophylaxis of depression in patients who have never had a hypomanic or manic episode, particularly if a family history of lithium-responsive mood disorder is present. Several recent reports demonstrate, that some depressed individuals who are unresponsive to tricyclic antidepressants may become responsive if lithium is *added* to the tricyclic regimen (De Montigny et al., 1981). The combination of lithium and a tricyclic antidepressant is also appropriate for treatment of depression in individuals with known bipolar disorder, in whom antidepressants alone may precipitate a swing into hypomania or mania. The daily dosage of lithium varies from person to person, but is usually determined by starting low (e.g., 300 mg three times a day), determining the patient's blood lithium level after four to five days, and then adjusting the dose to achieve a final blood level of between 0.8 mEq/l (milliequivalent per liter) and 1.2 mEq/l (for acute treatment) or between 0.4 mEq/l and 0.8 mEq/l (chronic prophylaxis). Similar dosages are appropriate when lithium and tricyclic antidepressants or lithium and monoamine oxidase inhibitors are prescribed in combination.

The kidney treats lithium as if it were sodium; therefore, any circumstances wherein total body sodium is reduced will cause the kidney to conserve sodium *and* lithium. As kidney excretion is the main route of elimination of lithium from the body, this conservation can rapidly lead to dangerous elevations of lithium and possible lithium toxicity. Therefore, patients must be cautioned against the use of diuretics (water pills), low-sodium diets, and situations of excessive perspiration. However, many older persons require diuretics as part of a medical regimen for control of hypertension or congestive heart failure; in these patients, lithium can be used safely if it is added to a diuretic regimen that is stable and remains so.

The side-effects of therapeutic dosages of lithium include nausea, fine tremor, and increased frequency and volume of urination. Following chronic ingestion of lithium, reversible hypothyroidism has been reported, as has microscopic kidney damage, the clinical significance of which is still under debate. Lithium toxicity, which may occur at as little as double therapeutic levels, is heralded by vomiting, disorientation and confusion, and lack of motor coordination, and may proceed to lethargy, stupor, coma, and, if untreated, death. Although it is common practice to monitor circulating levels of lithium by periodic examination of blood lithium levels, the level at which any individual may become toxic is quite variable. Therefore, blood tests cannot replace careful clinical observation of the patient as levels are raised.

In general, principles of lithium therapy are similar for older and younger patients, with the caveat that the older adult may require considerably smaller dosages to achieve therapeutic response as well as for the development of toxicity.

Second-Generation Antidepressants

In the past decade, several new pharmacologic agents with clinical efficacy in the treatment of depression have become available. These compounds are often referred to as "second-generation" antidepressants, as they are the first pharmacologically distinct antidepressants that have emerged since the tricyclics, monoamine oxidase inhibitors, and psychostimulants ("first-generation" antidepressants) were introduced in the 1950s. Although these compounds are not tricyclics, monoamine oxidase inhibitors, or psychostimulants, they have effects on synaptic availability of norepinephrine or serotonin, and are associated with the same side-effects and adverse reactions attributed to the first-generation compounds. In general, the second-generation drugs are of comparable antidepressant efficacy, both among themselves and relative to the older agents, with their main advantage being that they are claimed to have significantly fewer and less intense side-effects than the older agents. However, these claims are generally difficult to evaluate at this stage in their development, and studies in special populations, including the elderly, are few. The three second-generation antidepressants currently available in the United States are described below.

AMOXAPINE (ASCENDIN).　This agent is a derivative of a potent antipsychotic agent, loxapine, some of the pharmacologic properties of which it retains. Side-effects include most of those produced by tricyclic agents and effects on extrapyramidal structures of the central nervous system, which can produce a Parkinsonian syndrome, including difficulty initiating voluntary movement, muscular rigidity, tremor, and gait disturbance. Although definitive studies of amoxapine in the elderly are unavailable, the relatively high, age-related incidence of symptoms of Parkinson's disease in the untreated elderly suggests that this agent may be particularly unsuited for use in geriatric psychiatry until and unless some specific advantages are discovered.

MAPROTILINE (LUDIOMIL). This compound is similar to the secondary tricyclic agents in that it affects primarily norepinephrine re-uptake, and it has a similar profile of side-effects. There are no documented advantages to its use in the elderly, and a recent report from Great Britain indicates that maprotiline may be associated with a higher risk of grand mal seizures than most, if not all, of the alternative antidepressant agents. Until more data is available to resolve this issue, it seems advisable to reserve the use of maprotiline for patients who have not responded to other agents.

TRAZODONE (DESYREL). The only pure serotonin-reuptake blocker currently available, trazodone is the most promising of the second-generation agents for use in the depressed older patient. It is relatively free of anticholinergic effects and appears to have relatively lower cardiac toxicity than tricyclic antidepressants. Its major side-effect is sedation, which may be a problem in that its relatively short duration of action requires twice a day dosage. Postural hypotension and nausea have been observed in older individuals on trazodone and a few recent cases of priapism (prolonged or painful erection) have been reported. Otherwise, it is well tolerated and may turn out to be the treatment of first choice for the elderly depressive. At least one well-conducted clinical trial in elderly outpatients has shown trazodone to be as effective as imipramine and to produce significantly fewer side-effects (Gerner et al., 1980).

Electroconvulsive Therapy

This nonpharmacologic therapy, mentioned here only for the sake of completeness, remains the most effective and probably the safest treatment for the seriously depressed older patient. In this approach, an instantaneous electric current is used to induce a grand mal seizure in a patient who is anesthetized and partially paralyzed. Electroconvulsive therapy (ECT) has enjoyed a recent resurgence of interest in the psychiatric community, particularly among geriatric psychiatrists, for although antidepressant drugs are clearly effective when they can be tolerated, an alarmingly high proportion of elderly individuals cannot or will not suffer their side-effects in order to overcome a depressive episode. For these individuals, electroconvulsive treatment offers a high likelihood of cure in two to four weeks of three treatments a week.

Side-effects of ECT are usually limited to a few hours of mild confusion following each treatment, although in some cases more prolonged memory disturbance may develop during the course of treatment and persist for several months. These effects can be avoided by using unilateral, nondominant electrode placement (i.e., passing the current through the nondominant hemisphere of the brain only) and, in any case, are rarely of serious concern for patients or families. ECT is otherwise extremely safe; available mortality estimates suggest that ECT per se adds no additional risk of mortality to that associated with general anesthesia alone and does not cause sedation, orthostatic hypotension, anticholinergic effects, slowing of cardiac conduction, hypertensive crisis, or any of the other troublesome or dangerous side-effects of antidepressant medications. Nonetheless, ECT is expensive and requires special equipment and trained staff, and cannot be considered a routine first-line treatment at this time. The use of ECT should be restricted to patients in the following categories: 1) actively suicidal or homicidal; 2) unresponsive to other treatment, or 3) unacceptably high likelihood (or past history) of intolerance of side-effects of antidepressant medications.

Unfortunately, ECT has suffered the ill consequences of several generations of bad publicity, some well deserved, and remains controversial despite its clear efficacy and safety. Several comprehensive references are given at the end of the chapter (Fink, 1979; Weiner, 1979).

Other Psychoactive Drugs

Major tranquilizers (listed in Table 7.1), minor tranquilizers, and hypnotics are often prescribed for depressed patients. As these agents are *not* antidepressants, it is rarely appropriate to prescribe them as sole treatment, but they may be of value as adjuncts to antidepressant therapy. Major tranquilizers are primarily useful for control of hallucinations and delusions, in which situation they should be administered in doses sufficient to restore the patient's contact with reality before specific antidepressant agents are added. This sequence is important, because administration of an antidepressant alone to a psychotically depressed patient may lead to worsening of the psychosis, even as mood improves. High-potency, low-dose major tranquilizers are recommended for older patients, who are likely to be extremely sensitive to the anticholinergic side-effects of the lower potency agents. Major tranquilizers do not have a role in the psychopharmacotherapy of the nonpsychotic patient.

Minor tranquilizers listed in Table 7.1 may be useful for control of anxiety and muscle tension in the early phases of treatment with antidepressants. They are usually most effective when prescribed on an "as needed" basis, rather than on a regular daily basis; rarely are they needed after the patient begins to respond to the antidepressant. Short-acting agents without active metabolic products are most appropriate for use in the older individual.

Hypnotics ("sleeping pills") may be useful in depression in the early stages of treatment. Patients who are treated with sedating antidepressants, most of which can be given in a single bedtime dose, will rarely need additional chemical assistance with sleep; however, patients taking the more activating antidepressants may be helped by addition of a benzodiazapine hypnotic. If several days or weeks of hypnotic use are anticipated, elderly patients should be treated with short-acting agents that do not have active metabolites, such as temazepam or oxazepam.

PRINCIPLES OF PSYCHOPHARMACOLOGIC THERAPY

Figure 7.3 presents a recommended flowchart for the psychopharmacotherapy of the elderly depressed patient. In this schema, several possible branches related to the management of side-effects and adverse reactions have been omitted for purposes of comprehensibility. As it is acknowledged that equally appropriate alternative schemes could be proposed, this particular approach is presented mainly as an illustration of the concept of systematic, logical psychopharmacotherapy.

In general, psychopharmacotherapy should be conducted within the context of an ongoing psychotherapeutic relationship that can facilitate assessment of drug effects on perception, cognition, mood, behavior, judgment, and personality. The patient should be seen at least weekly for the first four to six weeks of treatment, or until a clear remission has occurred, at which time visits may be spaced out to once a month. In all instances, patients and their involved relatives and spouse should be informed in detail about potential side effects and adverse reactions before pharmacotherapy is initiated. Frail elderly patients or those with unstable cardiovascular disease, suicidal ideation, psychosis, or severe deterioration of self-care should be treated in a hospital, at least until maximum dosages of antidepressant are reached or life-threatening behavior is no longer evident.

Laboratory Tests in Psychopharmacotherapy of Depression in the Elderly

Presently, there are several laboratory tests that have potential value in the diagnosis and treatment of depression. These tests include the dexamethasone suppression test (DST), the thyroid releasing hormone (TRH) stimulation test, electroencephalographic sleep recordings, psychostimulant challenges, and measurement of serum levels in antidepressant treatment.

The DST is performed by administering a 1 mg or 2 mg tablet of dexamethasone, a powerful steroid hormone, at 11 PM, then drawing blood samples from the patient the following day (usually at 4 PM and 11 PM). The samples are analyzed to determine the serum concentration of

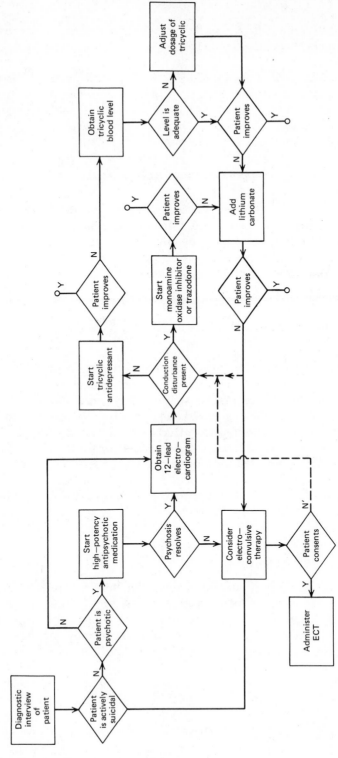

Figure 7.3 Flow scheme for psychopharmacology of depression in the elderly. (Note: Dotted lines represent return to scheme with different tricyclic or switch to MAOI.)

cortisol, an adrenal hormone. In about 96 percent of normal individuals, the serum cortisol will be suppressed to values below 5 μg/dl (micrograms per deciliter) at either the 4 PM or 11 PM measurement. This result occurs because the brain "reads" dexamethasone as cortisol and attempts to maintain a normal cortisol level by reducing the pituitary gland secretion of adrenocorticotropic hormone which in turn inhibits adrenal production of cortisol. About 50 percent of persons with neurovegetative depression have a 4 PM or 11 PM cortisol level equal to or above 5 μg/dl. Assuming that approximately 50 percent of the patients who are tested are depressed, a positive DST has about 94 percent reliability as a diagnostic test for depression, while a negative test cannot be interpreted (Carroll et al., 1981). However, there appear to be several serious limitations to the actual practical value of the DST as a diagnostic test, and they include a growing list of diagnoses in which false positive or false negative tests can occur. For example, some demented patients, some patients with personality disorders, and some anorexics apparently have false positive DSTs, while patients taking barbiturates may have negative tests. The relationship between the DST and several other clinical variables, such as depressive subtype, long-term treatment response, and prognosis are currently under investigation.

The thyroid releasing hormone (TRH) test is conducted by intravenously administering thyroid releasing hormone and then measuring blood levels of thyroid stimulating hormone at 15-minute intervals. It is based on principles analogous to those of the DST, and has been shown to be abnormal in some depressed individuals (Sternbach et al., 1982). Unfortunately, the specificity and sensitivity of the TRH test appears to be considerably lower than those of the DST, rendering the TRH test of even more questionable value at this time.

Electroencephalographic abnormalities found in some depressed people include decreased REM latency of about 45–50 minutes, and increased total REM sleep time (Coble et al., 1976). (REM latency is the amount of time between falling asleep and the first "rapid eye movement" stage of sleep, about 90–120 minutes in normal people). However, the practical value of electroencephalographic sleep recordings for the diagnosis of depression is also limited. Definitive knowledge of the prevalence and degree of these changes and their relationship to variables such as depressive subtype and other concomitant illnesses is not yet available and sleep recordings are expensive and require equipment and personnel not found in most treatment facilities.

Several investigators have examined the relationship between the depressed patient's responses to a test dose of psychostimulant medication and their subsequent long-term response to antidepressant therapy. Several studies (Maas, 1975) suggest that depressed individuals who experience transient mood elevation from psychostimulants may have a biochemical subtype of depression that is more likely to respond to imipramine and related tricyclic antidepressants than to amitriptyline; however, several recent studies have failed to confirm this relationship. Overall, the "state of the art" of pharmacologic challenge in the management of elderly depressed individuals also falls short of widespread clinical utility.

As gastrointestinal absorption, metabolism, distribution, and excretion of drugs can vary considerably among individuals, several investigators have studied the relationship between blood levels of antidepressant drugs and clinical response. As the blood level represents the final product of absorption and the other operations, it should be possible to eliminate some variability in drug response by determining a therapeutic blood level of a specific medication and then adjusting the ingested dose to achieve that level. This program has been successfully followed in the case of several drugs used in general medicine (for example, digitalis, dilantin, and aspirin) and in the case of lithium carbonate in psychiatry, wherein blood levels have been clearly related to therapeutic response. Unfortunately, the blood level-response relationship of the tricyclic antidepressants has been somewhat more elusive, although several studies agree that the chances of a good response to a tricyclic are somewhat increased if the blood level reaches 100 ng/ml (nanogram per milliliter) or greater (for the secondary tricyclics) or 200 ng/ml of combined tertiary molecule and secondary metabolite (for the tertiary tricyclics). Because of the statistical weakness of this finding and the well-known variability of blood level measurements among laboratories, tricyclic blood levels remain only a possibly useful rough measure at the present time.

Besides the inherent limitations of the laboratory tests, virtually none have been adequately studied in elderly patients. As it is well known that aging is accompanied by changes in endocrine function, electroencephalographic sleep architecture, and drug response, it is clear that more research is needed before those tests are useful in the management of the elderly depressed patient.

SUMMARY

Mood in elderly individuals, as in the young, appears to be a result of complex interactions between the individual's perception and interpretation of life events and his or her neurophysiological state, alterations in either of which sphere can produce positive or negative alterations in mood. In this chapter, the mood-altering potential and mechanisms of action of certain pharmacologic substances have been reviewed and basic principles of their use in clinical psychiatry have been suggested. While some drugs, even when prescribed appropriately, can cause significant mood disturbance, modern antidepressant agents, used judiciously and with proper respect for side-effects and adverse reactions, can make a major positive contribution to the treatment of the most disabling and life-threatening episodes of depressive illness in the elderly.

REFERENCES

Bielski, R.J., and Friedel, R.O. Prediction of tricyclic antidepressant response. *Archives of General Psychiatry*, 1976, 33:1477–89.

Carroll, B.J., Feinberg, M., Greden, J.F., Tarika, J., Albola, A.A., Haskett, R.F., James, N.M., Kronfol, Z., Lohr, N., Steiner, M., De Vigne, J.P., and Young, E. A specific laboratory test for the diagnosis of melancholia. *Archives of General Psychiatry* January 1981, 38:15–22.

Charney, D.S., Menkes, D.B., and Heninger, G.R. Receptor sensitivity and the mechanism of action of antidepressant treatment: implications for the etiology and therapy of depression. *Archives of General Psychiatry* 1981, 38:1160–80.

Coble, P., Foster, F.G., and Kupfer, D.J. Electroencephalographic sleep diagnosis of primary depression. *Archives of General Psychiatry*, 1976, 33:1124–27.

De Montigny, C., Grunberg, F., Mayer, A., et al. Lithium induces rapid relief of depression in tricyclic antidepressant drug non-responders. *British Journal of Psychiatry*, 1981, 138:252–56.

Fink, M. *Convulsive Therapy: Theory and Practice.* New York: Raven Press, 1979.

Gerner, R.H., Estabrook, W., Steuer, J., and Jarvik, L. Treatment of geriatric depression with trazodone, imipramine and placebo: A double blind study. *Journal of Clinical Psychiatry*, 1980, 41:216–20.

Katon, W., and Raskind, M. Treatment of depression in the medically ill elderly with methylphenidate. *American Journal of Psychiatry*, August, 1980, 137(8):963–65.

Maas, J.W. Biogenic amines and depression. *Archives of General Psychiatry*, 1975, 32:1357–61.

Robinson, D.S., Nies, A., Ravaris, C.L., Ives, J.O., and Bartlett, D. Clinical pharmacology of phenelzine: MAO activity and clinical response. In Lipton, M., DiMascio, A., Killam, K.F., (Eds.), *Psychopharmacology: A Generation of Progress.* New York: Raven Press, 1978.

Sternbach, H., Gerner, R.H., and Gwirtsman H.E. The thyrotropin releasing hormone stimulation test: a review. *Journal of Clinical Psychiatry*, January 1982, 43:1.

Weiner, R.D. The psychiatric use of electrically induced seizures. *American Journal of Psychiatry*, 1979, 136(12):1507–17.

8

Nutrients
and Nutrition

Ruth B. Weg

THE MAGIC OF FOOD

At the turn of this century, any consequences of malnutrition among middle-aged and older adults in the United States would probably have escaped notice for at least two reasons. First, the level of knowledge concerning the far-reaching, complex effects of nutrients was in its infancy and, second, the numbers of late middle-aged and elderly were relatively few. There were only 3 million persons (4 percent) over 65 in 1900 of a total of 76 million; in 1983, by comparison, there were 26.8 million elderly—about 11.5 percent of the total population of 232.1 million. With such growing numbers of older adults, the now well-documented effects of malnutrition on physical and mental status are important to the economic and human dimensions of the country.

The history of the human family is rich with stories of the real and symbolic meaning of food. Adam bit the apple and robbed the human family of innocence, making the human spirit know good and evil. Plant and animal potions—mandrake, orchid, and testes extracts, and birds' nest soup have been variously employed in the quest for love, sexuality, health, youth, vitality, long life, and immortality.

In the earliest times of the human family, there were wise or "witch" men who became the intermediaries between people and their gods (Camp, 1974; Trimmer, 1970). They were the healers who learned from the world of plants and animals that many plants had curative powers, that sick animals ate of these plants and became well. The shaman was a healer, a traveling medicine man whose efforts were directed at "curing" mental disorders, and shamans can still be found in Siberia and among some Inuit tribes. Healers combined appeals to certain gods, plants with curative powers, and astrological foretelling of the patient's future. The "natural

214

cure" was the significant basis for healing, although there was also much ritual and mystique—dancing around the patient, touching healing objects, incantations, and the use of direct physical contact to extract harmful spirits and demons.

A balanced daily intake of food was not the issue at the dawn of humankind's culture. Quantity of food was the concern—enough to sustain energy and body function for the rigorous life of primitive times. The appreciation of the nature of different plants as food with unique, curative, and therapeutic qualities beyond energy grew in breadth and depth with time. The Greek physician Hippocrates (approximately 460–377 B.C.), long considered the Father of Medicine, is said to have prescribed particular dietary regimens for his patients, convinced that foods in proper combinations were important to recovery from illness (Sebrell and Haggerty, 1980). Appropriate and "magical" plants were known even earlier; for example, the Ebers papyrus listed a wide variety of plants among the recommended remedies. Egypt was then a center of knowledge, and beginning in the seventh century B.C., Greeks studied medicine (and other arts) there. Medicine and healing were prevalent in India, Persia, and China as well. Ancient Chinese herbal concoctions of more than 4,000 years ago were apparently used after much experiment and observation; for example, treatment of asthma and bronchitis included the juice of a certain Chinese fir. This medication was no accidental witchcraft; in 1978 it was discovered that the alkaloid ephedrine, a bronchodilator used in pulmonary dysfunction, was in the juice. It was a Chinese physician in the eleventh century who said, "Experts at curing disease are inferior to the specialists who warn against disease. Experts in the use of medicines are inferior to those who recommend diet." (Tannahill, 1973) Consensus regarding the value of adequate nutrition as therapy and prevention may be coming full circle.

Contemporary societies are indebted to ancestral cultures for the identification of hundreds of plants and the suggestions for their use. The symptomatic relief of many diseases provided by these plants is the basis of modern pharmacology. In addition to the ongoing pursuit of more natural cures from plants everywhere in the world, there is the continuation of exploration concerning mechanisms and interaction of the plant derivatives with body chemistry and physiology. Today's use of plant medicinals and nutrients has left alchemy behind and is based increasingly on validation of experimental data and testing of theories. But the belief in magic persists and the deep-seated hope for everlasting youth and long life has nurtured the search in the miraculous and magical resulting in the multiplication of health food stores, mail order potency promises, guru mania, and the proliferation of health spas and clinics (Prehoda, 1968; Rosenfeld, 1976). Americans continue to spend between $5 billion and $10 billion every year on nutrition fraud and quackery (Davis and Davis, 1981).

Garlic is no longer used for strength as it was by the Egyptians who fed garlic to the workmen on the Great Pyramids; grasshoppers are not prescribed to relieve bladder disorders. A disease no longer requires a plant therapy that resembles patient symptoms (e.g., Diocorides, first century A.D., recommended the red juice of the alkanet as "the antidote to skin inflammation"). Very few medicinal herbs come from home-grown cottage gardens, yet millions of hard-earned dollars are spent on products of questionable origin and content that promise to revitalize the blood-stream, give sparkle to the eye, color to the lips and spring to the step (Camp, 1974, p. 82).

The new knowledge, experimental and clinical, which continues to develop about nutrition and health status, makes belief in the "magic" of food irrelevant to reality. Nutrients can and do make a difference in a number of cell and systemic functions and organismic health. What remains to be increasingly emphasized is public and professional education and the application of principles of adequate nutrition which could protect and support health promotion.

NUTRITION AS A SCIENCE

Even in the presence of the search for wondrous panaceas, the science of nutrition is dynamic and there are signs of its renaissance in academia, health-care professions and the government arena. The perception of nutrition is changing, reaching beyond sustenance and "after the fact" disease care to serious consideration as part of preventive health care. Medical schools are returning nutrition to a place in reorganized curricula.

A U.S. Senate Select Committee on Nutrition and Human Needs* (Butler, 1977) recognized the necessity to change the Westernized diet as a major factor in preventive medicine. It has been estimated that if Americans altered their diets and other life-style habits (Richmond, 1979), they could achieve better health and a reduction in mortality rates of up to 35 percent by 1990. As director of the National Institute on Aging in 1977, Robert Butler stated: "It is only through adequately nutritious diets that old people retain the capacity to remain active and productive." After a two-year review of worldwide studies, the National Research Council of the National Academy of Sciences announced that risk from breast, colon, and prostate cancer could be reduced by eating substantially less fat (News and Comment, 1982).

There is a growing literature in gerontology and geriatrics that describes the central role of nutrition in the later years for maintenance and promotion of mental and physical functional capacities. Nutrition and diet are investigated not only as therapy in the treatment of disorders but as

* Established in 1968, disbanded in 1977.

an integral part of a larger, preventive regimen in the middle and later years. Attention to prudent, appropriate nutrition (together with exercise and stress management) could be instrumental in the delay, minimization, and possible elimination of the chronic diseases that dehumanize the later years (Fries, 1980; Krehl, 1980; Watkin, 1981; Weg, 1979, 1980a, 1983).

THE RITUAL AND SOCIAL MEANING OF FOOD

Nutrition: More than Food

Nutritional status is more than food; it is the result of multiple interacting variables at any age, perhaps with greater impact in the later years. Nutritional adequacy is more than the food on the plate and more than the nutrient composition of a meal, important as they are. Factors such as transportation, availability of foods, economics, physical immobility, pathology, living situation, marriage, education, alienation, culture, ethnic, and genetic differences all play a role. In an even more direct way, aspects of individual life-style interact with nutrition: exercise, stress, alcohol, other drugs, social, and intellectual activities are affected by and affect nutrition.

Eating as Celebration and Comfort

That eating is a ritual and social activity is learned early in infancy and reinforced all through life. Religious and societal holidays, personal celebrations, birthdays and anniversaries, and the recognition of the end of life—all are marked by the preparation and eating of food. The breaking of bread and the fast together with others have religious and affectional connotations; to eat alone is often to feel desolate and deserted. Food preparation and serving is frequently learned, not only as necessities for living, but as acts of love for particular persons or groups.

Among elders, whose life space has generally narrowed because of various human and material losses, eating may become an important social and emotional experience. Nutritional programs set up under the Older American's Act were charged not only with improving the daily diet, but also with attending to the social needs for human intercourse and the enhancement of self-esteem (Natow and Heslin, 1980).

Today it is clear that no one food or nutrient is a panacea. No magical elixir has been found to keep the human family free from disease and mortality. The benefits of adequate nutrition have been demonstrated in coping with modern-day stress, the provision of energy and raw materials for maintenance of mind and body, supporting the capacity to fight disease and promote health, and, possibly, the extension of vigorous, later years.

HEALTH AND WELLNESS

The concept of wellness—a harmonious interaction of body, psyche, affect, and spirit within physical and human environments—has gained in theoretical and practical acceptance among health professionals and laypersons alike (Dychtwald, 1978; Farquhar, 1978; Hastings et al., 1980; Luce, 1976; Pelletier, 1977). Health is no longer definable as merely the absence of disease, but is more appropriately viewed as related to psychological, physiological, and spiritual well-being.

Multiple Components of Wellness

A number of interacting factors affect health status and wellness which differ in potential for individual and community control and management. They include 1) genetics, currently not under significant individual control; 2) environmental elements—air, soil and water pollution, pathogens, radiation, food handling, processing and production, generally under various governmental control and/or supervisory agencies; and 3) lifestyle. This last category is the most susceptible to personal control. It includes activity and exercise; stressors and their management; recreation, relaxation and sleep; work patterns; economic status; living arrangements; intellectual and emotional needs and behavior; the use of alcohol, tobacco, and other drugs; and finally, nutrition and diet. The concern in this chapter is with nutrition, a single but critical factor in dynamic interrelationships with the other variables in the framework of maintenance and promotion of functional health.

Nutrition and Wellness: The Disease Connection

The Westernized diet of the last 60 years is considered harmful to the nation's health, and particularly for the middle-aged and older subpopulations (Burkitt, 1982; Lawton, 1981; Richmond, 1979; Watkin, 1981; Weg, 1980a,b, 1983). Dietary intake is characterized by high intake of refined carbohydrates, processed foods, dairy products, and meat with saturated fat content and excess salt (see Table 8.1). Further, such a dietary pattern is low in fiber and whole grains, fresh fruits and vegetables. This pattern represents a rejection of the eating habits of the late 1800s and early 1900s, which included bulky, complex starches/sugars (whole grains, fibers, fruits, vegetables) and unprocessed fresh foods, in favor of one that has raised total fat consumption to 43–50 percent of total caloric intake, increased refined sugar in the diet by 50 percent to about 18 percent of daily calories. The Westernized diet is potentially inadequate in micronutrients (vitamins and minerals), energy, and protein of high biologic quality. Worldwide epidemiologic studies have implicated this diet in the major chronic diseases of contemporary civilization: cardiovascular and cerebrovascular disease (including atherosclerosis and hypertension)

TABLE 8.1

AMERICAN WESTERNIZED DIET AVERAGE DAILY INTAKE

	Percentage Daily Caloric Intake (2800–3000 Calories)
Carbohydrates	35–40%
Refined carbohydrates, Simple sugars	
Sugar, honey	15–25% of 35–40% (greater than 100 gm/day)
Fats	40–50%
High cholesterol intake	700–800 mg
High saturated fats	
Proteins	12–15%
Majority of animal origin (meat and milk products, egg yolk)	
Salt	10–20 gms

cancer, diabetes, and osteoporosis, all of which increase in morbidity and mortality in the middle and later years (Burkitt, 1982; Jarrett, 1982; Jowsey, 1978; Krehl, 1977; National Academy of Science, 1982; Weg, 1983). There have been few controlled studies with large numbers of people or experimental animals that have examined various dietary regimens for their effects. Animal studies do provide worthwhile clues and have elucidated mechanisms of action between diet and pathological changes (Harman, 1971; Walford, 1983; Sun and Sun, 1978; Young, 1978). Even more significant for people are the epidemiological data, which indicate that in countries where Westernized eating habits prevail, the incidence of these diseases of civilization is high—the United States, Sweden, and Finland being among them (Blackburn, 1977; Robertson et al., 1977; Turner, 1982). On the other hand, countries that generally have a dietary intake high in fiber, whole grain cereals, and fresh fruits and vegetables and low in salt and refined sugar and starch, experience a low incidence of these disorders (see Tables 8.1 and 8.2).

The American consuming public has apparently been growing responsive to recent emphases on fitness and health promotion. Since 1964 the diet (and other life-style variables such as sedentary habits and coping with stress) has undergone some measureable change—away from the high consumption of animal fats and oils, butter, liquid milk, cream, and eggs and toward an increase in whole grain cereals, complex carbohydrates, and vegetable oils. There are continuing data on age-specific cerebrovascular and coronary disease mortality rates that demonstrate a significant, continuous decline (Walker, 1977, 1983). (See Tables 8.3 and 8.4) Though

TABLE 8.2
PRUDENT DIET

	Daily Caloric Intake (1800–2400 Calories)
Carbohydrates	45–55%
Complex: whole grain cereal, breads, fruits, vegetables	
Refined/processed sugars	10% of total carbohydrates
Fats	
Fat, saturated/unsaturated	1:1 ratio or slightly in favor of unsaturated
Cholesterol	Maximum 300 mg
Proteins	12
Mixed sources[a]: animal, plant	
Salt	Maximum 2–3 gm

[a] lean beef, veal, lamb, poultry, fish; nuts, legumes, seeds.

cause and effect cannot be established for changing dietary habits and lowered mortality rates and, though nutrition cannot be the only life-style variable involved, the correlation is encouraging and strongly suggestive (Krehl, 1980; Turner, 1982).

Nutritional Status and Aging

In view of the gradually decreasing efficiency of systemic function with age, good nutritional status is even more significant. Any dietary deficiency

TABLE 8.3
DECLINE IN AGE-SPECIFIC CEREBROVASCULAR MORTALITY, 1963–1981[a]

Age Group (years)	Decline (%)
35–44	46.1
45–54	42.3
55–64	42.3
65–74	53.2
75–84	49.7
85+	44.4

Source: Walker, W.J. Changing U.S. lifestyle and declining vascular mortality: a retrospective. Abstracted by permission of The New England Journal of Medicine, 1983, 308(11):649–51.

[a] Decline calculated from figures from the National Center for Health Statistics (NCHS).

TABLE 8.4
DECLINE IN AGE-SPECIFIC
CORONARY MORTALITY,
1963–1981

Age Group (years)	Decline (%)
35–44	44.8
45–54	38.3
55–64	38.0
65–74	37.0
75–84	30.0
85+	25.6

Source: Walker, W.J. Changing U.S. lifestyle and declining vascular mortality. A retrospective. Abstracted by permission of *The New England Journal of Medicine*, 1983, 308(11):649–51.

or excess could exacerbate functional decline of already vulnerable systems. A particular consequence of long-time consumption of the Westernized diet that had been ignored or gone unrecognized for many years is the increased likelihood of subclinical malnutrition. The effects of such malnutrition are not the dramatic, classical signs of malnutrition—beriberi, pellagra, rickets, and scurvy—but, rather, the often insidious symptoms of general malaise—headache, fatigue, listlessness, insomnia, irritability, loss of appetite and body weight, failing memory, and anxiety and confusion (Clements, 1975; Exton-Smith, 1978; Weg, 1980a) These symptoms are still associated with growing older by health care professions and laypersons alike, a supposedly inevitable price for the added years of life. This prolonged, relatively low-level malnutrition affects cell and tissue metabolism and leaves the individual even more vulnerable and marked by diminished capacity for adequate response to infection, injury, emotional stress, and malignancy (see Table 8.5).

Listed below are the multiple effects beginning at the molecular and cellular levels that have been identified with protein, micronutrient and energy depletion:

· Cell generation time slowed, which retards wound repair.
· Decrease in ATP diminishes available energy for syntheses and catabolism.
· Inadequate energy stores impede maintenance of structural and functional integrity of cell.
· Diminished energy production leads to increased protein breakdown for energy, decreases pool of available amino acids.
· Damage in DNA leads to inappropriate information for protein synthesis.

TABLE 8.5
STAGES OF DEVELOPMENT OF NUTRITIONAL DEFICIENCY DISEASE

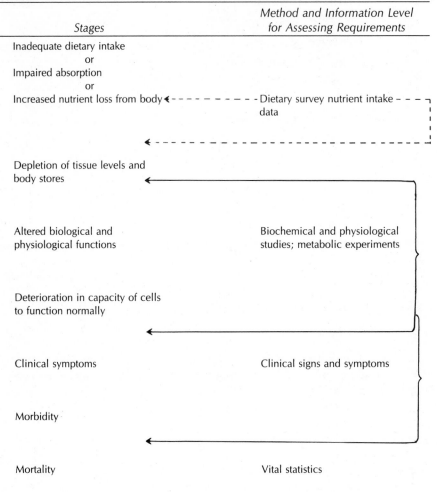

Stages	Method and Information Level for Assessing Requirements
Inadequate dietary intake or Impaired absorption or Increased nutrient loss from body	Dietary survey nutrient intake data
Depletion of tissue levels and body stores	
Altered biological and physiological functions	Biochemical and physiological studies; metabolic experiments
Deterioration in capacity of cells to function normally	
Clinical symptoms	Clinical signs and symptoms
Morbidity	
Mortality	Vital statistics

Source: From Beaton, G.H., and Patwardhan, V.N. In Beaton, G.H., and Bengoa, J.M. (Eds.), *Nutrition in Preventive Medicine*, Monograph Series, No. 62. Geneva: World Health Organization, 1976, pp. 445–81. Used with permission.

· Rapid degradation of cytoplasmic RNA results in decreased rate of protein synthesis.

· Immune or inflammatory response to microbial, toxic or genetic injury severely limited.*

* From Weg, R.B. "Changing physiology of age: changing Nutrition." In Slavkin, H.C. (Ed.), *New Horizons in Nutrition for the Health Professions. University of Southern California Journal Continuing Dental Education*, 1980, 1(2):38–70 (p. 42)

Nutrient requirements in the later years are being reevaluated. The attitude that careful dietary intake is significant only for the infant and child during the growing, developing years is no longer viable. Nutritional adequacy plays a role in disease prevention and health promotion at any age with particular emphasis for any identifiably at-risk group. Nutritional status is compromised during stress response, illness/disease, injury, surgery, bed rest, and bereavement. Inadequate and inappropriate nutrition deprives the organism of the following factors:

· A balance of processes and blood/tissue constituents in face of environmental and internal demands
· Prevention of significant structural and functional changes in cells, or prevention of premature decline in systemic function
· Maintenance of adequate immune response
· Capacity for stress response
· Promotion and maintenance of mental and physical vitality

Nutritional status is compromised during stress response, illness/disease, injury, surgery, bed rest, and bereavement, conditions that tend to increase with the years. It appears reasonable to assume that the elders who experience lowered systemic efficiency and stressful life experiences will also have different and/or greater requirements for particular nutrients than in their younger years (Weg, 1979; 1980a,b).

Malnutrition

In the past, malnutrition has generally been perceived as a disorder of poverty, undereating, and ignorance and considered most critical among infants and children. Today, malnutrition in the United States is more particularly identified as one of the most widespread and potentially destructive disorders of the later years (Posner, 1979). The causes of malnutrition are

1. Inability to prepare food (disability, inadequate facilities)
2. Inadequate living arrangements; lack of transportation
3. Social isolation—apathy, depression, diminished self-image
4. Depression
5. Poverty
6. Westernized diet
7. Ignorance regarding balanced, appropriate diet
8. Poor dentition, digestive dysfunction, or disease
9. Alcoholism or other drug abuse
10. Anorexia

Both undernutrition and overnutrition result in malnourished people, young and old. The limited nutritional surveys and related biochemical and functional data among older adults provide an unambiguous picture of a group of persons at nutritional risk (Ossofsky and Anderson, 1972; Weg, 1980 a,b).

Undernutrition may be the more significant of the two among elders. Greater than 50 percent of the older population appears to have dietary intakes that are less than recommended levels of nutrients (see Table 8.6), estimated as either borderline or frankly deficient (Beauchene and Davis, 1979; Natow and Heslin, 1980; O'Hanlon and Kohrs, 1978; Young, 1978, 1982a,b). Vitamin profiles of institutionalized elderly and healthy volunteers were compared and sublinical deficiencies were found: the vitamin B complex was characteristically low (Baker et al., 1979). Inadequate intake of a number of essential micronutrients has been noted: vitamins A, C, D, B_{12}, B_6, folic acid and minerals—calcium, zinc and iron. Low values have also been reported for vitamin B_1 (thiamin), B_3 (niacin), and proteins. It is speculated that the factors contributing to these deficiencies include natural sequelae to the Westernized diet described earlier; low calorie intake recommended for sedentary life-style of middle-aged and old without regard to the nutrient density of foods; lifelong poor dietary habits; emotional and physical trauma of the later years; limited income; move to unfamiliar housing; and illness or disease. Individual requirements for particular nutrients can, therefore, reasonably be expected to increase with the years and may vary with the nature of the challenge.

Overnutrition has been evaluated as a potential health risk among the middle-aged and young old since excess weight and obesity are correlated with chronic disorders—cardiovascular disease, hypertension, diabetes, osteoarthritis, renal and gall bladder disease, and increased surgical morbidity and mortality. Some observers estimate that two-fifths of older persons suffer from overweight and obesity, and they report a strong association between even moderate overweight and higher mortality (Posner, 1979). However, reviews of age and weight characteristics suggest that the weight gain considered typical of the middle and later years may actually slow with the years (Gordon and Shurtleff, 1973). Moreover, there is a very recent conclusion by Andres (1980) that emphasizes data indicating that extreme leanness is equally associated with elevated mortality. Andres contends that morbidity and mortality risk is heightened at both extremes, overweight and underweight. New height/age/weight charts have been published by Metropolitan Life Insurance to replace the 1959 tables and indicate the "desired" weights about 10–15 pounds greater (Lewin, 1981). There is continued controversy regarding the advisability of any poundage greater than "lean" in the middle and later years. Continued longitudinal studies will be necessary to support the Andres concept, which is based primarily on retrospective mortality data.

Hospital malnutrition has become a serious threat to health status and recovery from illness and surgery for the older patient. Studies indicate that malnourished older hospital patients experience exacerbation of

TABLE 8.6

FOOD AND NUTRITION BOARD, NATIONAL ACADEMY OF SCIENCES–NATIONAL RESEARCH COUNCIL RECOMMENDED DAILY DIETARY ALLOWANCES,[a] Revised 1980

Designed for the maintenance of good nutrition of practically all healthy people in the U.S.A.

	Age (years)	Weight (kg)	(lb)	Height (cm)	(in)	Protein (g)	Vitamin A (μg RE)[b]	Vitamin D (μg)[c]	Vitamin E (mg α-TE)[d]	Vitamin C (mg)	Thiamin (mg)	Riboflavin (mg)	Niacin (mg NE)[e]	Vitamin B6 (mg)	Folacin[f] (μg)	Vitamin B12 (μg)	Calcium (mg)	Phosphorus (mg)	Magnesium (mg)	Iron (mg)	Zinc (mg)	Iodine (μg)
Infants	0.0–0.5	6	13	60	24	kg × 2.2	420	10	3	35	0.3	0.4	6	0.3	30	0.5[g]	360	240	50	10	3	40
	0.5–1.0	9	20	71	28	kg × 2.0	400	10	4	35	0.5	0.6	8	0.6	45	1.5	540	360	70	15	5	50
Children	1–3	13	29	90	35	23	400	10	5	45	0.7	0.8	9	0.9	100	2.0	800	800	150	15	10	70
	4–6	20	44	112	44	30	500	10	6	45	0.9	1.0	11	1.3	200	2.5	800	800	200	10	10	90
	7–10	28	62	132	52	34	700	10	7	45	1.2	1.4	16	1.6	300	3.0	800	800	250	10	10	120
Males	11–14	45	99	157	62	45	1000	10	8	50	1.4	1.6	18	1.8	400	3.0	1200	1200	350	18	15	150
	15–18	66	145	176	69	56	1000	10	10	60	1.4	1.7	18	2.0	400	3.0	1200	1200	400	18	15	150
	19–22	70	154	177	70	56	1000	7.5	10	60	1.5	1.7	19	2.2	400	3.0	800	800	350	10	15	150
	23–50	70	154	178	70	56	1000	5	10	60	1.4	1.6	18	2.2	400	3.0	800	800	350	10	15	150
	51+	70	154	178	70	56	1000	5	10	60	1.2	1.4	16	2.2	400	3.0	800	800	350	10	15	150
Females	11–14	46	101	157	62	46	800	10	8	50	1.1	1.3	15	1.8	400	3.0	1200	1200	300	18	15	150
	15–18	55	120	163	64	46	800	10	8	60	1.1	1.3	14	2.0	400	3.0	1200	1200	300	18	15	150
	19–22	55	120	163	64	44	800	7.5	8	60	1.1	1.3	14	2.0	400	3.0	800	800	300	18	15	150
	23–50	55	120	163	64	44	800	5	8	60	1.0	1.2	13	2.0	400	3.0	800	800	300	18	15	150
	51+	55	120	163	64	44	800	5	8	60	1.0	1.2	13	2.0	400	3.0	800	800	300	10	15	150
Pregnant						+30	+200	+5	+2	+20	+0.4	+0.3	+2	+0.6	+400	+1.0	+400	+400	+150	*h*	+5	+25
Lactating						+20	+400	+5	+3	+40	+0.5	+0.5	+5	+0.5	+100	+1.0	+400	+400	+150	*h*	+10	+50

Source: From *Recommended Dietary Allowances,* 9th rev. ed. Washington, D.C.: National Academy of Sciences, The National Research Council, 1980.

[a] The allowances are intended to provide for individual variations among most normal persons as they live in the United States under usual environmental stresses. Diets should be based on a variety of common foods in order to provide other nutrients for which human requirements have been less well defined. See text for detailed discussion of allowances and of nutrients not tabulated. See Table 1 (p. 20) for weights and heights by individual year of age. See Table 3 (p. 23) for suggested average energy intakes.

[b] Retinol equivalents. 1 retinol equivalent = 1 μg retinol or 6 μg β carotene. See text for calculation of vitamin A activity of diets as retinol equivalents.

[c] As cholecalciferol. 10 μg cholecalciferol = 400 IU of vitamin D.

[d] α-tocopherol equivalents. 1 mg *d*-α tocopherol = 1 α-TE. See text for variation in allowances and calculation of vitamin E activity of the diet as α-tocopherol equivalents.

[e] 1 NE (niacin equivalent) is equal to 1 mg of niacin or 60 mg of dietary tryptophan.

[f] The folacin allowances refer to dietary sources as determined by *Lactobacillus casei* assay after treatment with enzymes (conjugases) to make polyglutamyl forms of the vitamin available to the test organism.

[g] The recommended dietary allowance for vitamin B₁₂ in infants is based on average concentration of the vitamin in human milk. The allowances after weaning are based on energy intake (as recommended by the American Academy of Pediatrics) and consideration of other factors, such as intestinal absorption; see text.

[h] The increased requirement during pregnancy cannot be met by the iron content of habitual American diets nor by the existing iron stores of many women; therefore the use of 30–60 mg of supplemental iron is recommended. Iron needs during lactation are not substantially different from those of nonpregnant women, but continued supplementation of the mother for two to three months after parturition is advisable in order to replenish stores depleted by pregnancy.

malnutrition and increased infection, anemia, general ill health, and higher mortality rates. Although some inquiries suggest that well-nourished hospital patients over 65 show no increased rate of abnormal findings than do well-nourished younger patients, it is also true that older patients are more frequently admitted with protein-calorie malnutrition (Biena et al., 1982). The significant effect of hospital food is more clearly understood when related to length of hospital stay. In one study there was a diminuition in nutritional status in more than 75 percent of patients who were admitted with normal values. There was an increased likelihood of malnutrition with time (during a 12 to 20 day stay) and a rise in mortality from 4 to 13 percent with a lengthened stay (Weinsier et al., 1980).

Drug-Related Nutritional Deficiencies

Polypharmacy, the frequent lot of many older people, may complicate as well as help the pathologies, levels of energy, and capacities. The elderly outnumber any other subpopulation in the number of prescription and over-the-counter drugs used. While drugs are often life-saving, they also too often contribute in illness and disease (iatrogenesis), invalidism, even death (Eckhardt, 1978; Weg, 1978). Drug effects on taste, appetite, intestinal motility, absorption and nutrient metabolism increase nutrient requirements. Hypovitaminoses and mineral deficiencies are the common signs of drug-induced nutritional disorders (Roe, 1976, 1978). Some examples of frequently used medications and the undesirable consequences among the middle-aged and old, will demonstrate the increased probability of micronutrient deficiencies.

Hypocholesterolemic agents (cliofibrate, neomycin) are efficient in the prevention of excess absorption of bile acids and the increase in cholesterol breakdown (and lowering serum cholesterol), but they also interfere with the absorption of vitamin B_{12}, carotene, xylose, iron, and nitrogen (Overton and Luckert, 1977). Alcohol and aspirin block vitamin C uptake; absorption of fat soluble vitamins A, D, E, and K is decreased by mineral oil; diuretics lower potassium (K^+) and manganese (Mn^{++}) levels; certain cathartics lower calcium (Ca^{++}) and potassium (K^+) absorption; and chronic use of some antacids result in thiamine deficiency.

Overall investigation of diet/drug interactions is limited, especially as it concerns older persons as subjects. In order to ensure optimal nutrition and support of capacities in the increasing older population, more studies are required to determine drug dosage, efficiency and response of the different subgroups among the elderly.

NUTRITION AND MENTAL HEALTH

Two recent decades, the 1960s and 1970s, will be remembered for the accumulation of evidence that nutritional status (together with other multiple, interacting factors, e.g., exercise, stress management, cigarette smoking) has significant impact on physical health and wellness, and the chronic diseases that accompany the late middle and older years. Although many details remain to be identified and clarified, the research continues to demonstrate specific relationships between diet and chronic disease, to develop improved therapeutics, and to design and implement preventive dietary patterns.

The 1980s appear likely to become the decade in which the suggested connections between foods and human feelings, memories, and moods will be thoroughly explored; a time during which mechanisms of food effects will be carefully uncovered; a period when appropriate dietary, preventive, and therapeutic manipulations (coupled with other useful approaches) can be tested and applied. Inquiry in brain research has moved beyond the important statement of Jarvik (1973): "the influence of nutrition and nutritional factors upon psychological functions associated with aging is only beginning to be realized" (p. 136).

Much about the etiology and mechanisms of brain function is still unknown. An active area of inquiry that relates to affective disorders in general, and depression in particular, is the biochemistry of synaptic transmission. Though many questions remain unanswered, knowledge and understanding have grown with significant impact in psychiatry and pharmacology (Hubel, 1979). A number of disorders are correlated with disturbances of synaptic transmission and drugs used appear to be effective by decreasing or increasing transmission, e.g., Parkinson's disease and depression.

Effects of Inadequate Nutrition on the CNS

Effects of inadequate, inappropriate nutrition for the development and function of the central nervous system (CNS) during gestation and childhood have been well documented. There is general agreement that apparently nutrition-related, permanent biochemical and structural brain damage can result from poor nutrition reflected in changes of sensorimotor and intellectual capacities (Nowak and Munro, 1977; Shoemaker and Bloom, 1977).

Animal investigations in the 1970s suggested that early malnutrition-related behavioral abnormalities were further enhanced by a deprived environment. Observations in human populations confirmed this probability; moreover, with an enriched environment, the behavioral changes may be reversible (Winick, 1980). Immature animals are thought to be most susceptible to effects of early undernutrition during a critical period characterized by rapid growth of neural and glial cells (Dobbing, 1970). When malnutrition occurs during slow growth (adolescence, adulthood), resultant changes in the human CNS are considered reversible (Winick, 1970). It is possible that even in the adult and later years, malnutrition could affect structural and biochemical CNS changes in elders similar to those seen in malnourished young in number, size, or ultrastructural aspects of the glial and neuronal cell populations.

The Older CNS

As discussed earlier in this chapter, people in their later years are particularly vulnerable to the consequences of nutritional inadequacies (deficiencies or excesses); subclinical malnutrition appears more common than anticipated. The notion that a normal or modified diet can alter brain metabolism appears to be based on direct, verifiable laboratory animal studies and on indirect, suggestive data from human trials (Davis et al., 1975; Fernstrom, 1979; Wurtman, 1982).

The adult nervous system, though considered to be less sensitive to dietary inadequacies than that of the young, can be damaged by nutrient deficiencies as well as toxic substances that may be ingested as or with food. Subclinical malnutrition as a frequent base and situational, stress-related, severe malnutrition as overlay, could indeed contribute to nutrition-dependent changes in the aging CNS. Malnutrition in the older adult is generally related to the micronutrients—vitamins and minerals. Vitamins that appear to play an essential role in brain function and are deficient in the diminished calorie or low nutrient density intake of older persons, include the B complex vitamins—vitamin B_1, B_3, B_6, B_{12}, folate, pantothenic acid, and perhaps riboflavin or B_2 (Dreyfus, 1979). Confusional states in 15 of 17 elderly were relieved with suitable multivitamin supplements that corrected vitamin B complex and C deficiencies (Mitra, 1971). There was a significant decrease in the severity of behavioral manifestations in psychiatric disorders of hospitalized elderly following dietary supplementation with vitamin B complex and vitamin C (Altman et al., 1973).

A number of factors can threaten vitamin sufficiency, among them inadequate dietary intake, alcoholism and other drugs, and disease. Alcohol not only distorts appetite and lowers food intake, but interferes directly with the metabolism of various B complex vitamins. The requirement for vitamin B_6 is increased under particular drug regimens, e.g., isonicotinic acid hydrazide in the treatment of tuberculosis and the antihypertensive hydralazine (Roe, 1978; Weg, 1983). The polypharmacy discussed in the earlier section plays an iatrogenic role in elder depression either in the initiation or exacerbation of an existing condition. Drugs, as treatment for a range of medical or psychiatric disorders, or as part of interaction between drugs, may be involved in the origin of depression (Salzman and Shader, 1978).

Some long-term debilitating conditions or diseases (Dreyfus, 1979) still the accompaniment of the later years for many elders, also contribute to severe nutritional disorders; they include malignancies, chronic infection, renal insufficiency, psychiatric disease, and severe stress.

The Biology and Physiology of Depression

The biological or physiological aspects of depression were assessed in the fifth century B.C. by Hippocrates, who explained this state as melancholia due to black bile (Stenback, 1980). Current research emphasizes the major role of the biogenic amines—norepinephrine, dopamine, and serotonin. Drugs and precursor substances that can modify the metabolism of these amines have also been demonstrated to exacerbate or relieve depression: levodopa, L-tryptophan tyrosine, monoamine oxidase inhibitors, and reserpine. Plasma levels of norepinephrine and serotonin (and their metabolites) are low in depressive individuals. An accumulation of intraneural sodium in neuronal receptor cells, found in some depressed persons has been reported to lower the resting membrane potential (Stenback, 1980).

Data from studies of depressed persons have been equivocal and controversial despite persuasive evidence for the catecholamine or indolamine hypotheses of depression. Difficulty in the establishment of clear-cut cause and effect and appropriate dietary or chemical therapy is due, in part, to the heterogeneity of etiology in depression and the similarity in symptoms (Akiskal and McKinney, 1975). Further, studies suggest that beyond the function norepinephrine has in the "reward" or pleasure diencephalic reinforcement system and its precursor dopamine in psychomotor function, deviations in their metabolism may be significant in the origin and course of depression. Deviations from normal in monoamine metabolism have been found even in those depressions with a minimum of disturbance in personality (van Praag, 1977). Changes in amine mediated neuroendocrine function have been described in post menopausal depressed women (Gruen et al. 1975). Further, Prange and coworkers (1975) suggest an hypothesis: a genetic predisposition to a low level of serotonin leading to reduced excretion of catecholamines which may cause the depression.

Depression and Nutrition Interaction

Perhaps one of the major difficulties in the diagnosis and treatment of depressive episodes and symptoms among the late middle aged and old is the lack of clear distinction between depressive disorders, physical illness, age-related grief, stress response, and malnutrition and their overlapping symptomatology (see Chapters 2 and 3).

An interactive relationship between depression and nutrition has been observed with both under- and overnutrition. Undernutrition and food deprivation may trigger depression that, in turn, leads to weight loss and anorexia. With time, the reciprocal effects are intensified and, unless interrupted, lead to illness or disease and possibly death. It is also true that overeating and weight gain increase feelings of helplessness, diminish self-image and self-control, and lay the groundwork for depressed behavior. Depressive disorders have also been noted repeatedly in psychiatric investigations among some younger and older adults to signal overeating and potential overweight or obesity (Atkinson and Ringuette, 1967; Halmi et al., 1980; Stunkard and Mendelson, 1967).

Undernutrition appears to be a consequence of life's status among many elderly people, a status characterized by social isolation, life changes (e.g., widowhood), alcoholism, poverty, mobility problems, medications, dental problems, and a range of mental and emotional disturbances. Refusal to eat is sometimes related to delusions or hallucinations about poisoners and poisoned food. Even in those situations where food costs can be managed, the purchased food may be of high calorie, low nutrient density, potentiating mineral, vitamin, and protein deficiencies (Garetz, 1976). Folate, in addition to a probable role in purine and protein synthesis, is necessary in the hydroxylation of tyrosine and tryptophan. Deficiencies of folate have been associated with depression and the mechanism appears related to folate's essential activity in catecholamine and indolamine metabolism (Dreyfus, 1979).

There are consequences from depression among the aging beyond dysfunctional behavior and exacerbated malnutrition (see Chapter 4). Ostfeld (1983) and others have found that with time, depression increases vulnerability to illness and death among elders, in relation to bereavement (Jacobs and Ostfeld, 1977), involuntary relocation (Kasl et al., 1980), and risk of cancer (Shekelle et al., 1981). At present, detailed investigation continues into the effects of depression in neuroendocrine and immune functions with subsamples of the study population (Ostfeld, 1983).

DIETARY MODULATION OF BRAIN FUNCTION: ALTERNATIVE OR ADJUVANT THERAPY

It is a little more than a decade since serious consideration of the nutrient effects on brain anatomy and function began. Drugs, electroconvulsive therapy, and psychotherapy have been the traditional choices for treatment of affective disorders. Since most of the effective drugs used in depression appeared to enhance neurotransmission of catecholamines or indolamines, the two biochemical models of depression were logical developments (Gelenberg et al., 1982; Maas, 1975).

Postmortem examinations of the brains of depressed suicide victims, which suggest central deficits of serotonin, lend some support to the monoamine theory of depression. Both 5HT and 5HIAA (5-hydroxyindole acetic acid) were in low concentration in the brainstem, particularly in the raphe nuclei (Birkmayer and Riederer, 1975; Lloyd et al., 1974). Ongoing antidepressant drug investigations continue to raise questions regarding the mechanism of action. Researchers at Yale University have discovered that a number of chemically varied antidepressants block the neurotransmitter histamine that adds yet another neurotransmitter—histamine—to the complex brain response (Kolata, 1976). Snyder (1978) maintains that serotonin and catecholamines still are involved and suggests that in blocking histamine receptors, the drugs may secondarily influence these neurotransmitters. Studies confirm changing levels and activities of the two monoamine transmitters, serotonin (5-hydroxytryptamine or 5-HT) and norepinephrine (NE). They are consistently invoked in regard to depressive illness (Kent, 1982). Some of the long-standing antidepressant drugs reinforce the role of the monoamines, e.g., amitriptyline and imipramine enhance central sympathetic nervous system activity by the inhibition of re-uptake of 5-HT and NE. Monoamine oxidase inhibitors such as isocarboxazid and tranylcypromine sulfate interfere with the activity of the enzyme monoamine oxidase, which catalyzes the breakdown of the monoamines. Serious side-effects of both groups of drugs may be more debilitating than the depression, and especially so for the elderly— e.g., confusion, nausea, headache, dry mouth, constipation, and increased heart rate. Researchers continue to develop and test more selective and purer uptake inhibitors that can be antidepressant with minimal side effects.

More recent findings support the suggestion that brain composition and function appear to be "responsive to changes in the quantity or quality of food eaten by organisms throughout their entire lifespans" (Lytle and Altar, 1979, p. 2020). Studies confirm that synthesis of serotonin and catecholamine neurotransmitters is, in part, controlled by their available amino acid precursors tryptophan and tyrosine (Anderson, 1981; Wurtman et al, 1980). There is now ample demonstration that dietary modifications affect brain function and behavioral response (rats) and result in altered communication among brain and spinal cord neurons with changes in neurotransmitter concentration and release by the nerve cells (Kolata, 1976). Studies of subclinical malnutrition in laboratory rodents also show significant changes in brain neurotransmission and function. Heightened synthesis of certain neurotransmitters is attributed to the increased plasma and brain levels of their nutrient precursors (Wurtman et al. 1977; Wurtman, 1982). A brain deficiency of 5-HT as a predisposing factor in endogenous depression has been confirmed in a study by van Praag and de Haan (1981). 5-HTP (the immediate precursor of 5-HT) was found to prevent the recurrence of future depressive episodes. They also found that lithium was more effective in the treatment of bipolar (manic-depressive) depression, but 5-HTP appeared more efficacious in unipolar illness. It is conceivable (though not yet demonstrated) that nutrients may also affect brain neurotransmission by modifying enzyme synthesis, intracellular transport or storage and release of neurotransmitters.

Monoamine Precursor Therapy

Other effective techniques were investigated that could increase the brain neurotransmitter levels and possibly avoid some of the negative side-effects from the aforementioned therapies. Oral or parenteral administration of the nutrient precursors of neurotransmitters ushered in an heretofore unheard of approach (Fernstrom and Wurtman, 1971). The blood-brain barrier, earlier thought to preclude dietary manipulation of any brain metabolite, has now been demonstrated in animal and human studies to function otherwise. Although all neurotransmitters may not be modulated by available precursors, three nutrient precursor substances have been under serious investigation since the early 1970s (Fernstrom and Wurtman, 1971; Wurtman et al, 1974).

Amino acids tryptophan, tyrosine, phenylalanine, and choline (a lipotropic vitaminlike factor found in lecithin) are the nutrient precursors to major brain neurotransmitters: tryptophan is synthesized into serontonin in certain neurons; L-tyrosine and L-phenylalanine are used in the synthesis of the catecholamine neurotransmitters dopamine, norepinephrine, and epinephrine in other neuronal cell populations; and in still other cells, choline is the substrate for synthesis of the neurotransmitter acetylcholine. Measurement of plasma and brain precursor levels of these substances following ingestion or other administration in study animals (rats) has provided encouraging information so that some clinical trials (human) have been undertaken. The results in the human studies are evaluated combining the information on plasma levels with affective quality and cognitive change. Such empirical and experimental evidence suggests that the altered biochemistry in particular brain sites can change brain function, more easily demonstrable in those persons with neurologic, metabolic, or affective disorders (Wurtman, 1982). Results of a study with normal male volunteers, using a double blind crossover design, which investigated the effects of additional oral tyrosine and tryptophan (with regular meals) led to conclusions concerning differential effects on brain and peripheral sympathetic activity (Benedict et al., 1983). These authors postulate "that dietary tyrosine supplementation in man causes an increase in brain catecholmaine activity which in turn leads to a decrease in sympathetic activity as evidenced by the decrease in plasma catecholamines" (p. 429).

Nutrition and Depression—Complex Relationships

That there exists a dynamic interaction between nutritional status and depression has been documented and discussed. Malnutrition, a widespread condition among the late-middle-aged and older populations, may initiate or exacerbate emotional and mental disturbances. In turn, depressive illness and other emotional or mental disorders may trigger or aggravate an already existing malnourished state. Social, societal, and other health-related factors impinge on both nutrition and depression and confound the diagnostic and therapeutic approaches. The data are nevertheless suggestive, even persuasive.

When the benefits and disadvantages of drug or electroconvulsive therapy for depression are carefully weighed, the effort and cost essential in the continued search for efficacious alternative, nontoxic therapies appear modest. Side-effects of traditional drug treatment, which can include confusion, weight gain, dry mouth, nausea, constipation, sexual problems, and at times untoward heart and kidney effects, resulted in a dropout rate of 50 percent in one study (Trafford, 1983). Recognition that different types of depression respond uniquely to particular therapies has intensified attempts in the use of varied therapies: psychotherapy, electroconvulsive, artificial solar-lite, sleep deprivation and nutrient precursors (Benedict et al., 1983; Trafford, 1983; Wurtman, 1982). In a report of the proceedings of the 1981 annual meeting of the New Clinical Drug Evaluation Unit of the Pharmacologic and Somatic Treatment Research Branch, National Institute of Mental Health, some important methodologic suggestions were made concerning research in neurotransmitter precursors for the treatment of depression (Gelenberg et al., 1982). In addition to widely recognized clinical research procedures in depression, it was noted that future research on precursors would be more useful if attention were given to "plasma amino acid levels, urine and possible cerebrospinal fluid (CSF) amino metabolites, careful control of diet, and attention to optimal level of drug dosages.

Difficulties in diagnosis of depression among elders arise from the similarity in symptomology among malnutrition, grief, early dementia, other systemic disorders, isolation or alienation, and the purposeful masking by the patient of affective disturbances with physical complaints that are supposedly more acceptable and expected in the later years. Moreover, the clinical subtypes of depression make it necessary to consider a variety of therapies, since particular subtypes respond to one or several nutrient precursors or combination of nutrient precursor and drug.

McCarty (1981) suggests that there be "nutritional insurance" supplementation as an integral part of preventive medicine and an important public health measure for all ages. Alfin-Slater and Jelliffe (1983) discuss the life-saving benefits and risks of total parenteral nutrition with institutionalized persons (hospitals, nursing homes, etc.) and note that nutrition, as part of hospital support services, may result in long-delayed recognition of nutrition in the prevention of disease as well as therapy regarding disease, surgery, radiation therapy, chemotherapy and any other debilitating treatment. They and others also hope for the integration of preventive nutritional principles as part of medical and psychiatric practice (Butler, 1977; Richmond, 1979; Weg, 1980a,b, 1983). (See Table 8.7).

TABLE 8.7

GUIDELINES AND MEAL PATTERNS FOR THE MIDDLE AND LATER YEARS

Daily Nutrition
Try, each day, for at least:

- 1 serving each meal of whole grain cereal, bread, or macaroni product
- 2 glasses of skim milk, or its equivalent, such as milk shake, soups, pudding, custard made with skim milk; ice milk; low fat cheeses such as cottage, hoop, or farmer
- 2 servings of meat or meat substitutes of high-quality protein: lean beef, veal, or lamb (preferably a maximum of 2 times/week), fish, poultry, peas, beans, legumes, nuts, seeds; eggs (not more than 3 times/week)
- 2 servings of fresh fruit including at least one that is especially rich in vitamin C— e.g. grapefruit, orange, cantaloupe, papaya, guava, strawberries
- 2 servings of vegetables, one of which should be a leafy, dark green type—e.g. spinach, romaine lettuce
- 6–8 glasses of liquids, including water. Weak tea or herb tea, decaffeinated coffee, skim milk, consomme, or other light, nonfatty soups, fruit juices, and watery fruits (watermelon) and vegetables all contribute to this total.

Note:

- Nonfat dry milk is useful as a protein supplement in soups, other fluid drinks, casseroles, or mixed into water for reconstituted milk.
- Eat a wide variety of foods. Use fresh foods whenever possible.
- Minimize or eliminate the use of refined sugar and salt.

Methods of Preparation

- Broiling is superior to frying. Frying increases the fat load of the meal, increasing empty calories, and makes food harder to digest.
- Baking is superior to boiling for preserving whatever vitamins exist. Boiling tends to lose vitamins of food to the water, which is usually discarded.
- Remove excess fat present close to skin of poultry, and on meats to insure the excellent source of essential amino acids without the potentially harmful fat food.

Note

- An average serving of bread is 1 slice.
- An average serving of cereal is $\frac{1}{2}$ to $\frac{3}{4}$ cup.
- An average serving of fruits or vegetables is approximately $\frac{1}{2}$ to $\frac{3}{4}$ cup.
- An average serving of cooked meat is 3 oz.

234

TABLE 8.7 *(continued)*

Meal Pattern Suggestions

Breakfast	*Lunch*

Fresh fruit
Egg or cereal[a] or both
Whole wheat toast or bread and margarine
Artificially sweetened jam or jelly occasionally
Skim milk, weak tea, decaffeinated coffee

Salad[b]
Main dish—meat or poultry or cheese
Green or yellow vegetable
Whole wheat bread or roll and margarine
Fresh fruit
Skim milk, weak tea, decaffeinated coffee

Dinner

Salad[b]
Main dish (meat, fish, poultry, or cheese)
Yellow or green vegetable
Baked potato
Whole wheat bread or roll with margarine

Dessert: fresh fruit and ice milk or plain cookies (no sugar icing or creamy filling)
Skim milk, weak tea, decaffeinated coffee

Source: Modified from Weg, R.B. *Nutrition and the Later Years.* Lexington, Mass.: Lexington Books, 1979, pp. 154, 155.

[a] Cereals, preferably whole grain and hot; if cold, nonsugared

[b] Salads: one (1) salad/day is generally adequate to provide its quota of vitamins, minerals, and fiber. Important that a mixture of leafy vegetables be included: dark green spinach and a variety of lettuce.

Snacks, e.g., carrots, celery, unsweetened grapefruit or apple juice, an orange or tomato, could make healthful additions to daily food intake, modified and selected according to individual caloric and specific nutrient needs.

Some people feel better, and use food more satisfactorily if total intake is divided into five or six small meals. This may be advantageous to digestion, to reducing over-eating tendency, or hunger pangs over a period of several hours.

Investigation of the dietary role in brain function is more than a pursuit for knowledge for its own sake, since the manipulation of dietary intake provides hope for intervention and individual control of brain function and disorders. Consequences of nutritional adequacy include support for emotional, mental, and physical functional capacities, and may contribute measurably to the diminution or prevention of human suffering and waste characteristic of brain deterioration and disease in the later years.

REFERENCES

Akiskal, H.S., and McKinney, W.T. Overview of recent research in depression. *Archives of General Psychiatry*, 1975, 32:285.

Alfin-Slater, R., and Jelliffe, D. More on total parenteral nutrition. *Los Angeles Times Home Magazine*, October 23, 1983, pp. 40, 43.

Altman, H., Mehta, D., Evanson, R.C., and Slettin, I.W. Behavioral effects of drug therapy on psychogeriatric inpatients. II: Multivitamin supplement. *Journal of the American Geriatrics Society*, 1973, 21:249–52.

Anderson, G.H. Diet, neurotransmitter and brain function. *British Medical Bulletin*, 1981, 37:95–100.

Andres, R. Influence of obesity on longevity in the aged. In Borek, C., Fenogleo, C. M., and King D. W. (Eds.), *Aging, Cancer and Cell Membranes*. New York: Thieme, 1980, pp. 238–46.

Atkinson, R.M., and Ringuette, E.L. A survey of biographical and psychological features in extraordinary fatness. *Psychological Medicine* 1967, 29:121.

Baker, H., Frank, O., Louria, D.B., Jaslow, S.P., and Third, I. Vitamin profiles in elderly persons living at home or in nursing homes, versus profile in healthy young people. *Journal of the American Geriatric Society*, 1979, 27:444.

Beauchene, R.E., and Davis, T.A. The nutritional status of aged in the U.S.A. *Age*, 1979, 2:23–28.

Benedict, C.R., Anderson, G.H., and Sole, M.J. The influence of oral tyrosine and tryptophan feeding on plasma catecholamines in man. *American Journal of Clinical Nutrition*, 1983, 38:429–35.

Biena, R., Ratcliff, S., Barbour, G.L., and Kumner, M. Malnutrition in the hospitalized geriatric patient. *Journal of the American Geriatric Society*, 1982, 30:433.

Birkmayer, W., and Riederer, P. Biochemical post-mortem findings in depressed patients. *Journal of Neurological Transmission*. 1975, 37:95.

Blackburn, H. Coronary disease prevention: controversy and professional attitudes. *Advances in Cardiology*, 1977, 20:10.

Burkitt, D.P. Diseases of affluence. In Rose, J. (Ed.), *Nutrition and Killer Diseases: The Effects of Dietary Factors on Fatal Chronic Diseases*. Park Ridge, NJ: Noyes Publications, 1982, pp. 1–7.

Butler, R.N. *Statement before the Select Committee on Nutrition and Human Needs*, U.S. Senate, September 23, 1977.

Camp, J. *Magic, Myth and Medicine*. New York: Taplinger, 1974.

Clements, F.W. Nutrition 7: Vitamin and mineral supplementation. *Medical Journal of Australia*, 1975, 1:575.

Davis, A.K., and Davis, R.L. Food facts, fads, fallacies, and folklore of the elderly. In Hsu, J., and Davis, R. (Eds.), *Handbook of Geriatric Nutrition*. Park Ridge, N.J.: Noyes Publications, 1981, pp, 8–15.

Davis, K.L., Berger, P.A., and Hollister, L.E. Choline for tardive dyskinesia. *New England Journal of Medicine* 1975, 293:152.

Dobbing, J. Undernutrition and the developing brain. In Himwich, W.A. (Ed.), *Developmental Neurobiology*. Springfield, Ill.: Thomas, 1970, pp. 241–246.

Dreyfus, P.M. Nutritional disorders of the nervous system. In Hodges, R.E. (Ed.), *Nutrition: Metabolic and Clinical Applications*. New York: Plenum, 1979.

Dychtwald, K. *Bodymind*. New York: Jove, 1978.

Eckhardt, M.J. Consequences of alcohol and other drug use in the aged. In Behnke, J.A., Finch, C.E., and Moment, G.B. (Eds.), *The Biology of Aging*. New York: Plenum, 1978, pp. 191–204.

Exton-Smith, A.N. Nutritional problems of elderly population. In Hawkins, W.W. (Ed.), *Nutrition of the Aged*. Quebec: Nutrition Society of Canada, 1978, pp. 66–76.

Farquhar, J.W. *The American Way of Life Need Not Be Hazardous to Your Health*. New York: Norton, 1978.

Fernstrom, J.D. Food and brain function. *Professional Nutritionist*, 1979, 11:5.

Fernstrom, J.D., and Wurtman, R.J. Brain serotonin content: physiological dependence on plasma tryptophan levels. *Science*, 1971, 173:149.

Fries, J.F. Aging, natural death and the compression of morbidity. *England Journal of Medicine*, 1980, 303:130.

Garetz, F.K. Breaking the dangerous cycle of depression and faulty nutrition. *Geriatrics*, 1976, 31:73.

Gelenberg, A.J., Gibson, C.J., and Wojcik, J.D.: Neurotransmitter precursors for the treatment of depression. Annual NCDEU Meeting, 1981, Abridged Proceedings. *Psychotherapeutic Pharmacology Bulletin* 1982, 18:7.

Gordon, T., Shurtleff, D. Means at each examination and inter-examination variation of specified characteristics: Framingham Study Exam 1 to Exam 10. In Kannel, W.B., and Gordon, T. (Eds.), *The Framingham Study: An Epidemiological Investigation of Cardiovascular Disease*. DHEW Pub. No. (NIH)74-478. Washington, D.C.: U. S. Government Printing Office, 1973.

Gruen, P.H., Sachar, E.J., Altman, N., et al. Growth hormone responses to hypoglycemia in postmenopausal depressed women. *Archives of General Psychiatry*, 1975, 32:31.

Harman, D. Free radical theory of aging: effect of the amount and degree of unsaturation of dietary fat on mortality rate. *Journal of Gerontology*, 1971, 26:451.

Hastings, A.C., Fadiman, J., Gordon, J.S. *Health for the Whole Person*. Boulder, Colo.: Westview Press, 1980.

Hubel, D.H. The brain. *Scientific American*, 1979, 241:45.

Jacobs, S., and Ostfeld, A.M. An epidemiological review of the mortality of bereavement. *Psychosomatic Medicine* 1977, 39:344.

Jarrett, R.J. Diabetes mellitus and nutrition. In Rose, J. (Ed.), *Nutrition and Killer Diseases: The Effects of Dietary Factors on Fatal Chronic Diseases*. Park Ridge, N.J.: Noyes Publications, 1982, pp. 107–15.

Jarvik, M. A survey of drug effects upon cognitive activities of the aged. In Eisdorfer, C., and Fann, W.E. (Eds.), *Psychopharmacology and Aging Advances in Behavioral Biology*, vol. 6. New York: Plenum, 1973, pp. 129–44.

Jowsey, J. Why is mineral nutrition important in osteoporosis? *Geriatrics*, 1978, 33:39–42, 47–48.

Kasl, S.V., Ostfeld, A.M., Brody, G.M., Snell, L., and Price, C.A. Effects of "involuntary" relocation on the health and behavior of the elderly. In Haynes, S.G., and Feinleib, M. (Eds.), *Second Conference on the Epidemiology of Aging*: *Proceedings*. National Institutes of Health, Pub. #80-969, 1980, pp. 211–35.

Kent, S. New treatments for depression. *Geriatrics*, 1982, 37:149.

Kolata, G.B. Brain biochemistry: effects of diet. *Science*, 1976, 192:41.

Krehl, W.A. The nutritional epidemiology of cardiovascular disease. *New York Academy of Science Annals*, 1977, 300:335.

Krehl, W.A. Role of nutrition in preventing disease. In Slavkin, H.C. (Ed.), *New Horizons in Nutrition for the Health Professions. University of Southern California Journal of Continuing Dental Education*, 1980, 1:72.

Lawton, A.H. *Nutrition Related Diseases of the Aged*. In Hsu, J., and Davis, R. (Eds.), *Handbook of Geriatric Nutrition*. Park Ridge, N.J.: Noyes Publications, 1981, pp. 266–77.

Lewin, R. Overblown report distorts obesity risks. *Science*, 1981, 211:258.

Lloyd, K.J., Farley, I.J., and Deck, J.H.N. Serotonin and 5-hydroxyindolacetic acid in discrete areas of the brainstem of suicide victims and control victims. *Advances in Biochemistry and Psychopharmacology*, 1974, 11:387.

Luce, G.G. *Your Second Life*. New York: Dell, 1976.

Lytle, L.D., and Altar, A. Diet, central nervous system, and aging. *Federation Proceedings*, 1979, 38:2017.

Maas, J.W. Biogenic amines and depression: biochemical and pharmacological separation of two types of depression. *Archives of General Psychiatry* 1975, 32:1357.

McCarty, M.F. Point of view—a role for "nutritional insurance" supplementation in preventive medicine. *Medical Hypotheses*, 1981, 7:171.

Mitra, M.L. Confusional states in relation to vitamin deficiencies in the elderly. *Journal of the American Geriatric Society*, 1971, 89:536.

National Academy of Sciences (National Research Council). *Diet, Nutrition, and Cancer*. Washington, D.C.: National Academy Press, 1982.

Natow, A.B., and Heslin, J. *Geriatric Nutrition*. Boston: CBI, 1980.

News and Comment. Report details diet-cancer connection. *Nutrition Action* 1982, 9.

Nowak, T.S., Munro, H.N. Effects of protein-calorie malnutrition on biochemical aspects of brain development. In Wurtman, R.J., and Wurtman, J.J. (Eds.), *Nutrition and Brain*, vol. 2, New York: Raven, 1977, pp. 193–260.

O'Hanlon, C., and Kohrs, M.B., Dietary studies of older Americans. *American Journal of Clinical Nutrition*, 1978, 31:1257.

Ossofsky, J., and Anderson, A.A. *A Nutrition Program for the Elderly*. Washington, D.C.: The National Council on the Aging, April 1972.

Ostfeld, A.M. Depression, disability and demise in older people. In Breslau, L.D., and Haug, M.R. (Eds.), *Depression and Aging: Causes, Care, and Consequences*. New York: Springer, 1983, pp. 244–55.

Overton, M., and Lukert, B. *Clinical Nutrition*. Chicago: Year Book Medical Publishers, 1977.

Pelletier, K.R. *Mind as Healer, Mind as Slayer: A Holistic Approach to Preventing Stress Disorders*. New York: Delta, 1977.

Posner, B.M. *Nutrition and the Elderly*. Lexington, Mass.: Lexington Books, 1979.

Prange, A.J. Pharmacotherapy of Depression. In Flack, F.F., and Draghi, S.C. (Eds.), *The Nature and Treatment of Depression*. New York, Wiley, 1975.

Prehoda, R.W. *Extended Youth*, New York: G.P. Putnam's Sons, 1968.

Richmond, J. *Healthy People: The Surgeon General's Report on Health Promotion and Disease Prevention*. Washington, D.C.: U.S. Department of Health, Education, and Welfare, 1979.

Robertson, T.L., Kato, H., Gordon, T., Kagan, A., Rhoads, G.G., Land, C.E., Worth, R.M., Belsky, J.L., Dock, D.S., Mityanishi, M., and Kawamato, S. Epidemiologic studies of coronary heart disease and stroke in Japanese men living in Japan, Hawaii and California: coronary heart disease risk factors in Japan and Hawaii. *American Journal of Cardiology*, 1977, 39:244.

Roe, D.A. *Drug-Induced Nutritional Deficiencies*. Westport, Conn.: Avi, 1976.

Roe, D.A. Drugs, diet and nutrition. *Contemporary Nutrition*, 1978, 3:1.

Rosenfeld, A. *Prolongevity*. New York: Alfred A. Knopf, 1976.

Salzman, C., and Shader, R.I. Depression in the elderly. I: Relationship between depression, psychologic defense mechanisms and physical illness. *Journal of the American Geriatric Society*, 1978, 26:253.

Sebrell, W.H., and Haggerty, J.J. (Eds.). *Food and Nutrition*, rev. ed. Alexandria, Va.: Time-Life Books, 1980, ch. 1, pp. 8–31.

Shekelle, R.B., Raynor, W.J., Jr., Ostfeld, A.M., Garron, D.C., Bieliaus-kas, L.A., Liu, S.C., Maliza, D., and Paul, O. Psychological depression and 17-year risk of death from cancer. *Psychosomatic Medicine*, 1981, 43:117.

Shoemaker, W.T., and Bloom, F.E. Effect of undernutrition and brain morphology. In Wurtman, R.J., and Wurtman, J.J. (Eds.), *Nutrition and Brain*, vol. 2. New York: Raven, 1977, pp. 147–92.

Snyder, S.H. Neuroleptic drugs and neurotransmitter receptors. *Journal of Continuing Education in Psychiatry*, 1978, 39:21.

Stenback, A. Depression and suicidal behavior in old age. In Birren, J.A., and Sloane, R. (Eds.), *Handbook of Mental Health and Aging*. New York: Free Press, 1980, pp. 616–52.

Sun, A.Y., and Sun, G.Y. Effect of dietary vitamin E and other antioxidants on aging process. In Roberts, J., Adelman, R.C., Cristofalo, V.J. (Eds.), *Advances in Experimental Medicine and Biology*, vol. 97. New York: Plenum Press, 1978, pp. 285–90.

Tannahill, R. *Food in History*. New York: Stein and Day, 1973.

Trafford, A. New hope for the depressed. *U.S. News and World Report*, January 24, 1983.

Trimmer, E.J. *Rejuvenation*. New York: A.S. Barnes, 1970.

Turner, R.W.D. Diet and epidemic coronary heart disease. In Rose, J. (Ed.), *Nutrition and Killer Diseases: The Effects of Dietary Factors on Fatal Chronic Diseases*. Park Ridge, N.J.: Noyes Publications, 1982, pp. 30–49.

van Praag, H.M. Significance of biochemical parameters in the diagnosis, treatment and prevention of depressive disorders. *Biological Psychiatry*, 1977, 12:101.

van Praag, H.M., and de Haan, S. Chemoprophylaxis of depressions: an attempt to compare lithium with 5-hydroxytryptophan. *Acta Psychiatrica Scandinavica*, 1981, 63:191.

Walford, R.L. *Maximum Life Span*. New York: Norton, 1983.

Walker, W.J. Changing U.S. life style and declining vascular mortality—a retrospective. *New England Journal of Medicine*, 1983, 308:649.

Walker, W.J. Changing U.S. life style and declining vascular mortality: cause or coincidence. *New England Journal of Medicine*, 1977, 297:162.

Watkin, D.M. Introduction: modern nutrition for those who are already old. In Hsu, J., and Davis, R. (Eds.). *Handbook of Geriatric Nutrition*. Park Ridge, N.J.: Noyes Publication, 1981, pp. 1–5.

Weg, R.B. Drug interaction with the changing physiology of the aged: practice and potential. In Kayne, R.C. (Ed.), *Drugs and the Elderly*. Los Angeles: Andrus Gerontology Center, University of Southern California Press, 1978, pp. 103–42.

Weg, R.B. *Nutrition and the Later Years*. Lexington, Mass.: Lexington Books, 1979.

Weg, R.B. Prolonged mild nutritional deficiencies: significance for health maintenance. *Journal of Nutrition for the Elderly*, 1980a, 1:3.

Weg, R.B. Changing physiology of age: changing nutrition. In Slavkin, H.C. (Ed.), *New Horizons in Nutrition for the Health Professions. University of Southern California Journal of Continuing Education*, 1980b, 1:38.

Weg, R.B. *Changing Years: Changing Nutritional Needs*. A position paper for General Foods, 1983.

Weinsier, R.L., Hunker, E.M., Krumdiek, C.L., and Butterworth, C.E. Patients during the course of hospitalization. In Cunningham, J.J. (Ed.), *Controversies in Clinical Nutrition*. Philadelphia: G. F. Stickey, 1980, pp. 44–52.

Winick, M. Nutrition and mental development. *Medical Clinics of North America*, 1970, 54:1413.

Winick, M. Nutrition and brain development. *Natural History*, 1980, 89:6.

Wurtman, R.J. Nutrients that modify brain function. *Scientific American*, 1982, 246:5.

Wurtman, R.J., Cohen, E.L., and Fernstrom, J.D. Control of brain neurotransmitter synthesis by precursor availability and food consumption. In Usdin, E., Hambun, D.A., and Barchas, J.D. (Eds.), *Neuroregulators and Psychiatric Disorders*. New York: Oxford University Press, 1977, pp. 103–21.

Wurtman, R.J., Hefti, F., and Melamed, E. Precursor control of neurotransmitter synthesis. *Pharmacology Review*, 32:315, 1980.

Wurtman, R.J., Larin, F., Mostafapour, S., and Fernstrom, J.D. Brain catechol synthesis: control by brain tyrosine concentration. *Science*, 1974, 185:183–84.

Young, V.R. Nutrition and aging. In Roberts, J., Adelman, R.C., and Cristofalo, V.J. (Eds.), *Advances in Experimental Medical Biology*, vol. 97. New York: Plenum Press, 1978, pp. 85–110.

Young, V.R. Nutrition. In Rowe, J.W. and Besdine, R.W. (Eds.), *Health and Disease in Old Age*. Boston: Little, Brown, 1982a, pp. 317–33.

Young, V.R. Plasma amino acids and proteins. In *Assessing the Nutritional Status of the Elderly—State of the Art*, Report of the Third Ross Roundtable on Medical Issues. Columbus, Ohio: Ross Laboratories, 1982b, pp. 35–38.

9
Exercise

Catherine M. Shisslak
James Utic

In studies to determine which factors are associated with successful aging, group activity and physical activity appear to be two of the strongest contributing factors (Palmore, 1979). Palmore observed that greater physical activity contributed directly to improved physical health and thereby indirectly to mental health and feelings of well-being among the elderly. Despite this finding, research related to the effect of physical activity and exercise on depression has been directed predominantly toward the young or middle-aged person to the exclusion of the older and elderly adults. This research, along with the few investigative endeavors dealing with the effect of exercise on depressed geriatric individuals, will now be discussed.

EXERCISE AND DEPRESSION

Generally speaking, physical activity, and particularly running, has been consistently cited as effective agents in reducing dysphoria among young and middle-aged individuals. Brown and colleagues (1978) investigated the relationship between thrice weekly exercise and depression in 167 college students. Students rated themselves on the Zung Depression Inventory before and after eight weeks of either wrestling, tennis, varied exercises, jogging, or softball. The softball players and joggers showed the greatest reductions. In addition, subjects who initially scored in the range of clinical depression showed a significant reduction in depression with activity. Brown et al. hypothesize that the antidepressant effect of exercise may depend to some degree on the intensity, duration, and frequency of the physical activity. Moreover, on the basis of a study of approximately 700 subjects, they concluded, "We recommend that any rational, safe and effective treatment regime for depression should include a prescription for vigorous exercise to bring about and maintain optimal effective functioning." Greist et al. (1978) found that running was at least as effective as psychotherapy of any duration in alleviating the symptoms of depression for individuals with moderate depression. In addition, Morgan and Pollock (1976) reported a significant reduction in depression in a group of 19 depressed subjects over a six-week endurance training period. Similar changes in a group of undepressed subjects were not observed. The relationship of exercise on depression in a "normal" adult population consisting of 67 college faculty members was also studied by Morgan et al. (1970). Five exercise groups (i.e., circuit training, jogging, swimming, treadmill, and bicycle exercise control were utilized). The researchers concluded that depression and physical fitness were not correlated in normal adult males. When the data were analyzed for those subjects scoring in the depressed range on the Zung Depression Scale at the outset of the physical activity study, however, a significant improvement in depression was apparent. Moreover, none of the subjects had fallen into the depressed range at the study's completion.

Other studies have provided further evidence of the dysphoric reducing effect of exercise. Kavanaugh et al. (1976) administered the Minnesota Multiphasic Personality Inventory (MMPI) to 101 patients 16 to 18 months after they experienced a myocardial infarction. He isolated a population of 56 with severe depression and engaged them in a regular running program. After following these subjects for four years, a significant improvement in the depression score (D) of the MMPI was found while other indexes remained unchanged. These researchers concluded that a correlation between improvement in depression and adherence to an exercise program was apparent. Folkins et al. (1972) found that a sample of college women were less anxious and depressed after taking a semester-long jogging course than before, while Post et al. (1973) noted improvement in their moderately depressed patients who adopted an exercise regimen. In examining the value of exercise on a psychiatric hospital unit, Conroy et al. (1982) found a six-week exercise program to produce substantial decreases in participants' reported depression, and nonsignificant trends toward a decrease in anxiety and an increase in their sense of accomplishment. The program did not, however, ameliorate many disturbing feelings such as anger and fear, nor did it elicit a wide range of positive effects such as cooperation and feelings of acceptance. The authors summarize the results stating, "Our findings certainly confirm other studies in the field that indicate positive effects of exercise on depression. Thus, it appears that a moderate amount of exercise helped relieve depression."

Unfortunately, a large portion of those experiments investigating the effect of exercise in depression have utilized running as the independent physical activity variable. As such, little information is available which is pertinent to geriatric populations, since running is often too vigorous a physical activity for elderly individuals. It is difficult to know, then, the effect exercise has on depression in geriatric populations because physical activity appropriate to this age group has not been utilized when making general statements about exercise's dysphoric reducing effect. As previously mentioned, the literature is lacking sufficient studies investigating the effect of exercise in reducing depression with geriatric populations as well as examining the effectiveness of different modes of age-appropriate physical activity, other than running, on minimizing depression.

Only two studies could be found in the literature which used a geriatric population to examine the effects of exercise on depression. Morgan et al. (1976) conducted a daily exercise routine of walking and stretching with elderly individuals and concluded, "most individuals middle aged and older, participating in regular exercise programs do, in fact feel better and experience a reduction in their dysphoria."

Bennett et al. (1982) conducted a study in which 38 subjects with the mean age of 75.7 years from both institutionalized and noninstitutionalized settings were used. Subjects at each site were assigned to one of the two groups either as an exercise group or control group. The exercise program consisted of two 45-minute sessions per week for eight weeks during which subjects participated in exercise designed to maintain or restore muscle tone, flexibility, and balance. Subjects in the control group were afforded similar social opportunities for the same period of time but did not participate in the exercise program. The Zung Self-Rating Depression Scale was administered to both groups before and after the exercise treatment intervention. The results from this study indicated that among those elderly who exhibited symptoms of depression, there was a significant decrease in their depression level following participation in the organized physical exercise program. No significant decrease in dysphoria was observed among the depressed nonexercise control subjects. Although these two studies provide important information, clearly additional research is needed to make more definitive statements about the effect physical activity has on depressed elderly individuals.

EXERCISE AND ANXIETY

The effects of exercise and anxiety have been explored in numerous studies. These investigations have examined the influences various forms of physical activity have on different populations of people. Overall, most of this research data suggests that exercise is, indeed, effective in reducing anxiety.

Morgan (1968), Byrd (1963), and Brunner (1969) were some of the first investigators to report that physical activity served to reduce anxiety and make participants "feel better." Morgan (1973) employed the State-Trait Anxiety Inventory (STAI) and evaluated state anxiety in 40 adult males before, immediately following, and 20–30 minutes following vigorous physical activity lasting approximately 45 minutes. The findings revealed a significant decrease in anxiety between the pretest and postexercise periods in both subjects falling within the normal range on anxiety, as well as in those classified as high anxious. Moreover, Morgan (1973) evaluated state anxiety with the STAI in 15 adult males before a vigorous workout, immediately following, and 15–30 minutes after the activity. It was found that significant decrements in anxiety occurred in both postexercise settings. Anderson and Morgan (1973) administered the STAI to 17 adult females before and following a treadmill exercise task. They reported that state anxiety decreased significantly in the group collectively, as well as in those subjects who were judged to be clinically anxious as measured by the STAI prior to exercise. An investigation by Mitchum (1976) found a significant decrease in State anxiety as a result of 15 minutes of racquetball activity by 20 adult males and 20 adult females. Similarly, Handlon et al. (1963) reported that bowling reduced anxiety in anxious subjects. In a more recent investigation by Wood (1977) a significant reduction in State anxiety was found for 62 college males, but not for 44 college females following a 12 minute run. Although significant decreases in State anxiety were reported for both high anxious males and females, low anxious males and females experienced a significant increase in State anxiety, although postexercise anxiety levels remained within the normal range.

Driscoll (1976) studied the acute effects of physical exertion versus that of a positive image procedure to reduce anxiety in college students before a major examination. It was concluded that individual exercise as well as the psychotherapy sessions were successful in reducing anxiety. In a further comparison of exercise with other frequently used anxiety-reducing techniques, Bahrke and Morgan (1978) examined the influence of acute physical activity versus that of meditation and relaxation in reducing anxiety. Analysis revealed that a significant reduction in anxiety occurred for each treatment. This occurred in both those subjects falling within the normal range for anxiety, as well as those subjects regarded as high anxious. The authors concluded that acute physical activity, meditation, and a quiet rest were equally effective in reducing anxiety.

Despite the numerous studies verifying the effectiveness of exercise in reducing anxiety, some contradictory findings have been cited. Most noteworthy is that presented by Pitts (1969), Pitts and McClure (1967), and Fink et al. (1969). They suggest that physical activity may not reduce tension or improve subsequent psychological states. Rather, these researchers postulate that physical exertion increases an exercise metabolite known as lactate, which ultimately increases anxiety. Additional research, however, has failed to support this hypothesis consistently.

Unfortunately, much of the work done in the area of anxiety reduction through exercise has not involved the study of elderly populations. Given today's longer life expectancy and the fact that many of the more severe mental health problems are most prevalent in the aged, additional research with geriatric populations seems warranted. Some studies, however, have been conducted investigating the anxiety-reducing effect of exercise on the elderly. DeVries and Adams (1972) reported that exercise has both acute and chronic effects on anxiety reduction. It was found that acute exercise of low intensity was effective in reducing muscle action potentials in older people. Moreover, the acute effects of exercise were compared to the neuropharmacological effects of the tranquilizer Meprobamate. The results indicate that acute exercise was more effective in reducing neuromuscular tension, in the muscle groups investigated, than was the drug. Wiswell (1980) concurs that low-intensity exercise done in chairs has a significant State anxiety-reducing effect in normally healthy subjects between the ages of 65 to 91. Reiter (1981) examined the effect of 10 special exercise sessions on 73 women, aged 65 to 90, to that of an alternative arts and crafts program in which 55 similar aged women participated. The results showed a significant reduction in State anxiety as well as an improvement in feelings of well-being following the exercise program. Furthermore, the exercise group reported feeling more relaxed and less tense, while experiencing improved sleep and vitality during the day. The arts and craft control group did not evidence any of these gains.

EXERCISE AND PERSONALITY CHANGE

The effect of physical fitness and exercise in changing an individual's personality has long been a debated question. Tillman (1965) maintains that basic personality structures do not change as a result of improved physical fitness. However, he holds that mood variables do appear to be altered by changes in fitness. In addition, Morgan (1976) discussed the "personality versus mood" dichotomy in terms of state versus trait variables and emphasizes that physical activity can significantly modify state variables such as anxiety and depression, but not trait variables such as extroversion or introversion. Several studies have been conducted that seem to support this notion. Folkins (1976) compared an exercise group to a control group and found that improvements in physical fitness were accompanied by significant decreases in two mood measures, anxiety and depression, for the exercise group. There was no change, however, for either group in relation to personality measures of adjustment, self-confidence, and body image. This pattern was also supported by Nowlis and Greenberg (1979) and Wilson, et al. (1980).

Despite the hypothesis that only mood states can be changed by physical activity, numerous studies have been conducted which refute this notion. Indeed, the literature suggests a certain interrelatedness of physical fitness and certain aspects of personality. Collingwood and Willett (1971) found significant increases in positive body attitude, positive self-attitude, self-acceptance, and decreases in real versus ideal self-discrepancy for five obese male teenagers involved in a three-week physical training program.

Ismail and Trachtman (1973) studied a group of 60 middle-aged men who jogged three times a week for four months using the Cattell 16/Personality Factor Questionnaire. High and low physical fitness groups were determined, with the low fitness group showing a significant increase in self-efficiency, imaginativeness, and emotional stability following completion of the jogging program. The authors state that the low fitness group approached the high fitness pretest scores on these dimensions by the end of their exercise program. They conclude that unfit normals begin to approach fit normals in certain psychological characteristics as a result of progressive exercise training.

Young and Ismail (1976) investigated personality differences in 90 subjects ages 21 to 61 who were classified as either "high fit" or "low fit." The results indicated that there was an increase in conscientiousness and persistence in adult men after a physical fitness program. In addition, it was found that regardless of age, the high fit group was more intellectually inclined, emotionally stable, composed, self-confident, easygoing, relaxed, less ambitious, and unconventional than the low fit group. Similarly personality changes attributed to exercise were noted by Jette (1975), who found a sample of habitual exercisers significantly more serious and tough minded than a group of nonexercisers.

Unfortunately, the majority of studies investigating the relationship of exercise on personality change have dealt with specific subsets of young athletes and not the elderly. For example, Darden (1972) found body builders to be more silent, reflective, and cautious than the overall population. Hartung and Farge (1977) observed 48 middle-aged runners to be more intelligent, imaginative, reserved, self-sufficient, sober, shy, and forthright than the general population. Participants in wrestling were found to be more tough minded than the norm, but karate participants did not differ from expected values (Kroll and Carlson, 1967). Differences among various stress-seeking athletes were evident of sport parachutists, race drivers, and professional football players. The parachutists and race drivers were similar in possessing qualities of self-sufficiency and independence, while the football players differed greatly in that they were more dependent and expressive. A study of long-distance runners by Burdick and Zloty (1973) found them to be significantly brighter, more imaginative, and forthright than the mean. Morgan (1974), however, stated that the personality characteristics of the long-distance runner were different from other successful athletes in that they were more reserved and introverted than athletes in other disciplines. Like other high-achievement athletes, however, they were similar in maintaining less anxiety and depression than the majority of nonathletes.

It is apparent that despite numerous studies in the area of personality change and exercise, many unanswered questions still remain. First, definitive evidence that changes in personality traits beyond that of mood alteration occur through physical activity has yet to be determined. Second, in those studies describing sports-related personality changes, there is no way of knowing if certain personality types select certain sports activities or if certain sports activities mold certain personality characteristics. These limitations hamper attempts to equate a specific physical activity, and exercise as a whole, with personality changes. Third, the generalizability of results gained from the research investigating exercise in personality change is limited due to the restricted subject sample typically used. Specifically, athletes and young to middle-aged adults comprise the subject populations for the majority of those studies being conducted. Little has been done with the elderly population. Even that research which has been done with geriatric populations is hampered by certain limitations. For example, Stamford et al. (1974) utilized an exercise program with nine male institutionalized geriatric mental patients while including a similar number of patients as controls. Four psychological tests were used in the pre- and post-testing to measure psychological changes due to exercise. Although the authors reported that all the subjects participating in the exercise group experienced a feeling of relaxation and well-being following training, a more specific account of personality changes was not done. In explaining the results, the authors stated that there "was a significant change on two of the four psychological tests," but they then failed to elaborate on how these test differences relate to alterations in personality.

Hammer and Wilmore (1973) found physically fit subjects more expedient and forthright. With additional exercise, the fit group became more trusting and anxious. A wide variety of different aged subjects were used in the study and the authors stated that age was not an important factor when appraising the effectiveness of the exercise program on psychological change. It appears, then, that psychological changes caused by exercise (i.e., expediency, forthrightness) can occur at any age. A major limitation existed, however, in that the oldest subject in the aforementioned study was 59 years old. Hence, generalization of this data to geriatric populations must be cautioned.

Perhaps the best study conducted thus far, in this area, incurred by exercise is that of Buccola and Stone (1975). Thirty-six males between ages of 60 to 79 participated voluntarily in the 14 week program of walk/jogging or cycling. Comparisons after the exercise period indicated that cyclers were more tough minded and overbearing, whereas there were no significant changes in the walk/joggers.

It seems evident that additional research is needed to clarify the confusing status of exercise on an individual's personality. Moreover, this need is accentuated when addressing the role exercise has on altering geriatric subjects' personality traits. Wiswell (1980) in reviewing the research conducted with geriatric populations summarizes: "It appears that 'old' refers to those individuals between the ages of 50 and 75 with no mention of possible benefits to individuals over the age of 75." To Wiswell's knowledge, there are no studies dealing with the psychological effects, either acute or chronic, of exercise training in normal persons over the age of 80. This is a major limitation because many of the more severe mental health problems are more prevalent in the very old age group.

EXERCISE AND PSYCHOBIOLOGY

There is sufficient evidence to suggest significant physiological adaptations to regular exercise that may prove beneficial to mental functioning. These include the improvement in cerebrovascular circulation which is brought about by regular endurance-type exercise, as well as increased neuroendocrine sensitivity and function, and finally a change of emotionality as previously outlined. More specific to the elderly, are the findings that suggest physical exercise may effect mental status in the elderly individual. Data from this area indicates that cardiovascular conditioning influences variables determining cerebrovascular sufficiency (Saltin et al., 1969; De Vries, 1970; Barry et al., 1966; Kjeilberg et al., 1949). Also, there is strong evidence that cardiovascular fitness improves the performance in older subjects on tests of digit span, general information, Ravens Progressive Matrices and Memory for Design, simple and choice reaction time, and attentional capacity (Stamford et al., 1974; Powell, 1974; Spirduso, 1980; Hawkins and Capaldi, 1982).

This evidence supports the fact that cerebrovascular insufficiency increases between middle and old age. The decline in mental functioning associated with cerebrovascular insufficiency may be attenuated by cardiovascular conditioning, which can enhance cerebrovascular sufficiency and reduce these age-related declines in mental functioning.

More direct studies of exercise levels in the elderly are related to cognitive performance (Powell, 1974). Kendrick and Moyes (1979) also found older subjects who scored high on activity scales to score equally high on cognitive performance tests as compared to low activity subjects.

Deterioration in psychological functioning does not seem to occur universally. Kendrick (1975) has challenged the myth that deterioration is inevitable. Birren (1965) and Szafran (1968) have shown that healthy, active individuals often show slight and few decrements in the later adult years. This research is fraught with problems, however. Powell (1975) has pointed out that although regular submaximal exercise may improve short-term cognitive functioning and long-term training may have a positive effect in maintaining cognitive status with advanced aging, there are reasons for caution. Severe exercise stress, particularly with the sedentary and untrained individual may have a detrimental effect upon cognitive functioning by reducing the cerebral metabolic rate of oxygen.

Scarborough (1977) demonstrated a positive correlation between levels of everyday activity, i.e., shopping, playing bingo, etc. and IQ for two subtests on the Kendrick battery. Another important study by Spirduso reported by Stelmach and Diewart (1977) looked at physically active men in two age groups, 20–30 years and 50–70 years, and contrasted them with inactive participants. They showed that both groups of young men processed information faster than the older groups, but that physically active older men were superior to the inactive older groups. Thus, an active life-style that stresses fitness is a prime factor in reducing the aging process. This is reflected in differential performance on such tests as simple reaction time, choice reaction times, and movement time tests.

Young and Ismail (1976) sought to determine the discriminate ability of selected biochemical compounds and personality characteristics between high and low fitness groups before and after an exercise program. Their subjects were between the ages of 21 and 61 years. The results showed two groups to be different in terms of physical fitness as shown by significant differences at pretest on measures of percentage lean body weight, blood pressure, VO_2max and physical fitness scores. Both groups underwent beneficial physiological changes from pre- to posttesting, although this was most pronounced in the low fit group. A multivariate discriminate function analysis showed that the highly fit individuals were more imaginative, adventurous, and trustful and lower on catacholimines, glucose, and cholesterol levels and higher on testosterone than low fit individuals. Thus, there is a strong interrelatedness between physiological, biochemical, and personality factors as related to established levels of fitness and changes thereof.

EXERCISE AND STRESS

Some researchers have proposed that moderate running by well-trained runners plays a significant role in reducing a stress response to subsequently introduced stressors. It has been demonstrated that regular aerobic exercise, with its requirements for sympathetic nervous system (SNS) activation and associated endocrine activity, leads to chronic reduction in the individual's experienced stress response to psychological stressors.

Another important benefit of exercise and subsequent relaxation is the potential for these interventions to assist older individuals in coping with stress both physically and emotionally. It has been hypothesized that an interaction of the following mechanisms may be the result of increasing resistance to stress: 1) Regular endurance activity may increase the efficiency and coordination of efferent signals from the brain. This change in efficiency may then improve nerve conduction and increase receptor responsivity. 2) Regular exercise may influence cellular metabolic processes and therefore require lower secretion rates of various hormones. 3) Regular exercise has the effect of improving peripheral vascular circulation and reducing vascular resistance. Thus the increased vasculature serves as a buffer system by which stressor substances are utilized, thereby reducing the effects of endocrine hypersecretion during stressful situations and exercise. 4) Acute effects of mild exercise, which would increase hormone utilization, and relaxation techniques, which could reduce hormone secretion, could influence the state of arousal, thereby affecting psychomotor efficiency (Wiswell, 1980). It has been hypothesized that exercise and relaxation may be important mediators in central control mechanisms to reduce the psychological impact of stress and further keep the body in metabolic balance (Wiswell, 1980)

NEUROTRANSMITTERS AND NEUROMODULATORS AS A RESPONSE TO EXERCISE

The physiological changes during exercise include changes in heart rate, blood pressure, and circulation. Substrate mobilization and utilization have also been attributed at least, in part, to changes in plasma, norepinephrine, and epinephrine. Exercise clearly affects plasma, norepinephrine, epinephrine (Christensen et al., 1979) and dopamine (VanLoon et al., 1979) and its effect is dependent on the duration and intensity of exercise (Christensen et al., 1979; Hartley et al., 1972; Robertson et al., 1979). Short-term high-intensity exercise such as vigorous stair climbing has been shown to result in a rise in both plasma, norepinephrine, and epinephrine (Dimsdale and Moss, (1980). The effect on norepinephrine is greater than on epinephrine, indicating a relatively greater contribution of the sympathetic nervous system. Hartley et al. (1972) examined the effect of short-term bicycle work at mild, moderate, and heavy work loads. Mild exercise had little effect on plasma norepinephrine, but moderate and heavy work loads resulted in significant elevations. Only heavy work significantly elevated epinephrine concentration.

Prolonged exercise results in a rise in both plasma norepinephrine and epinephrine (Christensen et al., 1979). The rise in norepinephrine is apparently associated with increasing heart rate and with the pulmonary oxygen saturation (Christensen et al., 1979).

Plasma dopamine concentrations are reportedly affected by exercise. VanLoon et al. (1979) reports significant elevations in plasma dopamine, as well as in norepinephrine and epinephrine, at heart rates of 150 percent of resting and at maximal. The functional significance of the rise in dopamine, however, is unknown.

The precise physiological role of the endorphins remains unclear, and little information is available concerning the interaction of endorphins and the stress of running. Pargman and Baker (1980) formed the hypothesis that endorphins are involved in producing the psychological adaptation called "the runner's high" apparently experienced by some distance runners. It apparently occurs in some distance runners who have been regularly running long distances for an extended period of time.

The postulated role of endorphins in producing the high is based largely on reports that endogenous and ejected endorphins produce an analgesic state (Bloom et al., 1976; Foley et al., 1979). The endorphins, in response to stress, typically produce a cataleptic state accompanied by a reduction in responsiveness to external stimuli. Whether this describes a state encompassed by the term *runner's high* is unclear.

A rise in endorphin levels in exercise would be necessary for the endorphins to play a role in a response mentioned or in others such as thermoregulation during exercise. Appenzeller et al. (1980) have demonstrated a statistically significant rise in serum beta endorphin levels as a result of long-distance running. This increase is intriguing and at least allows for speculation about the interaction of the endogenous opiatelike substance in exercise. The physiological significance of the rise, however, remains unclear and awaits further research. However, the implications of endorphin production as a side-effect in exercise in the elderly could obviate the effects of pain from other simultaneous conditions and potentially increase mood.

EXERCISE AND HEART DISEASE

Rehabilitation after myocardial infarction is directed at returning a patient to previous levels of physiological, vocational, and psychosocial functioning. Physical conditioning has been used as a major rehabilitation adjunct in achieving these goals. The obvious benefits from exercise relevant to these are 1) significant reduction of systolic blood pressure and heart rate at rest and comparable levels of submaximal work; 2) significant increases in peak oxygen uptake; 3) significant decreases in myocardial work at rest and submaximal work; 4) significant changes in body composition; i.e., reduced fat and increased muscle mass; 5) changes in central and peripheral circulation comparable with those observed in otherwise healthy physically active subjects; 6) improved life-style characterized by more regulated eating patterns, longer and more restful sleep, a more relaxed pace of life, and greater ease in handling daily conflicts at work and at home; and 7) improved sexual adjustment. Stern and Cleary (1981) have demonstrated in a middle-age and older group (30 to 64) with documented myocardial infarctions that low-level exercise is sufficient to stimulate positive psychosocial, sexual, and vocational changes. Others (Pollock and Schmidt, 1979) have demonstrated the benefits of exercise following myocardial infarction to enhance psychosocial and physical functioning.

EXERCISE AND THE ELDERLY

It can be said that an individual's psychological well-being is the result of an interplay between physical and mental health. From the data presented thus far, exercise and various physical activities have been reported to be important in the maintenance of one's mental and physical health. A major problem occurs, however, with the elderly in that exercise is not seen as very important in the lives of progressively older adults. Gordon and Gaitz (1977) examined age differences in physical activity with adult men and women. This was accomplished by analyzing differences in the level of activity ranging from passive and sedentary to vigorous and sensation-seeking, and secondly by establishing a typology of activities, including distinctions among noncompetitive, competitive, solitary, and group activities. The results indicated that with older age the level of activity was found to decrease, while the number of passive-solitary activities increased despite the greater opportunities for social leisure activities available in retirement. Moreover, the life satisfaction of older adults who had lower levels of activity was less than that of older adults who reported relatively high levels of activity and social involvement. However, with those individuals who expressed the greatest satisfaction due to high levels of physical activity, greater concern over the perceived physical health risk for such activity was also depicted. The question remains then, as to whether these perceived risks are justified, and how much and what types of physical activities elderly individuals can undertake to optimize psychological well-being. The remainder of this chapter will therefore be devoted to answering this question.

Perhaps part of the question as to whether the benefits of exercise are outweighed by the risks of increased physical activity in the elderly can be answered by historians. Investigators studying ancient societies with long life expectancies have found one interesting similarity among the various long-lived communities. These inhabitants, across all ages, had a very high level of physical activity. This finding has led some gerontologists to conclude that "exercise is the closest thing to an anti-aging pill now available." De Vries and Adams (1972) found that older people can recapture at least part of their youthful energy with special exercise programs. Specifically, they found that a vigorous six week regimen of toe touching, jogging, and swimming for one hour, three times a week transformed a volunteer group of more than 100 men ranging in age from 52 to 87 on several dimensions. Their hearts and lungs functioned better, the flow of oxygen through the body improved, and their blood pressure dropped. Moreover, the men reported that they were able to work longer and more efficiently, along with experiencing improved sex lives.

In addition to the beneficial consequences physical activity has had on older individuals' physical health, Joesting (1978), in a comprehensive review, found no reported studies which indicated that physical exercise had an adverse effect on mental health. Hence, perceived risks of high levels of physical activity leading to detrimental physical or mental health among the elderly has yet to be verified. Nevertheless, the question remains as to what types of exercise elderly individuals can realistically engage in. This question is confounded further by the inevitable physical limitations and restrictions that advanced age brings. Data compiled by the National Counsel of Aging (1978) states that while most older individuals have no serious physical activity limitation, the percentage of persons with *some* degree of limitation is substantial. Approximately 40 percent of the elderly are reported to be limited to some extent by health restrictions (i.e., heart condition, 52 percent; diabetes, 34 percent; asthma, 27 percent; and arthritis, 23 percent) in carrying out major activities. In addition, this report assessed restrictions in the general mobility of the elderly stating "most older persons—about 82 percent—do not suffer from serious handicaps in mobility, but the extent to which the elderly are limited in this regard is substantial when compared to other segments of the population." These facts suggest that the majority of those individuals over the age of 65 do not have serious limitations in the activities they can physically participate in, nor do they experience significant restrictions in their general mobility. Thus, while the vast majority of elderly individuals are physically capable of being involved and benefiting from exercise programs, a small but significant segment of geriatric individuals do possess physical limitations that minimize the overall effectiveness exercise can maintain in their lives. Despite this variance in the physical capabilities of the elderly, forms of physical activity can nevertheless be engaged in that would promote beneficial physical and mental health consequences no matter what the physical conditions of the elderly individual.

EXERCISE PROGRAMS FOR THE ELDERLY

Although the research to date on physical and mental health does not show consistent findings, it is safe to say that physical defect, illness, and immobility are related to poor mental health and social maladjustment. Thus, if exercise has a positive effect on improving physical and mental health, these changes may result in improved overall mental functioning. The major questions facing health professionals dealing with the elderly concern issues of motivating older individuals to exercise and what type of exercise or activity strategy best fits that individual. Variables that contribute to poor exercise motivation in a younger population may be quite different in the older population, especially for those individuals with some type of physical disability. For this reason it is very important to individualize an exercise program to the specific needs of the older individual. It should be stressed that, while running is still the most popular form of exercise, there are many alternative methods for both exercise and relaxation. An individual's feelings about the particular exercise and probability for performing this exercise are the most important variables to consider.

Despite the fact that most older persons do not consider themselves to be seriously handicapped in pursuing normal activities, limitations of activities nevertheless do emerge as a major consequence of both the chronic and acute health problems facing the older individual. Though most older persons have no serious limitations, the percentage of persons with some degree of limitation is substantial. It is more important, however, to evaluate the impact of these various health conditions on the daily lives of older persons by assessing not only their self-perceptions of health status but the extent to which their daily activities are limited in terms of general mobility. Most older persons—about 82 percent—do not suffer from serious handicaps in mobility.

The major cause of mobility limitation among the elderly are arthritis and rheumatism, impairment of the lower extremities, heart conditions, and strokes.

Females, who tend to constitute a larger subsample of the elderly population, are slightly more likely to have mobility limitations than males. Nonwhites and those in the lowest income category are the most limited in terms of mobility.

It should, therefore, be stressed that pre-exercise medical examination may both be important in terms of prescribing the limit of potential exercise, as well as to encourage and give permission to the elder individual to exercise. The necessity, however, is based on the intensity and expectations of the exercise program. If the exercise program is aimed at aerobic improvement, which would require a high level of exercise intensity whether it be walking, jogging, or swimming, a medical clearance is important. If, on the other hand, exercise is directed toward psychosocial involvement and low-intensity exercise the medical clearance may be less important. Wiswell (1980) stresses the idea that low-intensity exercise can have as dramatic an effect on mental health as aerobic conditioning in the elderly. Thus, whereas high-intensity exercise may contribute to both increased physiological status and psychological well-being, low-intensity exercise may, by adding to psychological well-being, reduce specific factors contributing to accelerated physical decline.

It is important when considering various forms of exercise for the elderly to consider two factors: how to get people started and, second, how to increase adherence to the exercise.

Regarding the former, Pollock (1978) has described the getting started process as exercise prescription. Exercise prescriptions are designed to enhance individuals of all ages in getting started, as well as continuing on an exercise regimen. Exercise prescriptions are based on present levels of fitness as well as the individual's own goals for exercise. The important questions are how much exercise is enough, as well as how much exercise and for what purpose.

Physical fitness programs are generally divided into three major categories: cardiovascular/respiratory fitness, physique, and motor function.

In assessing an exercise prescription for an individual, components of age, needs, or goals are crucial. Major goals in adult fitness programs, which include developing and maintaining cardiovascular/respiratory fitness, flexibility and muscular strength and endurance are expanded when looking at the elderly population. With the older individual, the initial level of fitness is crucial in considering the starting of an exercise program. The threshold for improvement is lower with an unfit individual as well as a sedentary older individual. As mentioned before, age should never be a deterrent for participating in endurance work. Several studies have shown that middle-aged and old athletes can perform high levels of work in their sixth and eighth decades of life. Other reports on athletes who exercise regularly show similar results. The difference, however, in beginning exercise programs for older individuals is that their initial level of fitness is lower, and the quantity and quality of work that they can tolerate is less. This means that the initial workload (intensity) should be moderate and the rate of progression slower for older individuals. Regarding low-intensity activities, such activities as walking, bowling, table tennis, badminton, and calisthenics may be quite appropriate. Finally, it is crucial to evaluate the individual's preference for a specific activity as this may be very important in enhancing adherence to that specific activity.

Up to this point, issues pertaining to the importance of exercise among the elderly have been discussed. What has not been examined, however, is compliance or adherence to a physical activity or exercise regime. In other words, how to keep an individual who finally decides to exercise, exercising regularly. Researchers have found that of those individuals who begin an exercise program, whether on their own or in a structured program, only half will still be exercising after three to six months. It can be speculated that among the elderly this "dropout" statistic is undoubtedly higher given the various physical limitations and health concerns these individuals come to experience. The question of exercise adherence, then, is crucial when dealing with geriatric populations. Several factors that have been found to be effective in enhancing exercise compliance will now be discussed.

One of the most important factors in increasing exercise adherence is environmental support. Heinzelmann and Bagley (1970) found that subjects with spouses to support their exercise habits were twice as likely to have good adherence than those whose spouses were either neutral or negative. In the case of the elderly where advanced age lends itself to being single, the emphasis on environmental support is often switched to that of friends, family, and workers of convalescent and activity centers. Support from these significant others is paramount to an older individual's compliance to physical activity. Environmental support, however, does not just mean acceptance of an older adult's physical activity, but more importantly, reinforcement for this action. Reinforcement, however, entails both the encouragement obtained from significant others in the individual's life to participate in physical activity, as well as the social reinforcement gained from exercising with other individuals. Although the former notion of reinforcement is relatively obvious, the latter idea of social reinforcement is not as well known. Social reinforcement during exercise nevertheless has been found to be particularly effective in increasing adherence. For example, Wilhelmsen et al. (1975) found significantly poorer long-term adherence in those individuals who exercised alone compared with those in a group. Similarly, Massie and Shephard (1971) discovered while only 47 percent of the participants in individual aerobic exercise programs were adherent, 87 percent participating in group exercise were adherent. Furthermore, in a sample of 195 exercisers, Heinzelmann and Bagle (1970) found that 90 percent of these individuals preferred exercising with others. It becomes apparent then, that the association with other individuals while exercising is, in itself, reinforcing and enhances adherence. Given this knowledge, it can only be hoped that more group oriented exercise programs can be implemented for the elderly. From structured settings, such as convalescent homes or golden age clubs where exercise can feasibly be conducted jointly, to individuals living alone who can, for example, go for morning walks with their neighbor, basic contact with other human beings produces reinforcement for engaging in physical activity and enhances exercise adherence. Moreover, once an exercise routine is established the effects of exercise will in itself be rewarding in that it will often result in improved health and better physical appearance.

Finally, other forms of contingency management have also been used to increase exercise adherence in the elderly, such as the use of token reinforcement procedures, behavior contracts, and group award presentations. These reward systems, however, should be individually tailored to the participant relative to the exercise engaged in.

A second factor that has been found to be effective in enhancing exercise adherence is the use of feedback. Providing information as to the progress, amount of time spent, as well as records of an individual's involvement in a physical activity are extremely effective in motivating the elderly exerciser to continue exercising. For example Katell et al., (1980) found that sedentary adults enrolled in an eleven-week jogging program in which instructors always ran with the participants giving feedback and praise on running form, pace, and so on were more successful (i.e., 80 percent adherence rate) in completing the jogging program than that of the control group. What has been found even more effective in increasing adherence than the feedback provided by others, however, is personalized feedback that is obtained and imposed by oneself. This, of course, involves goal setting by the elderly participant. Such self-imposed exercise goals produce motivation to continue exercising, as well as provide an award system when goals are actualized. Moreover, Martin (1981) found that exercise adherence was significantly better after a three-month period when participants determined specific exercise goals, than when these goals were fixed by an instructor.

When an individual does attempt to construct some exercise goals it is important that he or she does not set them unrealistically high or low. Given such extremes, the elderly participant is likely to lose interest due to either boredom (i.e., "This is too easy, and all of this exercise is silly anyway") or to that of frustration ("I'll never make my goal, I'm just not made for all this physical activity"). As previously mentioned, it is imperative that an individual's exercise goals be carefully tailored to his or her personality and the form of physical activity being conducted. It is generally found, however, that time-based goals (e.g., 30 minutes of walking, 20 minutes of stationary bicycling) are more effective than distance-based goals (e.g., a 3 mile walk, 40 toe touches) in promoting adherence to an exercise regime. In addition, the use of written records measuring daily exercise times, blood pressure, pulse, weight loss, and other variables provide important feedback to the elderly exerciser. Finally, the establishment of routines helps to facilitate exercise adherence. By making exercising a significant part of an older adult's everyday life, just like that of taking one's morning pills, adherence will be considerably enhanced.

Despite the increased interest in today's society to be physically fit and to "have the body you've always wanted," the physical fitness craze has not had a significant impact upon the elderly. Even though more older adults are engaged in some form of physical exercise than ever before, the vast majority of those over 65 are still largely sedentary. Misconceptions that exercise will cause more bodily harm than good, that "old people shouldn't be carrying on like that," are sufficiently prevalent among the elderly, their families, friends, and often the professionals that work closely with them (i.e., physicians, nurses). There is a need, therefore, to educate the elderly, and the population as a whole, concerning the beneficial physical and mental effects exercise can have. It is hoped that this can be accomplished both on a national level across all age groups via the media of television, books, magazines but also on a more focused level involving the caregivers who work closely with the elderly. For example, physicians are frequently consulted by the elderly when depressed or suffering from inevitable age-related physical complications. Physicians therefore play a major role in educating their elderly patients about the benefits of exercising and encouraging them to pursue such activity. Convalescent home staff cognizant of the benefits of exercise could incorporate an exercise program for residents as part of the everyday routine. Although change will be gradual, the motivating force toward making exercise a more integral part of the older person's life is largely dependent upon educating the public as to the realistic benefits physical activity can entail.

In addition to the need to educate the public further regarding the attributes of exercise, the need for further evaluation of exercise's effectiveness is warranted. Specifically, more research is needed to assess what types of exercise programs are the most effective with older adults; which exercise activities are best suited to certain people with certain limitations; what physical and mental consequences result from exercise participation, as well as a host of other unanswered questions. Clearly, further evaluation, assessment, and research on the effects of exercise can only help the rapidly growing geriatric population in the world today.

REFERENCES

Anderson, J., and Morgan, W.P. Influence of acute physical activity on state anxiety. In *Proceedings of National College Physical Education Association for Men.* January 1973, pp. 113–121.

Appenzeller, O., Standefer, J., Appenzeller, J., et al. Neurology of endurance training: V. Endorphins. *Neurology*, 1980, 30:418–419.

Bahrke, M.S., and Morgan, W.P. Anxiety reduction following exercise and meditation. *Cognitive Therapy and Research*, 1978, 2:323–33.

Barry, A., Daly, J., Pruett, E., et al. The effects of physical conditioning on older individuals. *Journal of Gerontology*, 1966, 21:182–191.

Bennett, J., Carmack, M., and Gardner, V. The effect of a program of physical exercise on depression in older adults. *Physical Education*, 1982, 21–24.

Birren, J.E. Age changes in speed of behavior: Its central nature and physiological correlates. In A.T. Welford and J.E. Birren (Eds.), *Behavior, Aging and the Nervous System*. Springfield, Ill.: Charles C. Thomas, 1965.

Blazer, D *Psychopathology of Aging*. Durham, N.C.: Duke University APFP Publications, 1978.

Bloom, F., Segal, D., Ling, N. et al. Endorphins profound behavioral effects in rats suggest new factors in mental illness. *Science*, 1976, 194:630–632.

Brown, R.S., Ramirez, D.E., and Taub, J.M. The prescription of exercise for depression. *The Physician and Sports Medicine*, 1978, 6(12):34–37.

Brunner, B.C. Personality and motivating factors influencing adult participation in vigorous physical activity. *Research Quarterly*, 1969, 40:464–69.

Buccola, V.A., and Stone, W.J. Effects of jogging and cycling programs on physiological and personality variables in aged men. *Research Quarterly*, 1975, 46:134–139.

Burdick, J.A., and Zloty, R.B. Wakeful heart rate, personality and performance— A study of distance runners. *Journal of Sports Medicine and Physical Fitness*, 1973, 13:17–25.

Byrd, O.E. The relief of tension by exercise: a survey of medical viewpoint and practices. *Journal of School Health*, 1963, 43:239–40.

Byrd, O.E. Viewpoints of bowlers in respect for relief of tension. *Physical Education*, 1964, 21:119–20.

Christensen, N.J., Galbo, H., Hansen, J.F., et al. Catecholamines and exercise. *Diabetes*, 1979, 28:58–62, (Supplement 1).

Collingwood, T.R., and Willett, L. Effects of physical training upon self-concept and body attitude. *Journal of Clinical Psychology*, 1971, 27:411–12.

Conroy, R.W., Smith, R., and Felthaus, A.R. The value of exercise on a psychiatric hospital unit. *Hospital and Community Psychiatry*, 1982, 33:641–645.

Darden, E. Sixteen personality factor profiles at competitive body builders and weight lifters. *Research Quarterly*, 1972, 43:142–47.

DeVries, H.A. Physiological effects of an exercise training regimen upon men aged 52–88. *Journal of Gerontology*, 1970, 25:325–336.

DeVries, H.A., and Adams, G. Electromyographic comparison of single doses of exercise and meprobamate as to the effects on muscular relaxation. *American Journal of Physical Medicine*, 1972, 51:130–41.

Dimsdale, J.E., and Moss, J. Plasma catecholamines in stress and exercise. *Journal of the American Medical Association*, 1980, 243:340–342.

Driscoll, R. Anxiety reduction using physical exertion and positive images. *The Psychological Record*, 1976, 26:87–94.

Fink, M. Anxiety precipitated by lactate. *New England Journal of Medicine*, 1969, 281:1429.

Foley, K.M., Dourides, I.A., Inturrisi, C.E., et al. Beta-endorphin: Analgesic and hormonal effects in humans. *National Academy of Sciences of the United States of America*, 1979, 76:5377–5381.

Folkins, C.H. Effects of physical training on mood. *Journal of Clinical Psychology*, 1976, 32(2):385–88.

Folkins, C.H., Lynch, S., and Gardner, M.M. Psychological fitness as a function on physical fitness. *Archives of Physical Medicine and Rehabilitation* 1972, 53:503–508.

Gerner, R.H. Depression in the elderly. In O.J. Kaplan (Ed.), *Psychopathology of Aging*. New York: Academic Press, 1979.

Gordon, C., and Gaitz, C.M. Leisure and lives: personal expressivity across the lifespan. In R.H. Binstock, and E. Shanas (Eds.), *Handbook of Aging and the Social Sciences*. New York: Van Nostrand Reinhold, 1977.

Griest, J.H. Running through your mind. *Journal of Psychosomatic Research*, 1978, 22:259–394.

Greist, J.H., Klein, M.H., Eischens, R.R., et al. Running out of depression. *Physical Sportsmedicine*, 1978, 6:49–56.

Hammer, W.M., and Wilmore, J.H. An exploratory investigation in personality measures and physiological alterations during a 10-week jogging program. *Journal of Sports Medicine and Physical Fitness*, 1973, 13:238–47.

Handlon, J.H., Byrd, O.E., and Gaines, J.O. Psychometric measurement of the relief of tension by moderate exercise. *Journal of California Physical Education Association*, 1963, 26:4.

Hartley, L.H., Mason, J.W., Hogan, R.P., et al. Multiple hormonal responses to graded exercise in relation to physical training. *Journal of Applied Physiology*, 1972, 33:602–606.

Hartung, G.H., and Farge, E.J. Personality and physiological traits in middle-aged runners and joggers. *Journal of Gerontology*, 1977, 32:541–48.

Hawkins, H.L., and Capaldi, D. Aging, exercise and attentional control. Submitted to *Journal of Gerontology*, 1982.

Heinzelmann, F., and Bagley, R.W. Response to physical activity programs and their effects on health behavior. *Public Health Reports*, 1970, 85(10):905–11.

Ismail, A.H., and Trachtman, L.E. Jogging the imagination. *Psychology Today*, 1973, 6:79–82.

Jette, M. Habitual exercisers: a blood serum and personality profile. *Journal of Sports Medicine* 1975, 3:12–17.

Joesting, J. The psychology of women runners: personal and professional perspectives. Paper presented at the meeting of the Southeastern Psychological Association, Atlanta, March 1978.

Johnsgard, K., Ogilive, B., and Merrit, K. The stress seekers: a psychological study of sports parachutists, racing drivers, and football players. *Journal of Sports Medicine and Physical Fitness*, 1975, 15:158–69.

Katell, A.D., Martin, J.E., Webster, J.S., and Zegman, M.A. Exercise adherence: impact of feedback, praise and goal-setting procedures. In Martin, J.E. (Chair), Exercise: Promoting Adherence and Physical Fitness, Symposium presented at the meeting of the Association for Advancement of Behavior Therapy, New York, 1980.

Kavanaugh, T.H., Shephard, R.J., and Tuck, J.A. Depression after myocardial infarction. *Canadian Medical Association*, 1975, 113:23–27.

Kavanaugh, T., Shephard, R.J., and Tuck, J.A., et al. Depression following myocardial infarction: The effects of distance running. Paper presented at New York Academy of Science, Conference on the Marathon, October 1976.

Kendrick, D.C. Activity and aging. *New Behavior*, 1975, 1:256–258.

Kendrick, D.C., and Moyes, I.C.A. Activity, depression, medication and performance on the Revised Kendrick Battery. *British Journal of Social and Clinical Psychology*, 1979, 18:341–350.

Kjeilberg, S., Rudhe, V., and Sjostrand, T. Increase of the amount of hemoglobin and blood volume in connection with physical training. *Iota Physiological Scandinavian*, 1949, 19:146–151.

Kroll, W. Sixteen personality factor profiles of collegiate wrestlers. *Research Quarterly*, 1967, 38:49–56.

Kroll, W., and Carlson, B.R. Discriminant function and hierarchial grouping analysis of karate participant's personality profiles. *Research Quarterly*, 1967, 38:405–411.

Martin, J.E. Exercise management: shaping and maintaining physical fitness. *Behavioral Medicine Advances*, 1981, 4:1–7.

Massie, J.F., and Shephard, R.J. Physiological and psychological effects of training—a comparison of individual and gymnasium programs with a characterization of the exercise "drop-out." *Medicine and Science in Sports*, 1971, 3(3):110–117.

Mitchum, M.L. The effect of participation in a physically exerting leisure activity on state anxiety level. Unpublished Master's Thesis, Florida State University, Tallahassee, 1976.

Morgan, W.P. Psychological considerations. *Journal of Health, Physical Education, and Recreation*, 1968, 39:26–28.

Morgan, W.P. Selected physiological and psychomotor correlates of depression in psychiatric patients. *Research Quarterly*, 1968, 39:1037–43.

Morgan, W.P. Psychological effect of chronic physical activity. *Medicine and Science in Sports*, 1970, 2:213–17.

Morgan, W.P. Influence of acute physical activity on state anxiety. In *Proceedings of National College Physical Education Association for Men*, January 1973, pp. 113–21.

Morgan, W.P. *Psychological Consequences of Vigorous Physical Activity and Sport in Introduction to Sport Psychology.* St. Louis: C.V. Mosby, 1976.

Morgan, W.P. Selected psychological considerations in sports. *Research Quarterly*, 1974, 45:374–90.

Morgan, W.L., and Pollock, M.L. Psychological characterization of the elite distance runner. Paper presented at New York Academy of Science, Conference on the Marathon, October 1976.

National Council on Aging. *Fact Book on Aging.* Washington, D.C.: The Council, 1978.

Nowlis, D.P., and Greenberg, N. Empirical description of effects of exercise on mood. *Perceptual and Motor Skills*, 1979, 49:1001–1002.

Palmore, E. Predictors of successful aging. *The Gerontologist*, 1979, 1965, 427–31.

Pargman, D., and Baker, M. Running high: Enkephalin indicated. *Journal of Drug Issues*, 1980, 10:341–349

Pitts, F.N. Biochemistry of anxiety. *Scientific American*, 1969, 220:69–75.

Pitts, F.N., and McClure, I.N. Lactate metabolism in anxiety neurotics. *New England Journal of Medicine*, 1967, 277:1329–36.

Pollock, M.L. How much exercise is enough? *The Physician and Sports Medicine*, 1978, 6:112–125.

Pollock, M.L., and Schmidt, D.H. (Eds.) *Heart Disease and Rehabilitation.* Boston: Houghton Mifflin, 1979.

Post, R., Kotin, J., and Goodwin, F. Psychomotor activity and cerebrospinal fluid amine metabolites in affective illness. *AMJ*, 1973, 130:67–72.

Powell, R.R. Psychological effects of exercise therapy upon institutionalized geriatric mental patients. *Gerontology*, 1974, 29:157–161.

Powell, R.R. Effects of exercise on mental functioning. *Journal of Sports Medicine*, 1975, 15:125–131.

Reiter, M.A. Effects of a physical exercise program on selected mood states in a group of women over age 65. *Dissertation Abstract International*, 1974, 1981, 52(5-A).

Robertson, D., Johnson, G.A., Robertson, R.M., et al. Comparative assessment of stimuli that release neuronal and adreno-medullary catecholamines in man. *Circulation*, 1979, 59:637–643.

Saltin, B., Hartley, H., Kilborn, A., et al. Physical training in sedentary middle aged and older man:II. *Scandinavian Journal of Clinical and Laboratory Investigation*, 1969, 24:323–334.

Scarborough, M. An investigation into the relationship between levels of activity and cognitive functioning in the normal community aged. Unpublished

Bachelors dissertation, University of Hull, Department of Psychology Library, 1977.

Spirduso, W.W. Physical fitness, aging and psychomotor speed—a review. *Gerontology*, 1980, 35:53–59.

Stamford, B., Hambacher, W.G., and Fallica, A. Effects of daily physical exercise on the psychiatric state of institutionalized geriatric mental patients. *Research Quarterly*, 1974, 45:34–41.

Stelmach, G.E., and Diewart, G.L. Aging, information processing and fitness. In G. Borg (Ed.), *Physical Work and Effort*. Oxford. Pergamon, 1977.

Stern, M.J., and Cleary, P. National Exercise and Heart Disease Project: Psychosocial changes observed during a low-level exercise program. *Archives of Internal Medicine*, 1981, 141:1463–1467.

Szafran, J. Psychophysiological studies of aging of pilots. In A.G. Talland (Ed.), *Human Aging and Behavior*. New York: Academic Press, 1968.

Tillman, K. Relationship between physical fitness and selected personality traits. *Research Quarterly*, 1965, 36:483–89.

VanLoon, G.R., Schwartz, L., and Sole, M.J. Plasma dopamine responses to standing and exercise in man. *Life Sciences*, 1979, 24:2273–2278.

Wilhelmsen, L., Sanne, H., Ehrfeldt, D., Grimby, G., Tibblin, G., and Wedel, H. A controlled trial of physical training after myocardial infarction. *Preventive Medicine*, 1975, 4:491–508.

Wilson, V.E., Morley, N.C., and Bird, E.I. Mood profiles of marathon runners, joggers, and non-exercisers. *Perceptual and Motor Skills*, 1980, 50:117–18.

Wiswell, R.A. Relaxation, exercise, and aging. In Birren, J.E., and Sloane, R.B. (Eds.), *Handbook on Mental Health and Aging*. Englewood Cliffs, N.J.: Prentice-Hall, 1980.

Wood, D.T. The relationship between state anxiety and acute physical activity. *American Corrective Therapy Journal*, 1977, 31:67–69.

Young, R.J., and Ismail, A.H. Personality differences of adult men before and after a physical fitness program. *Research Quarterly*, 1976, 47:513–19.

10

Psychotherapy

G. Maureen Chaisson-Stewart

Because of the scarcity of controlled studies to date, the efficacy of individual psychotherapy with the aged remains unproven. Consequently, it is not clear if and how the variable of old age influences the process and outcome of therapy. This research scarcity, in some measure, results from the difficulties in conducting such studies. Elderly research subjects are not as readily available in mental health clinical settings as are younger adults: they comprise 2 percent of all cases in outpatient clinics and 4 percent in mental health centers. Also, it has been difficult to make generalizations or draw meaningful conclusions because of the high degree of interindividual variability of personality characteristics and responsiveness to therapy in an aged population (Hoyer, 1978).

Yet, despite the dearth and difficulty of research on psychotherapy with the elderly, many therapists have dared to draw conclusions from their own empirical observations about the effectiveness of psychotherapy in older subjects. For a thorough review of the literature on psychotherapy with the aged, the reader is advised to review works of Rechtschaffen, 1959; Gottesman et al., 1973; Eisdorfer and Stotsky, 1977; Karpf, 1980; and Yesavage and Karasu, 1982.

This chapter will review information gleaned from the research literature about psychotherapy with the depressed elderly—the unique therapy needs of this group, and the approaches and techniques that reportedly are most effective.

Pessimism about the value of individual psychotherapy with the elderly that persists today in many circles can be attributed to the early influence of Freud (1924) who was skeptical about the successful analysis of the elderly for three reasons:

1. Limitations of the aged ego intellect: "Near or above the 50s the elasticity of the mental processes, on which treatment depends, is as a rule lacking—old people are no longer educable."

2. The unmanageable length of treatment that would be required: "the mass of material to be dealt with would prolong the duration of the treatment indefinitely."

3. The economic and long-term value of mental health in older persons: "With persons who are too far advanced in years it [psychoanalysis] fails because, owing to the accumulation of material, so much time would be required that the end of the cure would be reached at a period of life in which much importance is no longer attached to nervous health."

However, later psychoanalysts challenged this position. Based upon his observations of psychoanalysis with one 50-year-old patient, Abraham (1949) opined that the age of the neurosis is more important than the age of the patient. Jelliffee (1925) agreed with Abraham's thinking after completing psychoanalysis with several older patients. He stated that "Chronological, physiological, and psychological age did not go hand in hand." However, like Freud, these writers were more concerned with the suitability of the patient for orthodox psychoanalysis than with the consideration of modifications of this method.

Since then, the problem of "senile rigidity" has been reclassified by some as a problem of

1. The diminished capacity for new learning which is based upon irreversible physiological changes (Lawton, 1952)

2. The rigidity of personality types which are either
   a. Entrenched, due to continued practice of old habits
   b. Defensive, because of fear of change
   c. Compulsive, because of perfectionism

3. Diminished capacity for mental abstraction in consideration of concepts (Steuer & Hammen, 1983)

Besides personality and physiological variables influencing the responsiveness of the elderly to therapy, Yesavage and Karasu (1982) have noted that the internal and external resources that vary considerably between individuals are important factors to be considered:

some are intellectually alert and emotionally adventurous; others are obviously impaired. Some older persons have a number of choices open to them; others, because of varying economic, physical, and social factors, are relatively frozen in a given situation.

In view of these differences in the elderly population, they recommended that therapists use a variety of treatment approaches to the elderly.

FREUD'S QUESTIONS REFRAMED

The misgivings that Freud expressed about the use of psychoanalysis with older persons encompass questions with broader implications than just the suitability of the elderly for psychoanalysis. Reframed, the broader questions relevant to evaluating the merits of any type of psychotherapy with the depressed older person should be: Is psychotherapy effective with the elderly? What type of psychotherapy is most appropriate for an elderly population? And, what type of psychotherapy is most cost effective in a population with a limited remaining life span?

Is Psychotherapy Effective?

The rejection of the elderly as candidates for psychotherapy by Freud and present-day therapists may, in fact, be more related to countertransference and rejecting stereotypic attitudes of the therapist than to the actual potential of the elderly patient in therapy. Insistence that the older patient is too rigid to change may simply be a rationalization for the therapist's own anxiety about death and aging. A more extensive discussion of the therapist and patient attitudinal barriers to psychotherapeutic treatment can be found in Chapter 3.

Despite these barriers, some writers on the subject have expressed optimism about the value of psychotherapy for the elderly because of the overall beneficial effects on the mental and physical health of the patient as well as the emotional and economic relief it provides to family, friends, and community (Hammer, 1972).

Meerloo (1955) saw an openness rather than resistiveness to self-examination on the part of the elderly patient. He noted that there was less resistance because approaching death unconsciously presses the elderly to review life and compare early goals with actual achievements. "My impression is that because of the weakening defenses, there is a better and more direct contact with the unconscious. Older patients react more easily to interpretations and feel more easily relieved by relating present conflicts with those of the past." Agreeing with Meerloo, Grotjahn (1955) said, "A resistance against unpleasant insight is frequently lessened in old age."

Grotjahn was the first to place the emphasis on the *needs* of the geriatric patient which could be met in therapy. In so doing, he emphasized the need of the older person to cope with the reality that is changed by biological and social dependence and helplessness. Grotjahn's philosophy of using psychotherapeutic approaches that best meet the needs of the elderly is in tune with modern trends in psychotherapy.

What type of psychotherapy is most appropriate for an elderly population? Rather than concentrate on the responsiveness of the elderly to psychoanalysis, some authors have focused their discussion on the types of treatment that are appropriate to the elderly. Alexander and French (1946) noted that whereas the opportunities for change in the life situation are more restricted in the aged than they are in the young, and whereas therapy usually implies some form of change, prognosis for the elderly may not be as good as it is for the young. When options are restricted due to physical illness or disability, they proposed modifying analytic techniques to a more supportive type. In addition to supportive therapy Meerloo (1953, 1955) emphasized the patient's need for education, environmental modification and positive interpersonal relationship with the therapist. Weinberg (1951) suggested that the therapist be relatively active and direct in the treatment of older people. Other modifications to orthodox psychoanalytic methods which have been recommended are limiting treatment goals, supporting defenses, and intervening indirectly by modifying the environment.

In their review of individual approaches to psychotherapy of the elderly, Eisdorfer and Stotsky (1977) concluded that the differences between psychodynamic and cognitive approaches are smaller than might be supposed. Written reports indicate that often both techniques are modified to suit the status and needs of the patient and the requirements and limitations of the situation. Still, most of these reports tend to be anecdotal in nature, with outcome studies in short supply.

The needs of the elderly patient which were addressed in articles reviewed by Eisdorfer and Stotsky included understanding and sharing in a relationship, orienting to reality, building friendships, making adjustments to increased dependency, and increasing positive self-evaluative thoughts. Therapeutic approaches that were used to address these needs included cognitive therapy, behavioral modification therapy, and socioenvironmental therapy.

Other creative therapeutic approaches used and described in anecdotal reports by several authors cannot be classified easily into the foregoing three categories. One such pioneering effort developed by Lillian Martin in 1944 focused on positive thinking and inspirational literature. After retiring from an active career Dr. Martin founded the San Francisco Old Age Counseling Center in 1929. Her approach was directive and can be said to be a forerunner of the cognitive-behavioral techniques popular today. She used "homework assignments," behavior modifiers, and the self-help philosophy to recovery. She also believed that it was very important to obtain a holistic picture of the elderly person which included an assessment of assets and liabilities. The patient was given corrective slogans to practice, a technique similar to the cognitive-switching technique of cognitive therapy. Patients were encouraged to practice thought stopping and thought control at home. Her practice of using charts and quasireinforcement schedules concerning daily activities, budgeting, recreation, and future goals also resembles the goal-setting and pleasure participation skill development strategies commonly used in cognitive behavior therapies. She claimed that her approach was more successful than psychoanalysis. However, with no thereoretical framework, rationale, or convincing data to support her conclusions, the Martin method faded during the Great Depression and World War II.

Another treatment approach often quoted in literature is that of Goldfarb (1956). He believed in encouraging the natural dependency of the older patient upon the therapist for the purpose of creating an illusion within the patient that he has found a protective parent. In very brief interviews of 5 to 15 minutes Goldfarb and his associates attempted to create in the patient a feeling of having triumphed over the parent by obtaining small favors, thereby creating a feeling in the patient that he had won control of the resources of gratification. The brevity and, therefore, economy of these once-a-week sessions are attractive features, especially in nursing home settings where staff availability is severely constrained.

Life-review therapy has been strongly advocated by Butler (1960) and Butler and Lewis (1977). They felt that the review of one's past life was such a strong internal need that the elderly engage in this activity spontaneously without outside intervention. On this point they are in agreement with Grotjahn (1955), who believed that the task of integrating one's life and the acceptance of one's own death was a developmental task of old age. In the reminiscent therapy of Butler and Lewis, trained mental health professionals facilitate this process by actively encouraging patients to participate in a life-review process. Some of the techniques used in this therapy to capture memories of the past include written or taped autobiographies, reunions, reconstructing family histories, examining photo albums and scrapbooks, and encouraging the patient to document verbally or in writing his or her life's work. The exact therapeutic nature of this life-review process and its effect on the mental status of the elderly, however, remains unvalidated. Speculations about the therapeutic nature of life-review are derived more from theoretical explanations than from definitive outcome studies. It has been variously proposed that the approach is either an environmental modification, a confrontation of anxieties about aging and death, a revitalization of older people's experience, introduction of stimulation in an otherwise routine life (Karpf, 1980) or another form of the cognitive restructuring technique of cognitive therapy.

With the goal of making contact with withdrawn elderly persons residing in homes for the aged, Power and McCarron (1975) developed an "interactive-contact method" in which they used bodily contact and communication to gain the attention of the withdrawn person and to indicate to this depressed person that someone is interested in him and values him enough to make personal contact. Utilizing pre-post measures of depression (Brief Psychiatric Rating Scale and Zung Self-Report Depression Scale) the researchers were able to demonstrate significantly lower scores in the experiment group as compared to the control group after 15 weeks of half-hour, individual sessions with the subjects. In addition, the researchers noted that the friendly human relationships that were encouraged in the study strengthened the aged person's self-concept and amount of interaction with other members of the home. Not only was significant improvement noted in the experimental group, but a "deterioration trend" was seen in the control or nontreated subjects: their depression scores increased over time. The implication of this treatment approach is that when the elderly person's need for close human contact and social interaction remains unfulfilled, a progressive deterioration in mental health results. Follow-up results of this study indicate that the "socialized" experimental subjects were likely to continue to be socially involved.

Interpersonal psychotherapy (IPT) was evaluated by Rothblum et al. (1982) in clinical trials with depressed elderly. The focus of IPT is on

> improving the quality of the depressed patient's current interpersonal functioning . . . based on the premise that depression, regardless of the symptom pattern, severity, vulnerability, or personality traits, occurs in a psycho-social and interpersonal context and that understanding and renegotiating the interpersonal context associated with the onset of symptoms is important to the person's recovery and possibly the prevention of further episodes. (Rothblum et al., 1982)

The subjects for the study were men and women between the ages of 60 and 85 who had a diagnosis of moderate to severe major depressive illness according to the American Psychiatric Association's *Diagnostic and Statistical Manual of Mental Disorders,* Third Edition. The psychotherapy treatment consisted of weekly, 30–50 minute sessions with the treating psychiatrist. Subjects were randomly assigned in a double-blind manner to antidepressant treatment or pill-placebo treatment for six weeks. Although efficacy data on differential response to treatment was not yet available in the original research report, the results indicate a decrease in depressive symptomatology after the first and second weeks of treatment with a very gradual decrease thereafter. The problem areas that were defined in therapy to aid the therapist in formulating treatment goals for the patients were: grief (39 percent), role transition (39 percent), interpersonal disputes (56 percent), and interpersonal deficiency (28 percent). The chief difference noted by the researchers between younger adult patients and elderly patients was the prevalence of medical problems in the applicants for the study, which precluded psychotropic drug use. This finding alone suggests the importance of psychotherapy as a desirable treatment for depression in the elderly, one to be further developed and researched.

What type of psychotherapy is most cost-effective in a population with a limited remaining life span?

It seems reasonable to conclude that psychotherapeutic approaches which are most apt to be cost-effective in treating the elderly will have the following characteristics:

Acceptable and nonstigmatizing
Structured
Time-limited
Goal-oriented
Suitable and effective in a group approach
Teachable to non-mental-health-specialized providers and to the elderly
Demonstrated effectiveness

One psychotherapeutic approach that exhibits all of the desirable characteristics listed above and discussed below is cognitive-behavior therapy. It offers great promise as the psychotherapy of choice to treat the elderly. The patients who seem to respond best to this approach have sufficient intellectual ability to understand the basic concepts and sufficient motivation to participate actively in a process of analyzing and restructuring their depressogenic thought patterns and behaviors. Gallagher and Thompson (1981) have also noted that the most successful patient in cognitive therapy is one who is middle class, well educated, and verbal.

Acceptable and Nonstigmatizing

The educational thrust of cognitive behavioral therapy with its teaching of new concepts and skills and assignment of homework tends to appeal to the elderly. The elderly subjects in our study of cognitive group therapy tended to refer to the therapy sessions as their "classes," a notion reinforced further when they were encouraged and expected to bring spiral notebooks to "class" with them. The present cohort of elderly also tend to be attracted to the values of self-help and positive thinking integral to the approach. The opportunity that cognitive therapy offers to increase personal control, especially over one's mood state, is also appealing to this population. Because cognitive therapy appeals to their value system and is less stigmatizing in its educational image, it is likely to be more acceptable to the elderly than other types of psychotherapy that lack these characteristics.

Structure

Structure is important in the treatment of the elderly because it prevents misunderstanding and confusion (common problems in the elderly and in depressed individuals) about goals and time commitments. It also increases the efficient use of a short time for therapy in the limited remaining life span of the aged individual. Therapy is usually structured into three stages: diagnostic, working, and termination.

Data collected during the diagnostic stage includes 1) mood ratings, 2) an analysis of activities (including exercise), interests, social problem areas, support system strength, and observational data. When possible, the patient is observed at home and in interactions with others. When direct observation by the therapist is not feasible, observational data about the patient's behavior, mood state, social interactions, and activity, sleeping, and eating patterns can be obtained from the 24-hour nursing observations in an institutional setting or from family, friends, or associates who have frequent close contact with the patient. With the elderly especially, the data collected during the diagnostic stage should also include a medical history and physical exam (to rule out organic causes for depression); a drug history (to rule out drug-related causes for depression); and an evaluation of diet and nutritional status and eating patterns (especially related to socialization at meal times). Finally, the findings collected in the diagnostic stage are shared with the patient, to be used by both therapist and patient to collaboratively set short-term and long-range treatment goals.

Individual sessions are also structured so the patient knows what to expect and the time in therapy is well utilized. At the beginning of each session, the therapist and the patient collaborate in establishing an agenda. Agenda setting usually includes a brief resume of the patient's experiences since the last session and a review of homework assignments. The middle and major part of the session is spent in meeting the goals that both parties prioritized on the agenda. At the completion of the session the therapist solicits feedback from the patient concerning his perceptions and feelings about therapy, homework, or the therapist. Finally the homework assignment is determined collaboratively based upon the material discussed during the session.

Time-limited

Cognitive-behavior therapy is a short-term, time-limited therapy usually involving a maximum of 20 sessions over a 10–12 week period. The time-limited aspect of this therapeutic orientation, which perforce limits the cost, is also appealing to the third-party insurer, government agency, or the elderly, whoever pays the bill.

Goal-oriented

Cognitive-behavior therapy is goal-oriented. The therapist and patient work together in reducing the client's distress to a set of problems with attendant goals to solve the problems. There are sequential steps or goals for the overall treatment and goals for individual sessions. Goals are always jointly determined by both parties depending upon the stage of therapy and the patient's progress.

Clear goals help to focus therapy so that time is not wasted in unproductive whining, complaining, and emoting, the default mode that depressed patients quickly revert to when structure and goals are absent. Moreover, when therapy is time-efficient due to structuring and goal-setting, it is also apt to be more cost-effective. Goals are always open to revision during therapy and are most apt to require adjustment if the patient experiences unexpected personal crises requiring life-style changes (death in the family, illness, community changes) or if the patient, because of increasing insight, motivation and decision-making ability during therapy, himself makes significant life-style changes (change of job, divorce, relocation).

Another distinct advantage of goal-oriented therapy in work with the elderly is that such an approach is amenable to a multidisciplinary approach, especially in an institutional setting, where the entire staff can reinforce and facilitate the patient's achievement of the goals. A goal orientation ensures individualization of the therapy to meet the unique needs of the particular old person. By example and process, it teaches the patient how to set goals in the future. Finally, by documenting change, goal setting increases the patient's awareness of personal success and progress, both in and out of therapy.

Suitable and Effective in a Group Approach

A group approach can be more cost-effective because more patients can be treated with fewer personnel. Cognitive behavior therapy has been shown to be suitable and effective in a group approach. See Chapter 10 for a thorough discussion of this subject.

Teachable to Non-Mental Health-Specialized Care Providers and to the Patient

The principles and techniques of cognitive-behavior therapy can be taught to patients, thereby increasing their self-help abilities and control of negative mood states in the future. Service providers who are accessible to the elderly (such as staff of long-term care settings, senior centers, and public health nurses) but may lack the skills of a mental health specialist can be taught to use the principles and techniques of cognitive behavior therapy just as they can be taught the principles and techniques of crisis intervention. By incorporating these techniques into their daily interactions with the elderly, caregivers can provide a psychotherapeutic support system where there would otherwise be none, due to high cost or low accessibility.

Demonstrated Effectiveness

Cognitive behavior therapy has been demonstrated repeatedly to be at least as effective as drugs in treating depression in young and middle-aged adults. Since tricyclic antidepressants, widely prescribed since the late 1960s, are no panacea for depression (only 60–65 percent show definite improvement) and since their multiple side-effects and aggravation of pre-existing medical conditions in the elderly often preclude their use (see Chapter 3), there is additional impetus for promoting and researching the use of cognitive behavior therapy in the elderly.

Three controlled outcome studies, two of which used a group-treatment format, compared the effectiveness of cognitive therapy with other treatments for depression on a population of students. Data derived from these studies indicated that cognitive therapy exceeded the results obtained in waiting list, supportive treatment, or positive-experience control groups in facilitating relief of depressive symptoms (Shipley and Fazio, 1973; Taylor and Marshall, 1977; Gioe, 1975).

In studies of individual cognitive therapy with depressed psychiatric patients, cognitive therapy exceeded the results of waiting list, insight therapy, behavior therapy, nondirected therapy, and pharmacotherapy (Shaw, 1977; Rush and Beck, 1978; Schmickley, 1976).

In a summary review of approximately 50 studies of the use of cognitive and behavioral techniques in the treatment of depression, Rehm and Kornblith-Sander (1979) concluded that a relatively brief, structured behavioral or cognitive therapy method can have significant effects in ameliorating depression. The specific therapy techniques discussed by the authors in this review were 1) contingency management methods, 2) social skills training, 3) imagery-based procedures, 4) cognitive therapy, and 5) self-control techniques.

In 1978, Rush and Beck reported the results of a landmark study which showed that cognitive therapy was significantly more effective than imipramine in reducing acute depressive symptoms. Subjects in the study were depressed outpatients who were in their mid-30s. Subjects were self-referred psychiatric outpatients who satisfied research diagnostic criteria for depressive syndrome according to the Diagnostic Statistical Manual–II. At the start of treatment, all patients were moderately to severely depressed, by self-report (Beck Depression Inventory), by observer evaluation (Hamilton Rating Scales), and by therapist-rating (Raskin Scale). Patients were randomly assigned to either individual cognitive therapy or pharmacotherapy for 12 weeks of treatment. The cognitive therapy group members participated in twice weekly hour-long therapy sessions for a maximum of 20 visits. Subjects in the pharmacotherapy group received not less than 100 mg per day but not more than 250 mg per day of imipramine hydrochloride prescribed in 20 minute, once weekly visits for a maximum of 12 weeks. Therapists were psychiatric residents who had treated only two practice cases with supervision prior to the study. In implementing the cognitive therapy methodology, they followed the guidelines specified in Beck's treatment manual (Beck, 1976). To ensure standardization of the intervention, therapists were supervised on a weekly basis by three experienced clinicians and all treatment sessions were audiorecorded and spot checked for adherence to protocol. Repeated posttesting with the depression scales and observer ratings revealed that cognitive therapy resulted in a significantly greater improvement than did pharmocotherapy. Additionally, the dropout rate during active treatment was significantly greater with pharmacotherapy than with cognitive therapy ($p < .05$). Finally, while both groups maintained treatment gains over time, the cognitive therapy patients showed significantly lower levels of depression at 3 months ($p < .05$) and a trend toward lower levels at 6 months ($p < .10$). This study was the first demonstration that any psychotherapy was equivalent to or better than pharmacotherapy in the relief of depression.

The results of our research (Chaisson et al., 1984), investigating the use of cognitive group therapy with a sample of 46 depressed elderly recruited from the community, indicated that cognitive therapy, and not just a group experience, was the influencing variable in significantly decreasing the depression levels of the subjects. In comparing the mean change scores of the subjects in the pre, post levels of depression (using the Beck Depression Inventory) with the therapist's adherence to cognitive-behavioral approaches in therapy (as rated by observers using the Cognitive Therapy Scale; Young and Beck, 1980), we found a significant positive correlation ($r = .91$) between the two variables. Furthermore, despite the insufficient length of treatment (six sessions), the depression levels of subjects declined, although not significantly. Since the decline in depression levels of the subjects was significantly related to the cognitive therapy skills of the therapists, it is an encouraging sign that cognitive behavior therapeutic approaches may be effective in reducing depression in the elderly. More research of a similar nature should be done to confirm the effectiveness of these approaches. Incidentally, we also found that one public health nurse was able to reach competency level as a cognitive group therapist after participating in an intensive 10-week structured training program, a promising sign that other nurses can learn to implement these techniques with their patients.

In their research using cognitive-behavior therapy in a group approach, Steuer and Hammen (1983) observed that there were two main differences between the elderly and a younger population in their response to therapy. One was passivity, a tendency of the older patients to depend upon the experts to make recommendations. The authors attributed this tendency to the patient's prior experiences with a health care system that encouraged them to let the caregivers identify their problems and recommend solutions. To counter this tendency, the researchers taught the elderly subjects in the study how to actively generate and enact new behaviors for themselves.

The second tendency in the elderly patients was a prevalent belief in the social myth that they were "too old to change." This belief can become a significant barrier to accepting and responding to treatment and can breed feelings of futility and helplessness. For these reasons, it needs to be countered early in therapy. While it was slow to change, the researchers found that it was sometimes most effectively countered, not by cognitive restructuring but by social pressure from other group members to at least attempt new tasks or strategies. Social pressure, one of the many advantages of group therapy, is not present in individual therapy. (The other advantages of group therapy are discussed in great length in Chapter 11.) Finally, Steuer and Hammen noted that, given limited personal and social resources (described at length in Chapter 4) and the consequent restrictions in their alternatives in life, it is important for the therapist to be well-acquainted with community resources in order to assist the elderly to see and think about the future quality of their lives.

Cognitive-Behavior Theory

Cognitive-therapy is an approach that views depression as a disorder having emotional, behavioral, and cognitive components. The cognitive component involves distorted thinking, which in turn affects the emotional and behavioral components of the system. The attention devoted to cognitive variables in behavior therapy has grown steadily since the 1970s, resulting in a causal model for depression which identifies cognitions or conscious thinking as a mediational variable influencing behavior (see Chapter 4). The publications of Beck (1976) and Meichenbaum (1976), the appearance of the journal *Cognitive Therapy and Research* and the inaugural convention on "Cognitive-Behavior Therapy" in New York City in 1976 officially launched the cognitive-oriented revolution in psychology (Wilson, 1978).

Although there is no clearly agreed upon or commonly accepted definition of behavior therapy (Wilson, 1978), it is heavily based on three social-learning concepts of Bandura (1977). The first concept is that cognitive processes determine what environmental influences are attended to, how they are perceived, and how they effect action. The second concept of social-learning theory is that psychological functioning involves a reciprocal interaction between a person's behavior and the environment. In this concept a person is both the agent as well as the object of environmental influence. The third characteristic of social-learning theory is that by recognizing that cognitions have causal influence and emphasizing the reciprocal determinism of behavior, it highlights the human capacity of self-directed behavior change.

This "cognitive connection" within behavior therapy described by Ellis (1962) as rational-emotive therapy, Meichenbaum (1977) as cognitive behavior modification, and Beck (1976) as cognitive therapy has the following commonalities:

1. Humans develop adaptive and maladaptive behavior and affective patterns via cognitive processes.

2. In depression cognitive processes tend to be conceptually distorted and associated with perceptions of loss.
3. The resultant task of the therapist is that of diagnostician-educator who assesses maladaptive cognitive processes and subsequently arranges learning experiences which will alter cognitions and, in turn, behavior-affect patterns which result therefrom.

In this section, Beck's form of cognitive therapy, because of its proven efficacy in the treatment of depression, will be described. This therapy approach is well-described in the books *Cognitive Therapy of Depression* (Beck et al., 1979) and *Cognitive Therapy and the Emotional Disorders* (Beck, 1976). It is a short-term, time-limited form of psychotherapy usually involving a maximum of twenty sessions over a 10- to 12-week period. In the therapy process thoughts are treated as if they were hypotheses requiring validation. The therapist uses logic, persuasion, and evidence from the patient's past and present life to evaluate those "thought-hypotheses" in order to question beliefs and correct errors in logic and perceptions of reality. Conceptual distortions (as listed below) that are uniquely associated with depression are also identified and corrected.

Arbitrary inference
Selective abstraction
Overgeneralization
Magnification or minimization
Personalization

Over time the patient learns how to recognize and correct these thinking errors by himself or herself, thereby enabling the patient to continue thought-corrective therapy independently in the future. These distorted thoughts which are automatic, habitual, and self-derogatory are accessed through oral or written reports of the patient.

Thoughts that tend to take on a repetitive pattern are called "schemata." A schemata found in most depressed patients identified by Beck as the "cognitive triad" consists of negatively biased evaluations of self, the world, the past, and the future. Schema mold cognitions and act as screening agents in perceptions, differentiating, and coding stimuli that confront the individual. A person categorizes and evaluates his experiences through a matrix of schemas. A schema may be inactive at one time but can be activated by specific environmental inputs. They may become more global, being evoked by a wider range of stimuli as they become more active.

As depression worsens, the patient is less able to objectively evaluate negative interpretations and detect illogical thinking. Beck has noted:

Before the onset of a new depressive episode [people subject to recurrent depression] begin to show distortions in the way they interpret matters by failing to make the fine distinctions necessary to interpret reality correctly and, instead, misinterpret reality through a negative, cognitive screen. In a number of cases we have been able to arrest the onset of depression by pointing out to a person how he is beginning to misinterpret reality. (1974)

The theory that feeling-responses can be changed by a process of accessing and altering conscious meanings attached to stimuli is based upon the assumptions that 1) cognitions are automatic, habitual, involitional thought processes, 2) cognitions can be brought into conscious awareness through a series of structured, self-assessment exercises, 3) when individuals actively participate in identifying errors or distortions in their thinking they will correct their erroneous thought patterns, 4) corrected cognitions will alter emotional responses from abnormal to normal, 5) when individuals judge that their depressogenic automatic thoughts are based upon an accurate assessment of a stimulus, their depression will remain unchanged.

In stressing the importance of cognitions as a mediational variable in the development of depression, Beck recognizes that depression is a multiple-system disorder. Yet, he states, "Even if we state that some depression may stem from biological causes, we will still find that these depressive states do have a psychological phenomonology which can be approached psychotherapeutically" (Beck, 1974). However, proponents of cognitive therapy in addressing the psychosomatic aspect of depression make the assumptions that our thoughts, as part of the overall organic system, have the capacity to alter neuro and hormonal processes, which in turn control the immunological functions responsible for body surveillance. (See Chapter 4.)

Cognitive Therapy Compared to Psychoanalysis

Cognitive behavior therapy differs from psychoanalysis in the following areas as described in Table 10.1: main goal, therapist-patient relationship, activity of therapist, guideposts for therapy, and the main focus.

Techniques of Cognitive Therapy and Behavior Therapy Combined

In cognitive-behavior therapy the techniques of cognitive therapy are combined with behavioral techniques that are intended to correct maladaptive behaviors and increase life satisfaction in the following areas:

1. Communication, especially assertiveness
2. Behavioral productivity
3. Social interaction
4. Decision making and problem solving

TABLE 10.1

COGNITIVE BEHAVIOR THERAPY AND PSYCHOANALYSIS COMPARED

	Psychoanalysis	Cognitive Behavior Therapy
Main goal	Personality change	Concrete learning to change thoughts, feelings, and behaviors
Therapist-patient relationship	Therapist is superior. Patient is subordinate.	Therapist and patient collaborate as partners
Activity of therapist	Passive and transparent	Therapist active teacher and diagnostician
Guideposts for therapy	Diagnostic labels	Problems identified in a holistic assessment
Main focus	Unconscious thoughts	Conscious thoughts and behavior

5. Cognitive self-control

6. Goal setting, including time planning

An example of how some of these approaches are integrated into therapy is displayed in the flowchart in Figure 10.1. Following is a discussion of their relevance in therapy with the elderly patient.

COMMUNICATION, ESPECIALLY ASSERTIVENESS. The problems of communication breakdown and social isolation in an elderly population have already been discussed extensively in Chapter 4. Improving communication skills (especially assertion) through training helps the individual to 1) gain control over uncomfortable situations, thereby increasing their sense of personal power and self-confidence (Klerman, 1974) and 2) reduce interpersonal tension that results from blocked communication.

BEHAVIORAL PRODUCTIVITY. A cardinal feature of depressed persons is that they are notably inactive. They engage in fewer pleasant activities and exercise less. This is true of the elderly especially, since the frequency of involvement in pleasurable activities has been noted to decrease with age, even in those individuals who are not clinically depressed (Lewinsohn and MacPhillamy, 1974).

Positive reinforcement which is essential to the amelioration of dysphoria (Lewinsohn, 1976) is usually increased by contracting with the patient to alter the frequency, range, and quality of activities. By keeping a log of activities and mood-state ratings the patient can visibly note the improvement in mood state with increased activity over time, a relationship that has been demonstrated repeatedly through research (Lewinsohn and Libet, 1972; Lewinsohn and Graf, 1973). In institutional settings professionals have greater control over the old person's environment and can intervene directly to plan pleasurable events and programs. For the old

SKILL AREAS	PROBLEM AREAS	TREATMENT INTERVENTION	PRE–POST SCALED IMPROVEMENT CRITERIA
Communication 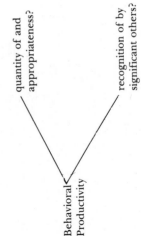	aversive marital interaction	Communication feedback training (± control) with regularly scheduled practice	(1) spouse report; (2) analysis of home conversation audio tape
	quantity and range of interaction sources constricted?	Regularly scheduled communication practice, content prompting and cueing with established sources, and initiation of verbal interactions with appropriate new sources	(1) frequency and duration of verbal interactions with both familiar and new sources; (2) client-satisfaction rating and communication interchanges with both familiar and new sources
Behavioral Productivity	quantity of and appropriateness?	Establish goal behavior that is acceptable to social environment as well as patient, construct graduated performance assignments using contingency management and successive approximations	(1) goal attainment scaling of objective and observable treatment goals; (2) feedback from significant other, when available; (3) record of objective events (e.g. work record, places visited, tasks accomplished, physical exercise)
	recognition of by significant others?	Conference with client and significant other to establish what are desirable behavior goals, teach both significant other and client contingency management	(1) feedback from significant other, when available; (2) client-report of feedback received from significant other re client behavioral productivity

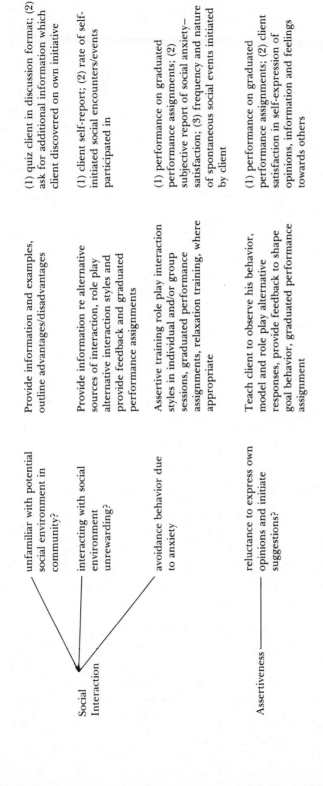

Social Interaction — unfamiliar with potential social environment in community?	Provide information and examples, outline advantages/disadvantages	(1) quiz client in discussion format; (2) ask for additional information which client discovered on own initiative
interacting with social environment unrewarding?	Provide information re alternative sources of interaction, role play alternative interaction styles and provide feedback and graduated performance assignments	(1) client self-report; (2) rate of self-initiated social encounters/events participated in
avoidance behavior due to anxiety	Assertive training role play interaction styles in individual and/or group sessions, graduated performance assignments, relaxation training, where appropriate	(1) performance on graduated performance assignments; (2) subjective report of social anxiety—satisfaction; (3) frequency and nature of spontaneous social events initiated by client
Assertiveness — reluctance to express own opinions and initiate suggestions?	Teach client to observe his behavior, model and role play alternative responses, provide feedback to shape goal behavior, graduated performance assignment	(1) performance on graduated performance assignments; (2) client satisfaction in self-expression of opinions, information and feelings towards others

Figure 10.1 Flow chart to facilitate therapeutic decision making in the behavioral treatment of depression. (From Lewinson, P.M. Therapeutic decision-making in the treatment of depression. In P. Davidson (Ed.), *Behavioral Management of Anxiety, Depression and Pain.* New York: Brunner/Maze;, Inc., 1976. Used with permission.)

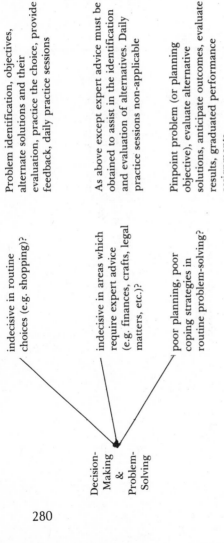

Decision-Making & Problem-Solving

indecisive in routine choices (e.g. shopping)?

Problem identification, objectives, alternate solutions and their evaluation, practice the choice, provide feedback, daily practice sessions

(1) lapsed time required for routine serial decision-making tasks (e.g. shopping, choosing clothes to wear); (2) daily decision-making frequency record by decision category (i.e. big/small decisions); (3) client and significant other report

indecisive in areas which require expert advice (e.g. finances, crafts, legal matters, etc.)?

As above except expert advice must be obtained to assist in the identification and evaluation of alternatives. Daily practice sessions non-applicable

(1) client record of contacting expert advice (e.g. legal aid society); (2) lapsed time required to make decision once all information available; (3) client report of anxiety associated with decision-making

poor planning, poor coping strategies in routine problem-solving?

Pinpoint problem (or planning objective), evaluate alternative solutions, anticipate outcomes, evaluate results, graduated performance assignments

(1) client report in form of problem solving/planning flow chart; (2) client satisfaction rating

Cognitive Self-Control

high-rate negative thought intrusions?

Establish thought delay, substitution and thought stopping, and geographical control techniques to control thought intrusions, rehearse positive ideational material (positive scanning), model positive self-evaluation

(1) rate chart of client's ability to suppress negative ideational material; (2) rate chart of client's ability to engage in positive scanning and positive self-evaluation

rehearsal of past events?

Suppress through thought substitution

(1) rate chart of client's ability to interrupt rehearsal of past events and substitute adaptive thoughts

concentration span?

Provide practice sessions on a variety of content areas with small but increasing time spans (temporal control), require reporting, provide feedback, daily assignments

(1) objective report of concentration span and content recall in watching T.V. or movies, reading papers, magazines or books, skill games (e.g. chess, checkers), etc.

Figure 10.1 (*continued*)

person who has few futuristic goals or long-range plans to mark his days and structure his life, daily events and simple pleasures (nature, animals, card games, visitors, scents, music, and aesthetic beauty of the environment) become the major source of pleasure and enhancement of the quality of life.

SOCIAL INTERACTION. Depressed persons are known to lack the social skills necessary to be accepted and positively reinforced in social situations. Instead, they tend to be rejected by others who avoid them as a depressing influence (Coyne, 1976). If interests and personal contacts are restricted, a phenomenon often occurring in old age, the individual is apt to have less to talk about and more discomfort in social situations. If sensory deficits (sight or hearing) or chronic illnesses (emphysema, aphasia, laryngectomy) handicap satisfactory communication, the individual is apt to withdraw. If illness causes one to be bedridden or homebound with few visitors or companionship, the individual is apt to experience social deprivation. The goal in therapy is to increase satisfying socialization which is incompatible with depression (McLean, 1976).

The process for facilitating social interaction usually involves

1. Survey of patient's social interests and areas of interpersonal difficulty
2. Survey of community or institution's resources relevant to patient's needs and interests
3. Employment of graduated performance tasks to promote social engagement that has been preceded by rehearsal
4. Review of task assignment to identify stress areas or deficiencies
5. Application of targeted social skills training to decrease deficiencies and reduce associated stress

PROBLEM SOLVING AND DECISION MAKING. Developing problem-solving skills improves that individual's ability to decrease the number of problems in their lives and the stress associated with said problems. Research shows that depressed people have difficulty coping, not with major life stress events, but with events that are in the range of everyday experience (Paykel, 1974). When Weissman and Klerman (1977) analyzed the content of interviews with 774 depressed females they found that the vast majority were preoccupied with concern with the management of routine problems (e.g., child management and interaction with spouse). The management of daily affairs can be especially problematic and stress-producing for elderly persons who have impaired memory. In one study aged subjects who were classified as memory impaired by objective testing (Crook et al., 1980) complained frequently about misplacing objects around the home, forgetting appointments, and recent events. Such daily microstressors increase risk for depression. However, memory deficits can be compensated for through the use of appropriate aids, such as, a pill-taking calendar or a well-trained handidog (Chaisson, 1983) and can be incorporated into the fourth step in the following list. In this regard, Brink (1977) has noted that the signal purpose of brief psychotherapy with the elderly, in the majority of cases, is to help patients cope with problems, not to reconstruct their personality. The following steps are usually involved in teaching problem-solving skills:

1. Pinpoint and identify the problem.
2. List alternative solutions.
3. Anticipate the outcomes of each of these alternatives in terms of cost, time, who is affected, short- and long-term effects.
4. Use organizational aids to assist in long-term planning and prevent decision crises. Examples of organizational aides are: daily time schedule, work and leisure planning calendars, budget.

COGNITIVE SELF-CONTROL.   Persons who are depressed experience an elevated frequency of negative thoughts, as was explained in the section on theory. Negative thoughts found frequently in older persons are as follows (Gallagher and Thompson, 1981):

Preoccupation with physical problems
Problematic thoughts about the past
Disappointments with adult children
Death of family members and friends
Changes in appearance with age
Loss of social roles
The need to care for an ill or impaired spouse or family member
Historical and social changes
Intense fear of low probability events—crime or accidents
Concern that sexual performance will not match that of youth

Following are the five steps the therapist usually follows in helping patients gain control over negative, depressogenic thoughts:

1. Use of the Triple Column Technique (described below) to become aware of habitual, depressogenic thought and monitor their effects on mood and behavior.
2. Suppression of negative thoughts and substitution of task-oriented or self-image-building thoughts and recording of frequency of negative thoughts over time and successful attempts to suppress them.
3. If the patient is unable to suppress dysfunctional thoughts, a switch is made to temporal control (for a specified time only) or geographic

control (thoughts suppressed while in a specific area, such as, desk, armchair, or leave the area temporarily).

4. Scanning of past events to increase identification of positive factors and decrease preoccupation with negative factors.
5. Develop ability to self-reinforce through positive self-talk and built-in reward systems for successful coping through thought-control attempts.

GOAL SETTING. Depressed patients react positively to tangible evidence of successful or superior performance (Loeb et al., 1971). But depressed persons usually have problems in setting and meeting goals. Typically, they set impossible goals and then, when they cannot meet them, their negative self-worth and self-depreciating thoughts are confirmed.

TRIPLE COLUMN TECHNIQUE. The Triple Column Technique (Rush and Beck, 1978) is often used to help the patient to identify and reality test upsetting cognitions. The patient records the events associated with unpleasant affect as well as the actual cognitions or automatic thoughts associated with the dysphoria. Next, the patient attempts to answer these cognitions using concrete evidence ("facts") to test the validity and reasonableness of each cognition. The evidence for and against each specific thought (e.g., "I'm a complete failure," or "Everyone is disgusted with me.") is examined. In this way, the patient learns to see his cognitions as psychological events or responses rather than as an accurate reflection of reality. The therapist helps the patient categorize his cognitions under relevant themes such as self-blame, inferiority, or deprivation. The patient learns that of the many ways to interpret life experiences he tends to persevere in a few stereo-typed, self-defeating patterns.

In therapy, the therapist initially selects a simple, easily done task, in order to allow the opportunity for successful completion on the part of the patient. As the patient's self-confidence, motivation, and energy level increase, the goals for each session and for homework assignments are gradually elevated in difficulty. In the physically incapacitated, disabled, or bedridden old person, the completion of simple tasks of personal hygiene and survival may be the beginning point in goal setting. Such efforts to increase the patient's independence and self-sufficiency do a great deal to enhance self-esteem and reduce depression.

Goals should also be age-specific. The practice of applauding the old for doing the things that are characteristic of young people subtly denigrates old age and the goals appropriate to that stage of life. "Thus, for example, we may applaud the old man who can still play three sets of tennis, run a marathon race or father a child or the old lady for looking as young as her daughter. However they are rarely applauded for that which should be a distinctive achievement for old age, such as a sense of wisdom and a non-striving peacefulness" (Meerloo, 1955b).

Goal setting also includes time management. Time that is structured with goals has increased value and provides something to look forward to. Time, when unstructured, accumulates with the "weight of fallen snow and moves with glacial slowness" (Sheehy, 1981).

THE MERITS OF THERAPY

In conclusion, there is a notable lack of controlled outcome studies measuring the therapeutic effects of one form of psychotherapy or comparing the differences between two or more types of therapy in treating depressed persons over 65. Yet, based on empirical observations and extensive clinical experience, several authors have reached similar conclusions: that the elderly are more responsive to therapy than we have thus far believed, that traditional analytic approaches need to be modified to address the unique developmental needs and limited remaining life span of elderly persons, and that therapy which is cost-effective, nonstigmatizing, and accessible is more likely to be accepted by the elderly. Cognitive-behavior therapy, which has demonstrated effectiveness as a treatment for depression in a young adult population, may prove to be the psychotherapy of choice with the elderly for several reasons. Being time-limited, goal-oriented, and structured, it is less costly than more traditional approaches. Also, its educational and self-help focus makes it less stigmatizing and more acceptable to the elderly. In many ways it mimics the Martin method of the 1920s, which was reported to be extremely effective in treating the elderly. Because its process and techniques are sufficiently structured, it is also conducive to replicable research and is teachable (especially to a variety of health care providers who are in settings where the elderly congregate or reside). Its foundation in learning theory, behavioral change, and stress management puts the accent on prevention: strengthening coping abilities and thereby reducing risk for depression in the future.

REFERENCES

Abraham, K. The applicability of psycho-analytic treatment to patient at an advanced age. In *Selected Papers of Psychoanalysis*. London: Hogarth Press, 1949, pp. 312–17.

Bandura, A. *Social Learning Theory*. Englewood Cliffs, N.J.: Prentice Hall, 1977.

Beck, A.T. The development of depression: a cognitive model in Friedman, R., and Katz, M. (Eds.), *The Psychology of Depression*. Washington, D.C.: Winston, 1974.

Beck, A.T. *Cognitive Therapy and the Emotional Disorders*. New York: International Universities Press, 1976.

Brink, T.L. Brief psychotherapy: a case report illustrating its potential effectiveness. *Journal of the American Geriatrics Society,* 1977, 25(6):273–76.

Butler, R. Intensive psychotherapy for the hospitalized aged. *Geriatrics,* 1960, 15:644–53.

Butler, R., and Lewis, M. *Aging and Mental Health: Positive Psychosocial Approaches.* St. Louis: C. V. Mosby, 1977.

Chaisson-Stewart, G.M., Beutler, L., Yost, E., and Allender, J. Cognitive group therapy: training therapists and treating the elderly. *Journal of Psychosocial Nursing and Mental Health Services,* 1984, 22(5):25–30.

Coyne, J.C. Depression and the response of others. *Journal of Abnormal Psychology,* 1976, 85:186–93.

Crook, T., Ferris, S., McCarthy, M., and Rae, D. Utility of digit recall tasks for assessing memory in the aged. *Journal of Consulting and Clinical Psychology,* 1980, 48:228–33.

Eisdorfer, C., and Stotsky, B. Intervention, treatment and rehabilitation of psychiatric disorders. In Birren, J., and Schaie, K.W. (Eds.), *Handbook of the Psychology of Aging.* New York: Van Nostrand Reinhold, 1977.

Ellis, A. *Reason and Emotion in Psychotherapy.* New York: Lyle Stuart, 1962.

Freud, S. On psychotherapy in *Collected Papers,* vol. 1. London: Hogarth Press, 1924, pp. 249–263.

Gallagher, D., and Thompson, L. *Depression in the Elderly: A Behavioral Treatment Manual.* Los Angeles: University of Southern California, Ethel Percy Andrus Gerontology Center, 1981.

Gioe, V.J. Cognitive modification and positive group experience as a treatment for depression. Doctoral dissertation, Arizona State University, Tempe, Arizona, 1975. *Dissertation Abstracts International,* 36:3039B, 1975. (University Microfilms No. 75-28, 219).

Goldfarb, A.I. Psychotherapy of aged persons. IV: One aspect of the psychodynamics of the therapeutic situation with aged patients. *Psychoanalytic Review,* 1955, 42:180.

Goldfarb, A.I. Psychotherapy of the aged: the use and value of an adaptational frame of reference. *Psychoanalytic Review,* 1956, 43:68.

Gottesman, L.E., Quarterman, C.E., and Cohn, G.M. Psychosocial treatment of the aged. In Eisdorfer, C., and Lawton, M.P. (Eds.), *The Psychology of Adult Development.* Washington, D.C.: American Psychological Association, 1973.

Grotjan, M. Analytic psychotherapy with the elderly. *Psychoanalytic Review.* 1955, 42:419.

Hammer, M. Psychotherapy with the aged. In Hammer, M. (Ed.), *The Theory and Practice of Psychotherapy with Specific Disorders.* Springfield, Ill.: Charles C Thomas, 1972.

Hoyer, W. Design considerations in the assessment of psychotherapy with the elderly. Paper presented at the meeting of the Gerontological Society, Dallas, Texas. November 1978.

Jelliffe, S.E. The old-age factor in psychoanalytic therapy. *Medical Journals Review,* 1925, 121:7–12.

Karpf, R.J. Modalities of psychotherapy with the elderly. *Journal of the American Geriatrics Society,* August 1980, 28(8):367–71.

Lawton, G. Psychotherapy with older persons. *Psychoanalysis,* 1952, 1(2):27–41.

Levy, Sandra M., Derogatis, L.R., Gallagher, D., and Gatz, M. Intervention with older adults and the evaluation of outcome. In Poon, L.W. (Ed.), *Aging in the 1980's,* Washington, D.C.: American Psychological Association, 1980.

Lewinsohn, P.M. Behavioral treatment of depression. In Davidson, P. (Ed.), *Behavioral Management of Anxiety, Depression and Pain.* New York: Brunner/Mazel, 1976.

Lewinsohn, P.M. and Libet, J. Pleasant events activity schedules and depression. *Journal of Abnormal Psychology,* 1972, 79:291–95.

Lewinsohn, P.M., and MacPhillamy, D.J. The relationship between age and engagement in pleasant activities. *Journal of Gerontology,* 1974, 29:290–94.

Lewinsohn, P.M. and Graf, M. Pleasant events and depression. *Journal of Consulting and Clinical Psychology,* 1973, 41:261–68.

Loeb, A., Beck, A.T., and Diggory, J.C. Differential effects of success and failure on depressed and non-depressed patients. *Journal of Nervous and Mental Diseases,* 1971, 152:106–14.

McLean, P.D. Therapeutic decision-making in treatment of depression. In P. Davidson (Ed.), *The Behavioral Management of Anxiety, Depression and Pain.* New York: Brunner/Mazel, 1976.

Martin, Lillian J. *An Handbook for Old Age Counselors.* San Francisco: Geertz Printing Company, 1944.

Meerloo, J. Contribution of psychoanalysis to problems of the aged. In Heiman, M. (Ed.), *Psychoanalysis and Social Work.* New York: International University Press, 1953, pp. 321–37.

Meerloo, J. Transference and resistance in geriatric psychotherapy. *Psychoanalytic Review,* 1955a, 42:72.

Meerloo, J. Psychotherapy with elderly people. *Geriatrics,* 1955b, 10:583.

Meichenbaum, D. *Cognitive-Behavior Modification.* New York: Plenum, 1977.

Paykel, E.S. Recent life events and clinical depression. In Gunderson, E.K., and Rahe, R.H. (Eds.), *Life Stress and Illness.* Springfield, Ill.: Charles C Thomas, 1974.

Power, C.A., and McCarron, L.T. Treatment of depression in persons residing in homes for the aged. *Gerontologist,* April 1975, pp. 132–35.

Rechtschaffen, A. Psychotherapy with geriatric patients: a review of the literature. *Journal of Gerontology,* 1959, 14:73.

Rehm, L.P., and Kornblith-Sander, J. Behavior therapy for depression: a review of recent developments. *Progress in Behavior Modification,* 1979, 7:277–318.

Rothblum, E.D., Sholomskas, A.J., Barry, C., and Prusoff, B.A. Issues in clinical trials with depressed elderly. *Journal of the American Geriatric Society,* November 30, 1982, 11:694–99.

Rush, J.A., and Beck, A.T. Cognitive therapy of depression and suicide. *American Journal of Psychotherapy,* 1978, 2:201–19.

Schmickley, V.G. The effects of cognitive-behavioral modification upon depressed outpatients. Doctoral dissertation, Michigan State University, 1976. *Dissertation Abstracts International,* 37:987B, 1976. (University Microfilms No. 76-18, 675.)

Shaw, B.T. Comparison of cognitive therapy and behavior therapy in treatment of depression. *Journal of Consulting and Clinical Psychology,* 1977, 45(4):543–51.

Sheehy, G. *Pathfinders.* New York: William Morrow, 1981.

Shipley, C.R., and Fazio, A.F. Pilot study of a treatment for psychological depression. *Journal of Abnormal Psychology,* October 1973, 82(2):372–76.

Steuer, J., and Hammen, C. Cognitive-behavioral group therapy for the depressed elderly: issues and adaptation. Unpublished paper, University of California, Los Angeles, 1983.

Taylor, F.G., and Marshall, W.L. A cognitive-behavioral therapy for depression. *Cognitive Therapy and Research,* 1977, 1:59–72.

Weinberg, J. Psychiatric techniques in treatment of older people. In Donohue, W., and Tibbits, C. (Eds.), *Growing in the Older Years.* Ann Arbor, Mich.: University of Michigan Press, 1951, pp. 61–70.

Weissman, M.M., and Klerman, G. Sex differences and the epidemiology of depression. *Archives of General Psychiatry,* 1977, 34:98–111.

Wilson, T.G. Cognitive behavior therapy. In Foreyt, J.P. and Rathjen, D.P., (Eds.), *Cognitive-Behavior Therapy.* New York: Plenum Press, 1978.

Yesavage, J., and Karasu, T. Psychotherapy with elderly patients. *American Journal of Psychotherapy,* 1982, 36(1):41–55.

Young, J., and Beck, A.T. The cognitive therapy scale. Unpublished paper, Mood Control Center, University of Pennsylvania, Philadelphia, 1980.

11

Group Therapy

Elizabeth B. Yost
M. Anne Corbishley

Since the mid-1940s, group work has become an increasingly popular form of treatment for the elderly. In fact, group counseling is considered by some to be the treatment of choice for the elderly because of the curative aspects of the group process (Waters et al., 1976; Finkel, 1980).

Of the 11 factors identified by Yalom (1975) as crucial to change in groups, five are particularly applicable to groups of older people. Two of the more important factors are socialization and group cohesiveness. Many elderly people suffer from intense loneliness. Friends and family die or visit less often, ability to travel to social events and to friends' houses is reduced by illness or inadequate transportation; thus are elderly people slowly stripped of meaningful relationships. Simply belonging to a group can decrease a sense of social isolation and can lead to the development of significant relationships among members. The group offers members an opportunity to revitalize and maintain social skills that may have become rusty through lack of use. Through the group, they can build a new network of ties and regain confidence in their ability to make friends. In addition, the group setting provides the opportunity for members to receive affection, which is especially important because withdrawal of affection has been shown to accelerate the process of senility (Etzioni, cited in Burnside, 1978).

Two other important curative factors are universality and the instillation of hope. Old age seems to be accompanied by so many problems (social, financial, physical) that people easily become overwhelmed. It is reassuring to find out in a group that such problems are common, that one is not alone (Mardoyan and Weis, 1981). Furthermore, when one's body is failing and friends are dying, when one is able to do less and less each day, it is difficult to see a ray of hope. Sometimes the group allows a person to see that others have partially solved similar problems.

A final important element of the group situation is altruism. Many older people are thrust from a lifetime of giving to others and of being needed by them into a situation where they have no meaningful work and are not needed by anyone. The group gives them a place to be helpful to others and to gain importance through giving.

Until the late 1960s, group therapy was considered unsuitable for depressed people, either in a homogeneous group of depressives or as members of groups with other problems and diagnoses as a focus (Hollon and Shaw, 1979). It was felt that their negative attitudes led them to compare themselves unfavorably with other group members and thus become more depressed. Furthermore, their low energy levels and withdrawn behavior did not lead to positive contributions to the groups and even had a negative influence on other group members. More important, group therapy was not effective in reducing the symptoms of depression or preventing relapse.

However, the therapies that were used in group settings were the traditional expressive, process-oriented, and nondirective therapies, which were not particularly effective with depressed individuals. Then, in the 1960s and 1970s, various types of therapy were developed that proved helpful to depressed patients. Generally, these therapies were active, structured, time-limited, problem-oriented, and contained a cognitive or behavioral component or both.

There is ample research evidence of the efficacy of various types of group treatment for depression. Subjects have ranged from mildly depressed college students to severely afflicted, hospitalized patients, and results show a fairly consistent pattern. Behavioral group therapy proves better than nondirective or nonspecific group therapy (Shaw, 1977; Fuchs and Rehm, 1977). Cognitive behavior therapy increases in effectiveness when combined with positive group interaction (Gioe, cited in Rehm and Kornblith, 1979) or with behavioral techniques (Taylor and Marshall, 1977) and is better than pharmacotherapy (Rush et al., 1977). It appears, therefore, that at this point there exist several effective group treatments for depression.

TYPES OF GROUPS CONDUCTED WITH THE ELDERLY

The many types of groups that have been conducted with the elderly fall into four basic categories, though many groups combine aspects of several categories. These categories are activity and interest groups, problem-oriented groups, groups to restore or maintain functioning, and therapy and growth groups.

Activity and Interest Groups

These groups may be largely physical in focus, as are dance and creative movement, fitness, body awareness, or sports groups (Corey and Corey, 1982). Or the content may be more intellectual, as it is in current events discussion groups, poetry reading and writing groups, story-telling groups (Linsk et al., 1975), or educational seminars. Many of the activity groups for the elderly center around arts and crafts. When these groups involve a group project, such as presenting a play or making toys for a children's home, there are extra benefits, as such projects promote interaction with the community and raise the status of the elderly people. Musical groups are especially beneficial, partly because music itself is powerful in releasing emotions, but also because music allows for both individual and group performance and accommodates all levels of ability.

In general, activity and interest groups restore people's self-confidence in their ability to perform, to produce, and to learn. These groups take elderly people out of a world that is usually far too narrow for comfort, and allow them to cooperate with others. In some ways these groups meet needs that were formerly met by the work world.

Problem-Oriented Groups

These are groups where members share a common problem that is designated as the focus of the group. Many of the problems relate to the changes that occur in old age. Preretirement and retirement groups, for example, deal with the difficulties involved in the transition from productivity to what is often viewed as a time of uselessness (Schlossberg, 1973). Some groups are formed to help members cope with specific health problems, such as stroke, glaucoma, poor nutrition, and deafness. Frequently these health groups are educational, with an emphasis, if it isn't too late, on prevention.

One of the most common problems among the elderly is widowhood, the greatest difficulty being loneliness. A group is an especially effective way to help people cope with the loss of a life companion because there is a chance to vent feelings of loss and fears about the future as well as an opportunity to reach out for support. The group is also a good source of practical information about the many tasks (e.g., writing a will) that face a widow or widower.

For elderly people who are leaving an institution after an extended stay, preplacement groups are of value to help them adapt to greater independence and the loss of institutional security (Corey and Corey, 1982).

Groups to Restore or Maintain Functioning

Several of the groups used to restore or maintain functioning can also be used as therapeutic or growth groups, but it is assumed here, that their main purpose is to prevent, or at least slow down further deterioration. In some cases, groups are able to reverse the process of senility and restore people to previous levels of performance. These groups may deal with people who are severely disabled (e.g., those with organic brain syndrome) or with elderly people who show only a few signs of deterioration.

People with organic brain syndrome exhibit poor memory, confused thinking, and slow reactions. They are often lethargic and unresponsive. However, Corey and Corey (1982) report that simple games, singing, and sensory stimulation increase the amount of talking and interaction among members. Most important, group members show clearly that they enjoy and value the group experience.

Another form of group for organic brain syndrome patients is known as reality orientation, first developed by Folson in 1968. The technique may also be used with elderly people who are only slightly disoriented and confused. The essence of the program is that it continue for 24 hours a day, during which all the people in contact with a patient frequently take time to orient the patient to time, place, and person. Group sessions also focus on reality and may include memory and concentration games and structured activities around daily concerns such as grooming. Response to these groups is said to be dramatic, with patients becoming more alert and independent (Taulbee, 1978).

For elderly people who do not have organic brain syndrome but who have withdrawn or given up, remotivation therapy has proved both useful and popular. Groups are highly structured, and visual aids are used extensively in order to promote interest in such everyday topics as pets and vacations. Remotivation is seen as a precursor to rehabilitation (Dennis, 1978).

Elderly people who are functioning at a slightly higher level than those who are withdrawn both enjoy and benefit from resocialization groups which are designed to encourage social interaction, relearn basic social skills, and reinforce appropriate social behaviors (Lazarus, 1976; Weiner and Weinstock, 1979–80). The technique of reminiscing can be used as part of a resocialization group or may be the sole purpose for which the group meets. Looking back over one's life is therapeutic because it validates an elderly person's life experiences, promotes a sense of commonality with one's peers, and combats depression (Lewis and Butler, 1974; Wolff and Meyer, 1973).

In an effort to foster pride and a sense of unity, Burnside (1978) has conducted age-specific groups, that is, groups where only those over, say, 90, can join. Such groups can encourage the very old to remain socially active. Members may even see themselves as an elite group.

Therapy and Growth Groups

Clearly, this category and the previous ones frequently overlap. Reminiscing, for example, can be enjoyable and beneficial regardless of the purpose of a group or of the level of functioning of its members.

In recent years there has been an increasing realization that the elderly can grow and change and are interested in enriching their lives and improving their relationships. Consequently, many different types of growth groups have been developed. There are, for example, problem-solving workshops (Toseland, 1977), sexual enhancement programs, assertiveness training groups, behavioral therapy groups (Gallagher, 1979, 1981), support groups (Petty et al., 1976), well-being "Here and Now" groups (Ingersoll and Silverman, 1978), and personal exploration and creativity groups (Bates et al., 1982). It is believed that, in some cases, use of outpatient therapy groups can prevent or postpone institutionalization (Duetsch and Kramer, 1977).

RESEARCH FINDINGS ON GROUP WORK WITH THE ELDERLY

Although a great deal of group work with the elderly is reported in the literature, these reports are primarily of two types: descriptive accounts (e.g., Berland and Poggi, 1979; Lazarus, 1976; Lewis and Butler, 1974; Murray et al., 1980) and case studies (e.g., Britnell and Mitchell, 1981; Duetsch and Kramer, 1977; Steuer and Hammen, 1983). There has been little controlled research on the efficacy of groups for the elderly.

Most descriptive accounts and case reports are enthusiastic about the benefits of group counseling to the elderly clients, and short-term gains in psychological functioning have been claimed to be associated with most interventions, However, some doubt is cast on these claims by the fact that methods of evaluation in such studies are both limited and subjective. In fact some authors use leaders' observations as their sole means of evaluating the efficacy of the group treatment. For example, Mueller and Atlas (1972) worked with a group of five noncommunicative and withdrawn elderly male patients in a county hospital. According to the authors "it was apparent" that after eleven 30 minute sessions, patients achieved greater social interaction.

The remainder of this discussion on research is confined to studies using more objective measures of evaluation. However, the reader should note that few of these studies employ control groups or otherwise meet the criteria for well-designed research efforts.

Institutionalized Subjects

Several researchers have investigated the effect of group counseling or therapy on elderly persons institutionalized in state and private psychiatric hospitals and in nursing homes (Elder-Jucker, 1979; Lindell, 1978; Lopez, 1980; Moran, 1978; Nashef, 1980; Tutaj, 1975). In these studies therapy lasted from 6 to 16 sessions and was helpful in a variety of ways to the institutionalized elderly, e.g., in increasing life satisfaction (Moran, 1978) and self-concept (Lindell, 1978) and in teaching social skills (Lopez, 1980). Although these studies do not focus directly on depression, one might assume that any program that resulted in positive gains for the participants, e.g., in life satisfaction or self-esteem, would also reduce depression.

Two recent dissertations specifically designed to reduce depression by means of group therapy in residents of homes for the aged reported unsuccessful results. In the one case (Tutaj, 1975) the reason may have been that a discussion of developmental stages was both too abstract and too passive a form of therapy for the group involved. In the other case (Elder-Jucker, 1979), the instruments used were not appropriate and there were probably too few therapy sessions.

More encouraging results were obtained by Nashef (1980), who worked with 62 hospitalized geriatric patients, comparing the effects of three dynamically oriented therapy groups to a waiting list control group. The groups met for 10 weeks for four 75-minute sessions weekly. Results indicated that patients in the experimental groups, as compared with the controls, significantly decreased their scores from pretest to posttest on anxiety, depression, and hostility as measured by the Zung Depression Inventory and the Multiple Affect Adjective Check List. These gains were maintained at one month follow-up. Treated patients, compared with the untreated, also significantly increased their scores on internality as measured by the Interpersonal Locus of Control, and on life satisfaction, as measured by the Life Satisfaction Indices. Ward behavior of experimental subjects was not significantly affected by group therapy.

Noninstitutionalized Subjects

Studies using noninstitutionalized elderly as subjects have found group counseling or therapy to be effective in teaching assertiveness skills (Toseland, 1977), in decreasing self-reported problems (Zgliczynski, 1978), and in increasing morale (Zgliczynski, 1978) and social engagement (Moss, 1976). An investigation by Weiner and Weinstock (1979) compared the effects of active and passive leadership on groups of older adults involved in a resocialization program. Fifty-eight women and nine men, mean age 73.1, were randomly assigned to a group led by an active leader, a group led by a passive leader, or a no-treatment control condition. Groups met for one-hour sessions, once a week for 12 weeks. The study assessed differential group progress in two ways: one scale indicated group tempo as determined by members' interaction with one another within each session, and a group evaluation scale was administered to members at termination of the 12 sessions. Results indicated that in groups with active leadership, the tempo was fast and vibrant, whereas the tempo of the passive leadership groups was slow and depressed. Group evaluation scores showed that the members in the active group expressed more satisfaction with the overall group experience than did the passive group.

However, as no validity or reliability data were reported for the Group Evaluation Scale, it is difficult to assess these results.

Depressed Elderly Subjects (Noninstitutionalized)

Several recent investigations have studied the effect of group counseling or therapy on elderly persons who are depressed. Petty et al. (1976) investigated the value of support groups for elderly persons, most of whom were mildly to moderately depressed. The 30 participants were divided into four groups, which varied in size from six to nine members. Each group met for 10 two-hour discussion sessions with a break for socialization. The primary goals of the groups included presentation of objective information about normal changes in old age, brainstorming to solve common problems such as memory loss, and development of more effective interpersonal skills to cope with these changes.

Pre- and posttests were designed to evaluate attitudes toward old age, satisfaction with daily activities, psychological and physical concerns and beliefs about the similarity of one's own concerns and those of other older persons. Comparisons of data from pre-and posttests indicated that group participants had come to believe with certainty that their problems were similar to those of others. Members also reported that they had engaged in new behaviors since the onset of the groups, such as improving safety conditions in their homes and interacting with their children in different ways. The authors concluded that group members had become more adept at both analyzing sources of physical and psychological discomfort and adopting new behaviors to cope with these concerns.

Although these results are encouraging, they need to be viewed with some reservation. The researchers give no information about the tests used to measure pre-post changes, or about the measurement of the members' initial depression. In addition, postgroup depression was not measured, so it is impossible to say what impact the group had. From the researchers' descriptions, it appears that much of the postgroup change was in the form of generalized self-reports. Thus it is not clear how much weight can be given to the results of this study.

Paradis (1973) also studied the manner in which elderly depressed persons were coping with age related problems. Ten moderately to severely depressed persons were given 15 weeks of supportive group therapy. Therapy sessions lasted 90 minutes and focused on coping with depression and related symptoms (e.g., sleeplessness, loss of appetite, other somatic complaints, lack of attention to physical appearance, and lack of socialization). At termination of therapy, six of the seven subjects who finished the study showed marked or very marked improvement in depression and attendant physical symptoms, in physical appearance and in socialization. Improvement was reported on the basis of detailed behavioral observations. Utilization of medical services decreased markedly during the 15 weeks of therapy and during the 15 weeks following therapy as compared with the 15-week period prior to therapy. For five of the members, gains were retained at three-month follow-up. There is value in this study in the inclusion of more objective criteria—i.e., observations of specific behaviors, rather than reliance on self-report alone. Major limitations, however, are the small number of subjects and the lack of a control group.

Two studies attempted to compare the efficacy of behavioral therapy to less structured therapy in relieving depression in the elderly. The first of these was by Ingersoll and Silverman (1978), who studied a group of elderly persons who were functioning independently in the community but were experiencing anxiety or depression resulting from age-related losses. The 17 volunteers (average age, 69), who had responded to announcements of a group for older adults experiencing tension, depression, memory lapses, or insomnia, were randomly assigned to one of two groups that met weekly for eight two-hour sessions with two cotherapists. The more structured "Here and Now" group focused on present problems and attempted to offer specific pragmatic help rather than trying to uncover past conflicts. Role-playing, modeling, and other behavioral techniques were used along with progressive relaxation to help clients cope with anxiety resulting from recent life changes. The "There and Then" group used reminiscing and a life review process to help clients establish a bridge between the past and the present.

Pre-post measurements were tests (unspecified) relating to self-esteem, anxiety and somatic behavior, therapists' progress notes covering participants' verbal and nonverbal behavior, and a debriefing telephone interview that occurred one week after termination. Only 10 of the original 17 members remained in the groups for the full eight sessions.

Results of this study were rather confusing. Most clients improved somewhat on most variables (e.g., self-esteem and anxiety), but, unexpectedly, both anxiety and somatic symptoms increased for some members of the behavioral group. Any improvements that occurred were small and insufficient to identify one group as more successful than the other. The authors suggest that careful screening is needed, as some types of therapy may not meet the needs of some elderly people. The small number of subjects and lack of a control group coupled with the high dropout and absentee rates cast some doubt on the results of this study that are already rather obscure.

In a similar study, working with 23 elderly depressed persons who applied for services at an outpatient clinic, Gallagher (1981) compared the efficacy of behavioral and nondirective group psychotherapy. Subjects were mildly to moderately depressed, having MMPI Depression Scale scores elevated at least two standard deviations above the mean. In all, there were four groups. Subjects were randomly assigned to one of the two treatment conditions: behavioral or supportive group therapy. Groups of approximately seven subjects were conducted by two experienced therapists who led one group in each condition. Groups met for 10 sessions of 90 minutes duration, held twice weekly for five weeks. Behavioral treatment followed Lewinsohn's model, which aims to improve social skills and increase the frequency of pleasant activities. In contrast, supportive treatment was quite unstructured and focused on helping clients to clarify and express their feelings, and to develop an atmosphere of group support.

The pre-post assessment battery included six measures of depression: Beck Depression Inventory, Zung Self-Rating Depression Scale, MMPI Depression Scale (D), the depression scale of the Hopkins Symptom Checklist (SCL-90), Dysfunctional Attitude Scale, and Cognitive Distortion Vignette Series. Results indicated that clients in both conditions improved considerably over time on self-report measures of depression and social behaviors and on observer ratings of interpersonal skills, regardless of which treatment group they were in. However, observer ratings of in-group verbal interaction indicated significantly greater improvement over time for behavioral subjects. In addition, during posttreatment interviews, behavioral subjects reported greater satisfaction with treatment and improved overall functioning.

This carefully conducted study lends support to the view that depressed elderly people can be helped by group treatment. However, as the author points out, the lack of substantial differences between the two groups may be due to the strong effect of social interaction on group members. This problem could be handled in future research by the inclusion of a control group.

Four groups of elderly depressed subjects were treated with cognitive therapy in a pilot study (Chaisson, et al., 1984; Yost et al., 1983). Based on scores from the Zung Self-Rating Depression Scale and the Beck Depression Inventory, 46 patients (aged 62 to 84) were identified as minimally, mildly, moderately, or severely depressed and randomly assigned to four groups led by trained cognitive therapists, whose competency in this type of therapy was also measured before and after treatment. Therapy lasted for six weekly two-hour sessions, and all groups showed a nonsignificant decrease in depression at posttest. In their discussion of the results of this study, Chaisson et al. (1984) point out that reduction in depression was related to therapist skill in cognitive therapy, indicating that the specific therapy, rather than just the socialization effect, was important. The researchers also felt that six weeks was too short a time in which to produce significant results.

Despite the limitations and inadequacies of many of the studies that assess the impact of group therapy on elderly people, several tentative conclusions can be drawn. Clearly, it is possible for the elderly to function well in a group setting and to both make and maintain changes in their lives. Apparently these changes are more likely to occur as a result of relatively structured groups of a behavioral nature, where both members and leader are active. It would seem important to build into the group some opportunity for socialization, as this is clearly one of the most therapeutic features of the group experience for this population. It is also apparent from several studies that groups may need to be conducted over a longer than usual number of weeks, perhaps because of such problems as absenteeism due to ill-health and other unavoidable difficulties. It seems that more than eight weeks of treatment may be necessary. Although some treatments seem to be more effective than others, it also appears that elderly people, particularly those who are not institutionalized, will respond to any supportive group situation, deriving comfort from the company of others and from a sense of the commonality of their problems.

CONDUCTING GROUP THERAPY WITH THE ELDERLY

The history of groups for the elderly clearly shows the benefits of group association for this age group. Kubie and Landau (1953) make several observations that would appear to apply to most group situations with the elderly. First, they note the value of encouraging members to take as large a part as possible in running the group. Things appear to run more smoothly, members are more cooperative and appreciative, and self-confidence increases when other elderly people, as opposed to the counselor or social worker make decisions about projects, disposition of funds, topics for discussion, and so forth.

A second important point made by Kubie and Landau (1953) concerns motivation, which can be a complex issue with this population. Elderly people are often slow to take up a new interest such as joining a group, and once involved, may not continue after a few sessions. This reluctance may be the result of health problems, lack of self-confidence, insufficient knowledge of what demands will be made of them, or even an avoidance of their own age group for fear of being viewed as old. For some, the fear goes deeper in that they refuse to view themselves as old and thus cut themselves off from a reference group that could provide support and a sense of identity. Despite these concerns and fears, a primary motivation for most elderly people in joining a group is social. Regardless of the purpose and content of a particular group, most elderly people are motivated to join by a desire to take part in what others are doing and by a desire to please and get the approval of the leader and of other group members.

In the case of the severely depressed, motivation is unlikely to be social, as these people are so withdrawn that the task of meeting others appears highly aversive. If they do attend a group, their motivation is more likely to be an urgent need for relief from their misery. They may, indeed, be there only partly of their own volition, as friends and family may have pressured them into seeking help.

A further powerful motivation of the elderly is altruism. They are likely to become more committed to a group when a project is undertaken for the benefit of others or when an audience is involved.

Leader's Attitude

The special concerns and characteristics of elderly people suggest that a group leader for this population must be especially sensitive to the needs of the group members and must be flexible in both leadership style and group methods. Some adaptation will be needed, as behaviors and techniques that are suitable for groups of younger people may not be so for groups of the elderly.

In addition, the leader needs to be well aware of the general societal view of aging people. Eisdorfer (1983) believes that society victimizes old people, viewing them as needy, dependent, and helpless. An effective group leader must both understand and repudiate this stereotype.

The leader's attitude that is perhaps of greatest importance is one of respect. Those in the helping professions often show great disrespect for the elderly by treating them like children, that is, by ordering them around, not consulting their wishes, using baby talk, assuming that they are incompetent, and filling their time with meaningless busywork. While it is true that people in advanced stages of senility may resemble children, most older adults are not senile, and it is far more common for helpers to underestimate rather than overestimate the potential of elderly people (Burnside, 1978). For the most part, the elderly show both dignity and courage in the way they cope with a time of life that can be difficult and disappointing (Levy et al., 1980).

A second important factor is the group leader's attitude to both old age and his or her own parents (Gatz et al., 1980). The leader who is apprehensive about aging and dying or who is upset by illness and debility will communicate these attitudes to the group members and can only do harm. The elderly have a normal human need for physical touch but few opportunities outside the group to experience it. Leaders must feel comfortable touching people who may have lost a lot of their youthful physical attractiveness (Murray et al., 1980).

It is also difficult for leaders to be effective with this age group if they have not resolved many of their relationship difficulties with their own parents (Mardoyan and Weis, 1981). There is a tendency for elderly people to treat younger therapists and helpers like their children, and it is very easy for old, intergenerational conflicts to arise again on both sides. In order to be able to maintain the necessary therapeutic objectivity, leaders need to resolve their own parental issues (Mintz et al., 1981).

A third important issue for group leaders to consider is that of values. Because of the age difference between leader and members it is natural for value differences to occur. For example, many of the elderly have what younger people call "old-fashioned" ideas on such subjects as sex, the family, and religion. The leader needs to understand that, unless the expressed purpose of the group is values clarification, it is not likely to be helpful to the group to focus on these differences. Elderly people have spent a lifetime developing a value system, and many have neither the time nor the desire to change. Group leaders, therefore, need to be alert to the potential disruptive effect of their comments on value-laden topics, and in general adopt an attitude of nonargumentative acceptance.

The differences between the leader and the members are revealed most clearly in language. In order to respect the elderly, group leaders should not assume that first name address is acceptable; the members should be asked what form of address they prefer. Overfamiliar comments and inappropriate humor can be shocking to people raised in an environment of more formal and restrained speech. Elderly people are likely to be confused by slang words and offended by swearing. Thus leaders may need to modify their language to some extent, though they should always be careful not to talk in a condescending or patronizing manner.

Fears of the Elderly About Therapy and Groups

For most of the present generation of elderly people, the idea of seeking help for problems other than physical ones is not familiar. They tend to retain the attitudes toward mental illness that were prevalent in their youth, and thus frequently believe that if you need the help of a counselor or a therapist you must be going crazy (Finkel, 1980). In addition, elderly people have little experience in belonging to counseling groups. They do not know what to expect or what will be expected of them, and often fear that they will get confused, be unable to follow what is happening (because of hearing problems, for example), and will appear stupid or, even worse, senile (Lago and Hoffman, 1977; Wolff and Meyer, 1979).

Present-day elderly people are less accustomed to discussing their feelings and private thoughts than are more psychologically sophisticated younger people, so feelings of fear and shame may be generated by the process or even the prospect of talking about their personal concerns (Lago and Hoffman, 1977). For elderly people whose social skills have atrophied, the act of speaking aloud in a group may be frightening. Concern and conflict may also arise over the seating in the group. Members may have a desire for close physical proximity, but the reticence and sense of privacy that is common to their generation can cause anxiety about such closeness (Burnside, 1978). These fears, which are special to the elderly, make them reluctant to seek help (Waters et al., 1976) and slow to trust others (Murray et al., 1980).

In order to address these fears, it is recommended that group members be interviewed individually before the group sessions start. This gives each person an opportunity to get to know the leader, to learn the purpose of the group, how sessions will be conducted, what is to be expected of members, and what benefits can be anticipated. A sensitive leader can explore each member's concerns and allay most fears before the first meeting (Lago and Hoffman, 1977).

Structure of Groups with the Elderly

Although cognitive abilities do not necessarily decline with age (Price et al., 1980), certain changes in functioning can occur either because of age or as a result of medication, and must be taken into account in the structuring of the group. For example, attention and processing styles change. Elderly people may not be able to focus their attention for as long, their minds may wander more easily, and they may take a longer time to organize their thoughts before they speak (Ford and Pfefferbaum, 1980). In addition, the ability to analyze and synthesize material may decline to some extent (Cerella et al., 1980). When we take these factors into account and also remember the fears of the elderly regarding therapy, it is clear that an effective way to conduct groups for older adults is according to an educational model (Bates et al., 1982). The classroom approach is not only psychologically acceptable but also provides the necessary structure that has been shown to produce increased performance on learning tasks (Lopez, 1980).

Specifically, explanations and directions should be clear and short, concepts should be presented as simply as possible, and time allowed for assimilation. The leader needs to be active and directive (Weiner and Weinstock, 1979). This means asking direct questions that relate precisely to the material at hand, attempting to involve all group members and presenting structured and relevant activities to the group. At the same time, it must be expected that, because of delayed response time, the pace of the group will be somewhat slow (Corey and Corey, 1982). In order to keep the group on track, the leader needs to ask for frequent feedback from members about what they are experiencing and learning (Kalson, 1982). Content needs to be specified, planned, and prioritized. A 1981 study by Gallagher demonstrated the superior effectiveness of behavioral over unstructured therapy.

In view of the almost universal need of elderly people for greater social contact, it is helpful to structure the group so that socialization is encouraged and facilitated. This may involve, for example, providing refreshments before or after sessions, arranging car-pooling, distributing lists of telephone numbers of group members (with their permission, of course) (Burnside, 1978).

In general, because of such factors as absenteeism and need for increased social interaction, progress in groups with the elderly may extend over more sessions than is usual with younger groups. However, the groups still should be time-limited, and sessions held frequently (Lago and Hoffman, 1977).

Process Issues

Special attention needs to be paid to certain aspects of the group process when one is conducting groups with the elderly. For example, the issue of confidentiality is important. Residents in hospitals or nursing homes have very little privacy and are often punished for misdemeanors by removal of privileges. For these people, self-disclosure could have disastrous consequences. Elderly people may have a stronger concern about maintaining privacy than do younger people. Thus it is important that group members discuss the issue of confidentiality and especially its realistic limits (Burnside, 1978).

Another process issue is that of confronting and probing. The elderly neither enjoy nor benefit from groups where they are expected to expose and explore their deepest and most painful emotions and concerns. They often need support and encouragement more than they need confrontation. Any probing or confronting that the leader feels is appropriate should be done gently and with caution (Corey and Corey, 1982).

Group cohesiveness can also present difficulties. On the one hand, the elderly are often very supportive of their peers, whom they may view as fellow sufferers, and are also gracious in their appreciation of the group leaders' efforts. On the other hand, members may be socially isolated and in great need of individual attention, and thus may behave in a demanding and egocentric fashion in the group. Group cohesiveness can also be affected by the high absentee rate and frequent turnover (Lazarus, 1976). In addition, many of the elderly have moved from positions of power and responsibility to a state of comparative ineffectuality. Those who feel strongly the loss of control may unwittingly use the group as a place to recapture some control or a position of prominence (Burnside, 1978).

It is important that part of the group process be an allowance for complaining, storytelling, and general social interaction (Corey and Corey, 1982). The group may be the only social outlet for members, whose need to talk must be respected.

The therapist-client relationship has rather different limits than is usual with younger clients. The elderly tend to want the leader to share personal details and respond with interest and warmth, thus creating a sense of intimacy that may be inadvisable for other groups but is very appropriate for the elderly. A valuable part of this process is the giving and receiving of affection, in the form of touching, hugging, smiling, and verbal expressions. It is here that the leader needs to be a model to the group, encourage the expression of concern and affection, and ensure that no one gets left out. Particularly in need of warmth and signs of physical caring are people whose illness or handicaps may have made them feel or look less attractive than before.

A final aspect of group process concerns the termination of the session. It is important that there be little or no unfinished business at the end of each session. Elderly people have an understandable concern with the rapid passage of time and the possible imminence of death, and consequently do not feel comfortable leaving things incomplete. They also know that illness may force them to miss the next session and thus they may never see the end of a particular issue (Kalson, 1982).

Practical Considerations

The physical condition of many elderly people requires that those conducting groups consider various practical issues. In the first place, group members need to be carefully screened in terms of their illness, their medication, and their level of functioning in relation to the purpose of the group. Some medication, for example, may produce delusions or severe agitation, which could be disruptive in a discussion group. The presence of a severely regressed person in a group of well-functioning elderly people could be discouraging to everyone.

Attendance is likely to be erratic because of illness or problems posed by dangerous weather conditions (e.g., icy streets) or the need to rely on others for transportation. However, lack of attendance should not be ignored. It is encouraging to members when the leader calls if they missed a session, explaining what happened in the group meeting, and demonstrating support and concern for their continued involvement (Corey and Corey, 1982). The leader may be the only person in their lives who takes the time to call.

The meeting place for group sessions needs to be chosen carefully and modified if necessary. Elderly people feel the cold, so the room should be warm enough and draft-free. Slippery floors and lightweight scatter rugs are hazardous, and deep, soft arm chairs can be almost impossible to get out of for a person with leg and back problems. Harsh lights, insufficient light, and irrelevant noises are all more distracting to the elderly than to younger people.

The time of the session is a matter of concern. Evening is usually not suitable as those on medication are ready for bed, and outpatients are often afraid to leave their homes at night. Immediately after lunch is a time of rest for many elderly people. Access to transportation also influences when people can come to a group; the leader may need to take some responsibility for helping with transportation. Unlike younger people, the elderly may not drive and may not be able to walk to a bus stop. Length of time of sessions should match the energy level of the participants, 90 minutes usually being a good length.

Special Demands on the Leader

It is apparent from what has been said thus far, that the leader of a group of elderly people is in a special position, one that can be very demanding of the leader's time, energy, and skills. For one thing, the leader has a more complex role than is usual in groups with other populations. For the elderly, the group leader is a friend, one of their few social contacts, a link with the real world; the leader is a model of social skills and of how to give affection and reinforcement; the leader may be, in turn, both parent and child to the members, monitoring their physical well-being, and bearing the brunt of any negative emotion they may feel toward their own children.

Group members themselves can be demanding, anxious, and slow to warm up. They may have deficient interpersonal skills and be hypochondriacal. In addition, the health and group functioning of group members may deteriorate visibly from week to week. Some members may be hospitalized or even die during the course of the group. In any case, loss and death will tend to be topics of frequent discussion.

In the face of all this, it is not surprising that group leaders can easily become depressed and start to believe that, as age cannot be halted nor the social system changed, their influence in the lives of group members is negligible and their efforts futile. The slow pace of the group can also be discouraging. Sometimes a leader who is young, healthy, and has had little experience with loss may find it hard to empathize with members and may become impatient. Or the leaders may go to the other extreme and provide so much support and sympathy that members are encouraged to remain dependent or even to regress.

Because the task of leader is so difficult, various recommendations are made to help reduce the impact of the demands of the role. First, groups need to be small, with six to eight members. A cotherapist can be very useful to share the responsibility and may be needed with more than five members (Altholz, 1978). Because of the complex social, medical, and psychological difficulties of the elderly and because of the generation gap between members and leader, a special training program is recommended where leaders can acquire knowledge about the population and also explore their own age-biases and parental issues (Wolff and Meyer, 1979). Corey and Corey (1982) suggest that group leaders not work full-time with the elderly and find other avenues for staying vital and enthusiastic. They also believe that it is important for leaders to limit their expectations of both the group and themselves, taking the attitude that *any* progress is good, and the leader cannot fix everything. Finally it is suggested that leaders who must work full-time with this population (e.g., in a nursing home) get support and ongoing supervision from someone who works in a different environment and is therefore more likely to be objective and capable of providing a fresh look at the group (Goldfarb, 1971).

Advantages to Working with the Elderly

People who have worked with the elderly frequently give eloquent testimony to the rewards they derive from contact with this population (Burnside, 1981; Corey and Corey, 1982). Any extended relationship with old people introduces one to the variety and richness of their experience. The younger person gains a sense of historical perspective and frequently a better understanding of his or her own parents (Britnell and Mitchell, 1981). Also, the elderly can become role models of how to cope with loss and suffering (Lewis and Butler, 1974). Younger therapists thus get a chance to face the prospect of their own eventual decline (Berland and Poggi, 1979) and learn how to approach that time of life with courage and dignity. Most elderly people are deeply appreciative of any efforts to help them and respond to such help with kindness and enthusiasm. Although there may be some special problems in working with this age group, most older people have a great deal to offer. It can be both a privilege and a very rewarding experience to work with them.

APPLICATION OF COGNITIVE BEHAVIOR THERAPY

Of the various new approaches to the treatment of depression, cognitive behavior therapy is one of the most effective. The reader will recall from the previous chapter that this therapy focuses on changing negative thinking patterns which are assumed to be responsible for the negative emotions associated with depression.

There are three main reasons that cognitive behavior therapy is particularly appropriate as a treatment for depression in the elderly. In the first place, this therapy deals with the potentially depressive aspects of life peculiar to old age. Second, it attacks directly the particular negative beliefs that both produce and maintain depression in the elderly. Third, the method by which the therapy is conducted requires the clients to act in ways that would tend to extinguish depressive attitudes and behaviors.

Potentially Depressive Life Situation

As has been noted previously, old age is to some extent characterized by loss—loss of health and mobility, of friends and family, of role satisfaction, and of autonomy. In addition, poverty frequently forces old people to follow an inadequate diet and to live in unattractive and even unsafe surroundings. In many cases, the changes and losses come suddenly and accumulate rapidly so that elderly people have little time to make adjustments. Obviously, there is enormous potential for feelings of confusion, helplessness, and loneliness, and it is easy to see how a state of clinical depression could develop.

Cognitive behavior therapy addresses these problems directly by encouraging group members to examine the sorrows and frustrations of their lives. Rather than focusing on venting feelings or problem solving, the therapy assesses the ways in which members think about their situations and teaches them how to avoid or change thinking patterns that lead to depression. For example, if a best friend dies, it is neither true nor helpful to think, "Now I am totally alone in the world." A less depressive thought might be, "I'm sad because I've lost a friend but I still have family and other friends." Similarly, an increase in blood pressure may be disturbing and have serious implications, but it is likely to lead to depression to think: "It's all over. I'm as good as dead. I might as well give up now." It would be more positive to think, "I'll have to take it easier in some ways because of my elevated blood pressure, but there are still lots of things I can enjoy." Thus, cognitive behavior therapy does not ignore the fact that much of life can be distressing for the elderly, but tries to teach the skills that will enable elderly people to take as optimistic and realistic an attitude as possible. Lazarus and DeLongis (1983), in discussing their data on stress, coping, and adaptation, emphasized that one must take into account not only the events themselves, but the significance of those events to the people involved.

Depressive Beliefs

Certain beliefs common to many old people make them vulnerable to depression. Many elderly people, for example, share the negative societal stereotype of old age (Bennett and Eckman, 1973). Some believe, in the absence of evidence, that they can no longer think clearly and fear that they are becoming senile. They have expectations of themselves that they cannot meet. For example, they expect that as mature adults they should be able to cope well with any crisis or change that occurs and they are bitterly disappointed in themselves when they do not respond as well as they would like to (Schlossberg, 1973). At times, elderly people forced to live below the poverty line blame themselves for their inability to manage their money (Gottesman et al., 1973). There is also some evidence that old people tend to view their environment as complex and dangerous and they see their role in this world as one of passively conforming to external demands (Neugarten, 1973).

In addition to faulty beliefs about the present, elderly people may also bring into old age beliefs from the past that are no longer appropriate. Riker (1979) thinks that elderly people should be encouraged to examine troublesome parts of their value systems, since the transition to old age involves new goals and developmental tasks with which parts of the old value system may conflict. For example, a value that measures human worth by productivity could make a person see retirement in a completely negative light. A particularly important aspect of the elderly person's past is the extent to which it differs from the reality of old age. A person whose life was rich in resources might develop expectations that in old age he or she would continue to find life satisfying and supportive. For this person, isolation and poverty would be more stressful than they would for someone who had lived an unrewarding life and expected little from old age (Schlossberg, 1979).

In all of these beliefs, there may be an element of truth, but frequently there also exists a larger element of exaggeration, scanty evidence, lack of information, or unrealistic expectations. It is this element that is the target of cognitive behavior therapy.

Therapeutic Methods

The way in which cognitive therapy is conducted makes it useful in combatting the attitudes and behaviors that tend to develop easily in old people and can lead to depression. The model requires a collaborative relationship between client and therapist. This means that the client participates in deciding the direction of therapy, in choosing techniques, and in designing homework assignments. The therapist continually asks for feedback from the client to ensure that the client is involved in what is happening. This collaborative aspect is of value in reducing the tendency of older persons to be dependent and compliant, to feel helpless and out of control of their lives.

Another aspect of the model is the highly structured nature of the therapy. Specific, clear-cut, limited goals are set. Assignments focus on one therapeutic principle at a time and are usually quite simple, without being childish. The structure of the therapy tends to minimize mental confusion, a result that is of value when dealing with people whose ability to concentrate, to analyze, and to synthesize may have diminished because of age or medication. Also, the belief of many elderly people that they are too old to change can be more easily challenged by a model that deals, not with large personality changes, but with small alterations in daily habits and thoughts.

Cognitive therapy frequently uses behavioral techniques that require the client to increase activity levels between sessions. The value of this procedure can be understood when one considers that decreased activity has been associated with the development of depression and that elderly people are often very inactive because of illness and other problems associated with age.

The model also uses "experiments," that is, the testing of the validity of a belief against reality. The client is the one who actually carries out the experiment and thus receives direct feedback from others and from the environment. Elderly people are often somewhat isolated and tend to lead directionless lives. The experiments promote involvement with the world and provide a sense of perspective that can help the elderly assess their situation and set realistic goals.

One feature of this model is the heavy use that is made of questioning. In a study of the effects of questioning on groups, Linsk et al. (1975) reported that elderly people responded to questions with increased interest and participation.

Finally, the very emphasis on cognitions can be particularly appropriate for elderly people because their reduced levels of physical and social activity leave them with a great deal of time for thinking. Cognitions therefore assume an important role in their lives. There are also some indications that elderly people prefer cognitive therapy to insight therapy (Steuer, 1982).

There are some features of the cognitive behavior therapy model which may require modification for some elderly people. Recording forms need to be of an appropriate clarity and visibility. Instructions and concepts may need to be presented in smaller segments and repeated frequently. For the less educated and less psychologically sophisticated, it may be necessary to focus more on the behavioral than on the cognitive interventions (Steuer and Hammen, 1983).

Bennett and Eckman (1973) distinguish between adjustment (putting up with or resigning oneself to a new situation) and adaptation (fitting comfortably into and deriving benefit from a new situation). According to them, both adaptation and survival are affected by a person's attitudes. Obviously, therefore, a therapy such as cognitive behavior therapy that concerns itself chiefly with attitudes and beliefs, is likely to help with adaptation to old age.

A Method for Conducting Cognitive Behavior Therapy with Groups of Elderly

The following plan, based on Beck's model of cognitive behavior therapy, has been developed for use with groups of the elderly. Because this method is structured and combines an educational approach with one-to-one therapy, it is particularly appropriate for older adults. Needless to say, it is assumed that the group leader will not allow the highly organized nature of the plan to supplant such therapeutic elements as empathy and support.

After an initial session to get acquainted and explain the nature of Cognitive Behavior Therapy and of the group, each session will, more or less, follow the same outline (as shown in the box) for a total of twenty 90-minute sessions.

Cognitive Group Therapy Plan

I. *Review Homework*	40 minutes
A. Set agenda.	
B. Review homework from last week:	
1. Successes	
2. Failures	
II. *Lecture and Call for Action*	40 minutes
A. Lecturette (5–10 minutes).	
Choose appropriate topic from lecturette list.	
B. Call for action (30 minutes).	
Ask patients to apply topic to their own lives.	
(This is an opportunity to do cognitive	
therapy with individual group members.)	
C. Assign general homework.	
D. Ask for feedback.	
III. *Assign Homework*	10 minutes
A. Review homework assignments:	
1. General. (For everyone. Related to	
lecturette and assigned during	
Call for Action.)	
2. Specific. (For group members who did	
individual cognitive therapy	
during this session.)	
B. Ask for feedback	

At the start of the session, the group members and leaders, together, set an agenda for the session, to include special concerns that have arisen and any deviations from the regular session plan. This should take just a few minutes.

The first major segment, lasting about 40 minutes, deals with the homework that members were assigned the previous session. Each group member should be given a chance to report and the focus of the first round should be on successes, with the leader providing strong reinforcement for even a small amount of progress and for honest attempts to complete homework. The second round deals with failures or problems that arose with homework, and it is here that the leader has the opportunity to do one-to-one therapy with one or two members, while the rest of the group listens and provides input when requested by the leader.

The second segment also lasts about 40 minutes and constitutes the formal, educational part of the session. In the course of the 20 sessions, the leader teaches the concepts of cognitive therapy to the group, in the form of weekly lecturettes. Each lecturette should be short, simple, appropriate to the group and confined to one aspect of the model. For example, the leader may explain, in one of the earlier sessions, how thoughts affect feelings. Lecturettes should follow a logical order from week to week. A list of suggested topics is given in the accompanying box but for complete explanations of the concepts and for ideas of other topics, the reader should consult *Cognitive Therapy of Depression* by Beck et al. (1979). Once the leader has given the lecturette, group members are asked to apply the concept to their own lives. Here again, there is an opportunity for one-to-one therapy. This time the group members are in a position to contribute a great deal, as they have just learned the concept presented in the lecturette and can, therefore, understand the therapy that is being conducted. As age-peers, the group members can be particularly valuable in helping challenge one another's negative thoughts and suggesting more realistic and optimistic ways of looking at events.

Lecturette Examples

Activity and Depression
1. Pleasant activities
   A. The relationship of pleasant activities to depression
   B. How to rate pleasant activities
   Homework: Keep a record of your pleasant activities.

2. Mastery activities
   A. The relationship of mastery activities to depression
   B. How to rate mastery activities
   Homework: Keep a record of both your pleasant and mastery activities.

3. Schedules
   A. The value of schedules
   B. How to plan a weekly schedule
   Homework: Plan a skeleton schedule and keep to it.
               Note your pleasant and mastery activities on the schedule.

4. Increasing social activities
   A. The value of social activities, friends, and a support system.
   B. Common mistakes
     1. Waiting to be asked rather than asking
     2. Focusing on negative aspects of a person rather than positive
     3. Not forgiving past slights
     4. Requiring that a person be perfect before spending time with him or her
   Homework: Extend one extra invitation or make one extra phone call above what you would normally do.

Automatic Thoughts and Negative Thinking
5. Automatic thoughts
   A. The relationship between thoughts and feelings
   B. How to record automatic thoughts
   Homework: Record your automatic thoughts on Daily Record of Dysfunctional Thoughts, three column (Beck et al., 1979).

6. Countering automatic thoughts
   A. Countering automatic thoughts can elevate mood
   B. From your Daily Record of Dysfunctional Thoughts (DRDT) choose one thought and try to think of another response to that event that is not so negative.
   Homework: Complete DRDT, four column, including the rational response column

7. Types of negative thoughts
   A. Negative opinion of yourself
   B. Self-criticism and self-blame
   C. Negative interpretation of events
   D. Negative expectations of the future
   Homework: Using last week's Daily Record of Dysfunctional thoughts, identify which of these four categories your thoughts fit into.

8. Overgeneralization
   A. Definition and examples of overgeneralization; the relationship of this error to depression
   B. Think of one example where you overgeneralized from one negative event to another that was only slightly similar.
   Homework: On this week's DRDT look for examples of overgeneralization that lead to negative feelings.

9. Ignoring the positive and misinterpreting positive events
   A. Definition and examples of ignoring and misinterpreting the positive; the relationship of these errors to depression
   B. Think of one example where you ignored or misinterpreted a positive event
   Homework: On this week's DRDT look for examples of ignoring the positive and misinterpretation of positive events that lead to negative feelings.

10. Dichotomous thinking
    A. Definition and examples of dichotomous thinking; its relationship to depression
    B. Think of one instance in which your manner of thinking was dichotomous
    Homework: Think of an event in your life that was adverse. Try to think of several benefits of that event, however small they might be.

11. Catastrophizing
    A. Definition and examples of catastrophizing; its relationship to depression
    B. Think of a concern you have that could be a problem in the future but which, in fact, has a low probability of ever happening
    Homework: On this week's DRDT, identify a thought on which you catastrophized.

Altering Negative Thinking

12. Alternative explanation
    A. Explanation and examples of how alternative interpretations can change mood
    B. For one of the events on your DRDT, think of an alternative explanation that is less upsetting to you.
    Homework: On this week's DRDT look for examples of events that could have alternative explanations.

13. Reattribution
    A. Explanation and examples of how depression can be reduced when responsibility for negative events is realistically assigned
    B. Think of a situation where you took more than your share of the blame for things going wrong
    Homework: This week, any time you blame yourself for anything at all, ask yourself, "Realistically, how much of this is my fault?"

14. Reality Testing
    A. Explanation of how the judgments of depressed people need to be checked against reality
    B. Select one of your DRDT examples for reality testing. In collaboration with your therapist, set up an experiment to test your belief
    Homework: Carry out this experiment to examine the evidence for and against your belief.

Toward the end of this segment, the leader assigns general homework to all group members that is relevant to the lecturette of that day. The leader then elicits feedback from members about the lecturette and the homework and deals with any anticipated difficulties.

Finally, in the last 5–10 minutes of the session, the leader reviews the specific homework that may have been assigned throughout the session to members who did individual therapy and clarifies for all members what is required for the next session. Again, the leader requests feedback on the whole session by asking such questions as "What was the most important thing you got out of today's session?"

REFERENCES

Altholz, J.A.S. Group psychotherapy with the elderly. In Burnside, I.M. (Ed.), *Working with the Elderly: Group Processes and Techniques.* North Scituate, Mass.: Duxbury, 1978.

Bates, M., Johnson, C., and Blaker, K.E. *Group Leadership: A Manual for Group Counseling Leaders,* 2nd ed. Denver, Colo.: Love, 1982.

Beck, A.T., Rush, A.J., Shaw, B.F., and Emery, G. *Cognitive Therapy of Depression.* New York: Guilford, 1979.

Bennett, R., and Eckman, J. Attitudes toward aging: A critical examination of recent literature and implications for future research. In Eisdorfer, C., and Lawton, M.P., (Eds.), *The Psychology of Adult Development and Aging.* Washington, D.C.: American Psychological Association, 1973.

Berland, D.I., and Poggi, R. Expressive group psychotherapy with the aging. *International Journal of Group Psychotherapy,* 1979, 29(1):87–108.

Britnell, J.C., and Mitchell, K.E. Inpatient group psychotherapy for the elderly. *Journal of Psychiatric Nursing and Mental Health Services,* 1981, 19(5):19–24.

Burnside, I.M. (Ed.). *Working with the Elderly: Group Processes and Techniques.* North Scituate, Mass.: Duxbury, 1978.

Burnside, I.M. *Nursing and the Aged.* New York: McGraw-Hill, 1981.

Carman, M.B. Effects of emotional innoculation and supportive therapy on stress incurred from nursing home placement. *Dissertation Abstracts International,* 1977, 37, 4132B.

Cerella, J., Poon, L.W., and Williams, D.M. Age and the complexity hypothesis. In Poon, L.W. (Ed.), *Aging in the 1980s: Psychological Issues.* Washington, D.C.: American Psychological Association, 1980.

Chaisson, M., Beutler, L., Yost, E., et al. Treating the depressed elderly. *Journal of Psychosocial Nursing,* 1984, 22(5):25–30.

Corey, G., and Corey, M.S. *Groups: Process and Practice,* 2nd ed. Monterey, Calif: Brooks/Cole, 1982.

Dennis, H. Remotivation therapy groups. In Burnside, I.M. (Ed.), *Working with the Elderly: Group Processes and Techniques.* North Scituate, Mass.: Duxbury, 1978.

Duetsch, C.B., and Kramer, N. Outpatient group psychotherapy for the elderly: an alternative to institutionalization. *Hospital and Community Psychiatry,* 1977, 28:440–42.

Eisdorfer, C. Conceptual models of aging: the challenge of a new frontier. *American Psychologist,* 1983, 38(2):197–202.

Elder-Jucker, P.L. Effects of group therapy on self esteem, social interaction and depression of female residents in a home for the aged. *Dissertation Abstracts International,* 1979, 39, 5514B.

Finkel, S.I. Experiences of a private-practice psychiatrist working with the elderly in the community. *International Journal of Mental Health,* 1980, 8 (3–4):147–72.

Folsom, J.C. Reality orientation for the elderly mental patient. *Journal of Geriatric Psychiatry.* 1968, 1:291–307.

Ford, J.M., and Pfefferbaum, A. The utility of brain potentials in determining age-related changes in central nervous system and cognitive functioning. In Poon. L.W. (Ed.), *Aging in the 1980s: Psychological Issues.* Washington, D.C.: American Psychological Association, 1980.

Fuchs, C.Z., and Rehm, L.P. A self-control behavior therapy program for depression. *Journal of Consulting and Clinical Psychology,* 1977, 45:206–15.

Gallagher, D. Behavioral group therapy with elderly depressives: an experimental study. In Upper, D., and Ross, S.M. (Eds.), *Behavioral Group Therapy, 1981: An Annual Review.* Champaign, Ill.: Research Press, 1981.

Gallagher, D.E. Comparative effectiveness of group psychotherapies for reduction of depression in elderly outpatients. *Dissertation Abstracts International*, 1979, 5550B–5551B.

Gatz, M., Smyer, M.A., and Lawton, M.P. The mental health system and the older adult. In Poon, L.W. (Ed.), *Aging in the 1980s: Psychological Issues*. Washington, D.C.: American Psychological Association, 1980.

Goldfarb, A.I. Group therapy with the old and aged. In Kaplan, H.I. and Sadock, B.J. (Eds.), *Comprehensive Group Psychotherapy*. Baltimore: Williams and Wilkins, 1971.

Gottesman, L.E., Quarterman, C.E., and Cohn, G.M. Psychosocial treatment of the aged. In Eisdorfer, C. and Lawton, M.P. (Eds.), *The Psychology of Adult Development and Aging*. Washington, D.C.: American Psychological Association, 1973.

Hollon, S.D., and Shaw, B.F. Group cognitive therapy for depressed patients. In Beck, A.T., Rush, A.J., Shaw, B.F., and Emery, G. *Cognitive Therapy of Depression*. New York: Guilford, 1979.

Ingersoll, B., and Silverman, A. Comparative group psychotherapy for the aged. *Gerontologist*, 1978, 18(2):201–206.

Kalson, L. Group therapy with the aged. In Seligman, M.E.P. (Ed.), *Group Psychotherapy and Counseling with Special Populations*. Baltimore: University Park Press, 1982.

Kubie, S.H., and Landau, G. *Group Work with the Aged*. New York: International Universities Press, 1953.

Lago, D., and Hoffman, S. Structured group interaction: an intervention strategy for the continued development of elderly populations. *International Journal of Aging and Human Development*, 1977–78, 8(4):311–24.

Lazarus, L.W. A program for the elderly at a private psychiatric hospital. *Gerontologist*, 1976, 16(2):125–31.

Lazarus, R.S., and DeLongis, A. Psychological stress and coping in aging. *American Psychologist*, 1983, 38(3):245–54.

Levy, S.M., Derogatis, L.R., Gallagher, D., and Garz, M. Intervention with older adults and the evaluation of outcome. In Poon, L.W. (Ed.), *Aging in the 1980s: Psychological Issues*. Washington, D.C.: American Psychological Association, 1980.

Lewis, M.I. and Butler, R.N. Life-review therapy: Putting memories to work in individual and group psychotherapy. *Geriatrics*, 1974, 29(11):165–173.

Lindell, A.R. Group therapy for the institutionalized aged. *Issues in Mental Health Nursing*, 1978, 1:77–86.

Linsk, N., Howe, M.W., and Pinkston, E.M. Behavioral group work in a home for the aged. *Social Work*, 1975, 20(6):454–63.

Lopez, M.A. Social skills training with institutionalized elderly: effects of precounseling, structuring and overlearning on skill acquisition and transfer. *Journal of Counseling Psychology*, 1980, 27(3):286–93.

Mardoyan, J.L., and Weis, D.M. The efficacy of group counseling with older adults. *Personnel and Guidance Journal*, 1981, 60(3):161–163.

Mintz, J., Steuer, J., and Jarvik, L. Psychotherapy with depressed elderly patients: research considerations. *Journal of Consulting and Clinical Psychology,* 1981, 49(4):542–48.

Moran, J.A. The effects of insight-oriented group therapy and task-oriented group therapy on the coping style and life satisfaction of nursing home elderly. *Dissertation Abstracts International,* 1979, 40, 1377B–1378B.

Moss, Eric P. A study of the relationship between group counseling, social activities, and aspects of life adjustment of older, sheltered workshop clients. *Dissertation Abstracts International,* 1976, 37, 979B.

Mueller, D.J., and Atlas, L. Resocialization of regressed elderly residents: A behavioral management approach. *Journal of Gerontology,* 1972, 27(3):390–392.

Murray, R.B., Huelskoetter, M.M.W., and O'Driscoll, D.L. *The Nursing Process in Later Maturity.* Englewood Cliffs, N.J.: Prentice-Hall, 1980.

Nashef, A.A. The effects of group therapy on the affective states, social distance, interpersonal locus of control, life satisfaction, and ward behavior among the institutionalized aged. *Dissertation Abstracts International,* 1981, 42, 384B.

Neugarten, B.L. Personality change in late life: a developmental perspective. In Eisdorfer, C. and Lawton, M.P. (Eds.), *The Psychology of Adult Development and Aging.* Washington, D.C.: American Psychological Association, 1973.

Paradis, P.A. Brief out-patient group psychotherapy with older patients in the treatment of age-related problems. *Dissertation Abstracts International,* 1973, 34, 2947B–2948B.

Petty, B.J., Moeller, T.P., and Campbell, R.L. Support groups for elderly persons in the community. *Gerontologist,* 1976, 16(2):522–528.

Price, L.J., Fein, G., and Feinberg, I. Neuropsychological assessment of cognitive function in the elderly. In Poon, L.W. (Ed.), *Aging in the 1980s: Psychological Issues.* Washington, D.C.: American Psychological Association, 1980.

Steuer, J.L., and Hammen, C.L. Cognitive-behavioral group therapy for the depressed elderly: Issues and adaptations. *Cognitive Therapy and Research,* 1983, 7(4):285–296.

Taulbee, L.R. Reality orientation: a therapeutic group activity for elderly persons. In Burnside, I.M. (Ed.), *Working with the Elderly: Group Processes and Techniques.* North Scituate, Mass.: Duxbury, 1978.

Taylor, F.G., and Marshall, W.L. Experimental analysis of a cognitive-behavioral therapy for depression. *Cognitive Therapy and Research,* 1977, 1:59–72.

Toseland, R. A problem-solving group workshop for older persons. *Social Work,* 1977, 22(4):325–26.

Tutaj, G.A. The effectiveness of group counseling in alleviating depression among the aged. *Dissertation Abstracts International,* 1975, 36, 2653A.

Waters, E., Fink, S., and White, B. Peer group counseling for older people. *Educational Gerontology,* 1976, 1:157–70.

Weiner, M.B., and Weinstock, C.S. Group progress of community elderly as measured by tape recordings, group tempo, and group evaluation. *International Journal of Aging and Human Development,* 1979–80, 10(2):177–85.

Wolff, A.R., and Meyer, G.W. Counseling older adults: suggested approaches. In Ganikos, M.L. (Ed.), *Counseling the Aged*. Falls Church, Va.: American Personnel and Guidance Association, 1979.

Yalom, I.D. *The Theory and Practice of Group Psychotherapy*, 2nd ed. New York: Basic Books, 1975.

Yost, E.B., Allender, J., Beutler, L.E., and Chaisson-Stewart, G.M. Developments in the treatment of depression among the elderly. *Arizona Medicine*, 1983, 40(6).

Zgliczynski, M. Multimodal behavior therapy with groups of aged. *Dissertation Abstracts International*, 1979, 39:4159A.

12
Voluntarism

Barbara R. Heller
Marian Emr
Arthur J. Engler

The sense of self that an individual develops in early life becomes a basic part of personality and a means of adapting to the environment. Self–esteem develops from one's own achievements, activities, and sense of mastery. This sense of self is a critical element in determining life satisfaction as well as the degree to which an individual can tolerate rejection, failure, physical illness, and stress (Weiner et al., 1978).

When an individual is faced with role loss, physical illness, financial insecurity, and other stresses that can accompany aging, there is a decreased opportunity for the continued sense of mastery that is an essential ingredient of self-esteem (Weiner et al., 1978). It is therefore no surprise that depression, along with feelings of worthlessness, is the most prevalent psychological problem found in older people. Indeed, Beverley (1975) found that survival of an elderly individual was related not only to good physical health but also to the individual's self-view and sense of continued usefulness.

Unlike many cultures that value their aged, American society values self-reliance, independence, and many of the characteristics associated with youth. Success is measured by each of these factors as well as by a person's role in the labor force, which is one of the principal markers of a person's value in society. Blau (1973) aptly stated the problem facing the elderly in America today: "Society ignores older people—their accumulated experiences, their skills, and most of all, their desire to perform useful roles that would sustain their self-respect and earn them the respect of others. The . . . old are excluded from society's productive or generative

No official endorsement by the National Institute on Aging or the Department of Health and Human Services is inferred.

system. They are 'free' of responsibility for anyone but themselves, and this demoralizes them." Given that more and more people are living for decades after they retire, society must reevaluate its definition of productivity and success.

THE FUNCTION AND IMPORTANCE OF VOLUNTARISM

Involvement in voluntary activities may be one way to ward off the negative effects of societal attitudes on the precarious self-concept of the elderly. Gerontologists, however, have been divided over the actual benefits of voluntary activities in terms of life satisfaction, morale, and happiness. Several researchers have suggested that health, socioeconomic status and a variety of other factors are associated with life satisfaction among the elderly (Adams, 1971), more so than voluntary activities (Bull and Aucoin, 1975; Edwards and Klemmack, 1979). A longitudinal study by Graney (1975) found that activities such as socializing with friends, talking on the telephone, and going to church were more likely to affect morale and happiness.

On the other hand, activity theorists speculate that people who participate in voluntary associations have greater life satisfaction and a better self-concept than those who do not. Sainer and Zander (1971) claim that voluntarism can solve some of the common problems of aging by instilling a feeling of continued usefulness and self-respect, filling large blocks of unused time, and neutralizing the negative effects of loneliness in old age. Sainer and Zander further suggest that some volunteer programs have developed new roles for older people which, in turn, help maintain self-esteem. Havighurst (1961) concluded earlier that continued social participation, either in paid work or free time activities, offer the aged "opportunities for pleasure, to be creative, . . . to have self respect, . . . to be of service to others, and to give prestige and popularity."

Studies have shown that most aged want meaningful work which provides them with prestige and gratification (Morris et al., 1964). Riessman (1965) found that initially, helping others might be more beneficial to the giver than to the receiver. This could, however, lead the helper to become more efficient, better motivated, and eventually, more helpful.

A number of studies have identified the potential benefits of voluntary activities for older individuals. Peppers (1976) found that life satisfaction scores were higher for the retired elderly whose activity levels increased than for those whose activity levels either remained constant or declined. In this particular study, however, the aged who increased their activity levels may have been able to do so because of good health and adequate finances.

In another study, Hirsch and Linn (1977) compared 50 elderly hospital volunteers with 50 nonvolunteers in the community. The volunteers reported greater life satisfaction, self-esteem, and will to live, and less depression despite the fact that there were no differences in recent life events, anxiety, or locus of control between the two groups. The investigators also found that the volunteers had significantly less disability and took fewer medications. Not knowing whether this was a cause or an effect of voluntary activity, the investigators adjusted their findings to account for differences in health status as well as incomes between the two groups. Volunteers still had significantly greater life satisfaction and will to live. This suggests that encouraging elderly who are in reasonably good health to join some structured program and help others will increase their own quality of life.

Pritchard and Tomb (1981) also identified a number of the benefits that can result when older adults become involved in organized volunteer programs. While some of these help the individual—such as improved intergenerational communications and enhanced quality of life in retirement—others help society. Pritchard found that elderly volunteers helped counteract negative attitudes toward aging, or ageism, and also provided useful services to educational institutions.

Older persons possess a number of special qualities that make them valued members of society. Among them are life experience, skills learned through work or leisure-time activities, and the ability to cope, to accommodate life's demands (Swartz, 1978). Volunteer work offers elderly persons the opportunity to share these experiences while providing more tangible services. In 1982 Butler and Lewis noted that most elderly individuals have a strong desire to leave a legacy and to share their accumulated knowledge and experience with the young. They also have a unique sense of the entire life cycle, an enhanced creativity and curiosity, as well as a sense of fulfillment in life.

In 1975 Payne and Mazur noted that "volunteering is becoming a prestigious social role for the elderly as many agencies and organizations incorporate older volunteer positions into their formal structure." In this way, the volunteer role replaces lost work roles, group memberships, and other solidarity ties because it is judged a meaningful activity by the community; provides social identity, a social future, and an acceptable self-concept; allows the individual to continue several life roles; and reduces social loss.

The benefits of voluntarism to society and the individual obviously are closely linked. As Schindler-Rainman and Lippitt (1975) reported, "most volunteer activity not only represents a significant contribution of energy and skill and individual resources to the functioning of democracy, but also makes a significant contribution to the volunteer's own psychological health and self-actualization."

MOTIVATION AND INTEREST—PREDICTORS
AND PATTERNS

A number of factors contribute to volunteer motivation. According to Schindler-Rainman and Lippitt (1975), high volunteer morale and motivation are linked to the opportunities 1) to participate in problem solving and significant decision making, 2) to relate particular individual interests and need to responsibilities as a volunteer, and 3) to provide meaningful service to others. It also seems important that there be a "contract" clarifying responsibilities and expectations between the volunteer and the agency and adequate records of the volunteer's activities, as well as opportunities for evaluation and advancement, a regular mechanism for feedback and recognition, and training.

The participation of the elderly in voluntary organizations also seems to depend, in part, on the function of those organizations. Among the accepted functions are goal attainment, socialization, support to an established institution, allocation of power, social integration, and social change (Amis, 1974).

Several studies have examined the specific differences between the elderly who volunteer and those who do not. Dye and colleagues (1973) identified two factors that differentiate these two groups: gender and past pattern of organizational participation. Morris et al. (1964) found that characteristics differentiating volunteers from nonvolunteers included previous experience as a volunteer, educational level, and state of health. Monk and Cryns (1974) focused on six attributes that can best predict a person's interest in volunteering: age, education, belief in one's capacity to serve others, interest in senior citizen activity, scope of social interests, and home ownership. These investigators concluded that "while over-all stated interest in social participation is on the rise, it searches for modes of expression that impose upon the individual minimum levels of risk and self-investment."

In 1981 a survey by Louis Harris and Associates provided information on rates of the elderly's participation in voluntary activities. This study showed that 23 percent of Americans over age 65—5.9 million people—reported doing volunteer work. Harris also found that, among the elderly, 31 percent with incomes between $10,000 and $20,000, 45 percent of the college educated, 24 percent of the whites, 17 percent of the blacks, 25 percent of the employed, and 24 percent of the unemployed all reported doing some type of volunteer work. The work usually involved physical or mental health services; transportation; civic affairs; psychological and social support services; giveaway programs; and programs oriented toward helping families, young people, or children. In the same study, another 10 percent of the elderly population said they would like to volunteer but were not able to because of poor health, lack of time or transportation, or family responsibilities.

A number of studies have focused on four factors that seem to influence voluntary activities among the elderly: age, gender, ethnicity, and socio-economic status. In 1976(a) Cutler examined the curvilinear pattern of age differences in membership that had been reported in earlier studies. Cutler analyzed data from two different studies after removing the effects of income and education. Results showed that membership levels increased through the ages of 35 and 44 and then either remained generally stable or increased through age 75. Put another way, if older persons had the same socioeconomic characteristics as younger and middle-aged persons, they would probably have membership levels as high or higher than those of middle-aged persons.

Replicating Cutler's work, Knoke and Thomson (1977) also found a curvilinear pattern of association membership after discounting the effects of socioeconomic status. The difference between these two studies was that Knoke and Thomson did not recognize church memberships per se. They felt that church membership should not be counted since it measured the individual's religiosity, not voluntarism. Instead, the individual's participation in a voluntary association *within* the church ought to be counted. Hendricks and Hendricks (1977) also found evidence of a curvilinear pattern. They discovered that affiliations approximate a normal curve, reaching a peak between the ages of 36 and 50 years, remaining at a plateau until age 60 through 69, and then slowly declining.

Research by Babchuk and colleagues (1979) suggested that greater numbers of persons 65 and over are continuing to take an active role in organizational life. They noted no sharp drop even among individuals over 80 years old. The very elderly, however, are less likely to be very active in their organizations or to have multiple memberships. Wan et al. (1982) reported that males and females aged 60–74 were more likely to volunteer than those over 74 years of age.

Another study by Cutler (1976b) proposed that the aged of the future may participate in more voluntary associations than today's aged simply because they will have more leisure time, better health and economic security, and higher levels of education. In this study Cutler attempted to determine age profiles in 16 voluntary associations and to establish baseline data to monitor future membership trends. Results showed that the aged were more likely than the young to belong to fraternal and church-related groups. Participation leveled off with age in labor unions; professional and academic societies; school service groups; youth groups; veterans' groups; service clubs; and literary, art, and music discussion/study groups. The most popular voluntary associations for the aged of 1955 were still attractive to them in 1974–75, although there were some variations by sex.

Work by Cutler (1977) and others refutes the disengagement theory by showing that age appears to be accompanied by stability and continuity in levels of voluntary association participation. When middle-aged and older persons are followed as they age, rather than compared to younger individuals, there is no evidence that association membership decreases.

Gender is a second factor that seems able to predict participation in voluntary activities. Cutler (1976b) found that at all ages men were more likely to belong to labor unions and women were more likely to belong to church-related, school service, or discussion groups and hobby or garden clubs. Also, separated or divorced persons were the least likely to be doing volunteer work, but the most interested in becoming involved in it (Wan et al., 1982).

Other studies have focused on differences in voluntary association membership and participation among ethnic groups. Williams et al. (1973) proved ethnicity to be an important variable in predicting participation and found that blacks had the highest levels of social participation, Mexican-Americans had the lowest levels, and other whites were somewhere in the middle. Clemente et al. (1975) found that aged blacks have higher rates of participation in voluntary associations regardless of health or socioeconomic status. This difference may be due, in part, to the greater participation of aged blacks in church-related groups (46 percent as opposed to 28 percent for whites). Aged whites, on the other hand, are more likely to belong to and participate in ethnic organizations and senior citizen clubs.

The findings of Cutler and others indirectly support the conclusion that lower levels of voluntary activities among older adults compared to younger adults may be largely due to socioeconomic compositional differences between the age groups. Social class can also affect participation in voluntary organizations. Trela (1976) examined the relationship between social class and both "age-graded" (designed exclusively for the aged) and non-age-graded voluntary association membership in 320 older people. Social class differences did not seem to affect how many groups an individual belonged to, whether or not an individual joined a group, or participation or attrition over a six-year period. The investigators found, however, that the kind of organization was likely to be affected by social class. Higher class aged were more likely to belong to "age-graded" groups.

Social factors can also dissuade elderly from volunteering. A program of neighborhood one-to-one volunteer activity by urban low-income aged blacks proved to be unsuccessful despite participants' eagerness, because of the high crime rate involving the elderly in the area in which they were to serve (Faulkner, 1975).

THE IMPACT OF VOLUNTEER SERVICES: OVERVIEW OF PROGRAMS AND MODELS

ACTION, the national volunteer agency, includes three programs for elderly volunteers: the Foster Grandparent Program, the Senior Companion Program, and the Retired Senior Volunteer Program (RSVP). Together, these programs involve more than 323,000 persons over age 60. They serve in some 1,000 local projects and devote an annual total of more than 76,000,000 hours of service to their local communities (ACTION News, 1982).

It was not until the 1960s, though, that the strengths and vitality of the elderly were formally recognized in the United States. The Foster Grandparent Program, established in 1965, became the first government-sponsored volunteer program for the elderly. The 1971 White House Conference on Aging gave new impetus to volunteer opportunities for the elderly. The Foster Grandparent Program was followed in 1971 by the Retired Senior Volunteer Program and in 1973 by the Senior Companion Program.

As the economic foundation of human services becomes more and more unstable, the need for volunteers in social service programs is becoming critical. The elderly of this country are well equipped to meet some of these needs by virtue of their life experiences.

Foster Grandparent Program

The Foster Grandparent Program utilizes the services of some 16,000 low-income people over age 60 in the United States, Puerto Rico, and the Virgin Islands. These elderly use their skills to assist handicapped children and benefit by adding to their own incomes. Volunteers work 20 hours each week and are paid a nominal hourly wage. They are reimbursed for transportation and receive a meal each day that they work (Tenenbaum, 1979).

When the Foster Grandparent Program was first established, volunteers worked exclusively in institutional settings. More recently, the program has begun to provide some services in the home. In Pittsburgh, for example, a group of foster grandparents work with families who have histories of child abuse and neglect, alcoholism, or emotional and physical illness. Their aim is to stabilize the family so that it can continue to function as a unit. Oftentimes, this helps avoid institutionalization.

Ashby (1981) reported the positive experiences of aged Native Americans in the Foster Grandparent Program in the State of Washington. These elderly teach children how to fry bread and to make quilts and blankets; they also teach them about the meaning of totem poles and other cultural lore. According to one volunteer in Ashby's study, "Our own children moved away and we didn't get to watch our grandkids grow up. Now we have our foster grandchildren—they're our family now."

Senior Companion Program

This program is newer and smaller than the Foster Grandparent Program. It also provides volunteer opportunities for low-income persons over age

60 who receive the same pay and benefits as do foster grandparents (Tenenbaum, 1979). Currently, there are about 3,000 senior companions who provide care and companionship to 6,000 frail elderly people.

Retired Senior Volunteer Program

RSVP volunteers are retired or semi-retired people over age 60. This is the largest ACTION group, with over 350,000 volunteers serving in nearly 700 programs that provide elderly persons with interesting work and opportunities for socializing. Volunteers serve in courts, schools, libraries, day-care centers, hospitals, nursing homes, economic development agencies, and other community service centers.

Kallan (1978) looked at a sample of RSVP participants in an attempt to identify which areas of the program were satisfying. People were more likely to continue to serve when they were assigned to community agencies, were recruited by senior center staff or other volunteers, and received meals while at work. The investigators did not consider that these were major factors in the decisions made by volunteers, however. Except for health status, there were no significant differences between people who continued to volunteer and those who dropped out.

In 1978 Rath examined the backgrounds and current activities of elderly volunteers in community-based and residential programs. The investigator was interested in studying the differences between volunteers working with children (as in the Foster Grandparent Program) and those working with older adults (as in the Retired Senior Volunteer Program). She found that the most integrating theme was the element of continuity. In other words, the past experiences of individual volunteers helped explain their present choices. Such factors as sibling rank, type of social interactions with and responsibilities for siblings, and affinity as adults toward children who were or were not relatives, were differentiating factors. Also, older adults who volunteered for activities involving "relationship skills" seemed to have predominantly positive outlooks toward their own aging. Rath concluded that such studies might be useful in identifying the most appropriate candidates for volunteer programs.

Peace Corps

In addition to volunteer programs specifically designed for the elderly, a number of established programs include older individuals among their ranks of volunteers. Approximately 6,850 Peace Corps volunteers serve in 62 countries in Latin America, Africa, Asia, and the Pacific. Of these, 306 are between the ages of 51 and 70, and 29 are between 71 and 80.

Volunteers generally serve for two years and receive a monthly allowance for rent, food, travel, and other necessities. In addition, a readjustment allowance is set aside monthly and payable upon completion of service (Tenenbaum, 1979).

Volunteers in Service to America (VISTA)

About 15 percent of all VISTA volunteers are 55 years of age or older. These volunteers assist the poor in the United States for one-year terms of service. Benefits are smaller than in the Peace Corps (Tenenbaum, 1979).

Mass Membership Organizations

There are many mass membership organizations in the United States. Some of these groups are specifically geared toward the aged and provide volunteer service opportunities for their members. The National Council of Senior Citizens has over 4 million members, 3,500 affiliated clubs in the United States, and is involved primarily with political action. The National Retired Teachers' Association/American Association of Retired Persons (NRTA/AARP) sponsor community service programs, and provide social benefits to approximately 15 million members. The Gray Panthers (officially named the Coalition of Older and Younger Adults) has no official membership but has a mailing list of 5,000 interested individuals. This is an advocacy group that speaks out on issues related to social justice and health care reform, and monitors government activities. The Retired Professional Action Group was formed by Ralph Nader to investigate and report consumer problems and also deals with class-action suits. The Senior Advocates International are active in social, political, and community affairs. The National Association for Retired Federal Employees is a lobbyist group, especially geared to supporting improved pension benefits for its members.

Tax Aides

The National Retired Teachers' Association/American Association of Retired Persons has instituted a program to assist the elderly in coping with the complicated and ever-changing task of dealing with income tax. In 1978 more than 7,500 volunteers helped well over 500,000 low-income and elderly persons file their taxes (Tenenbaum, 1979).

SCORE and ACE

Since 1964 retired business executives have responded to almost a half million requests for assistance in legal and tax services as part of the Service Core of Retired Executives (SCORE), a program sponsored by the Small Business Administration. Today there are 6,000 SCORE volunteers who staff regional SBA offices and do on-site counseling in every facet of business management in over 300 chapters in each of the 50 states as well as Puerto Rico. Active Corps of Executives (ACE) was established as a supplement to SCORE. The only difference is that the 2,600 ACE volunteers are still active in the business world.

Regional Programs

Over the past several decades, model volunteer programs have been developed in various parts of the country. Many of these programs are specifically designed to allow elderly individuals to help others who are less fortunate than themselves. In 1978 Bolton and Dignum-Scott described a program developed by the University of Nebraska Center on Aging. As part of this program, older volunteers were trained to counsel other elderly persons who might need information on physical health, mental health, and other services.

Blumenfield (1978) described a New York-based program in which senior citizens provided a variety of services to their peers by acting as counselors/assistants in a community hospital. This program was very useful to those who volunteered, who found a productive way to use their time, and to those who received the services. The availability of older people to provide companionship and perform a variety of unpredicted services proved very helpful.

Heller et al. (1981) described the development of the Seniors Helping Seniors demonstration project conducted under the auspices of the State University of New York at Farmingdale. The purpose of this project was to test the feasibility of using older adult, nonprofessional volunteers in home health care programs. A major thrust of the project was to build a model for recruiting and training of a core of elderly volunteers to act as peer caregivers within the community.

Seligman (1973) wrote about Jerusalem's Elderly-to-Elderly Mutual Help Project. As volunteers in this program, partially handicapped elderly persons visited the homes of bedridden or housebound elderly. The visitors regained a sense of purpose in life, and the people they visited felt that someone cared they were alive. Many of the visited responded so well that they eventually became visitors themselves. The visitors were given a small token wage, which proved to have a psychological as well as a practical value.

Such programs obviously provide more than a way for older people to pass the time. In 1979 Edwards and Klemmack designed a community college model for training older volunteers in Florida to render human services. At the end of the training program, the volunteers felt more positive about themselves emotionally, economically, intellectually, and physically.

A number of programs are designed to utilize the skills older people have developed during the years they have spent in the labor force. These include Project ASSERT, a program sponsored by the National Research Center on Vocational Education, which mobilizes journeymen and other retirees from trades, crafts, semiskilled, and technical occupations as support personnel for occupational, technical, and career education and training programs in postsecondary institutions (Sheppard, 1981). The International Executive Service Corps is made up of experienced executives who serve as advisors in developing countries. The Executive Volunteer Corps is a New York City group made up of specialists in a variety of fields. Members of the Society of Retired Executives give advice and consultation and are involved in the research activities of a variety of organizations. The Senior Medical Consultants are retired physicians who provide educational opportunities in smaller hospitals. The Literacy Volunteers of America tutor others in basic reading and English as a second language (Tenenbaum, 1979).

SELF-CARE, SELF-HELP, AND OLDER PERSONS

In the Elderly-to-Elderly Mutual Help Project, partially handicapped individuals learned to help themselves by helping others. In 1975 Friedman reported the experiences of a group of relatively impaired, institutionalized elderly who volunteered to provide needed emotional support and orientation to new residents at the Philadelphia Geriatric Center. During weekly meetings, old and new residents discussed common problems. The meetings not only solved many problems, they also allowed for social interchange and support. Both this program and the Mutual Help Project contrast with other programs that use the "well elderly."

Ruffini and Todd (1979) also described a program in which the volunteers learned to help themselves. The Senior Block Information Services included among its volunteers large numbers of elderly living in a dispersed setting in the city of San Francisco. This program was designed to: 1) provide information and referral services, 2) encourage increased interaction among the aged, and 3) provide structure for the development of leadership and self-help among the elderly. The program began in 1973 and eventually involved 400 elderly volunteers, who delivered monthly newsletters and provided referral and counseling services to approximately 10,000 aged. This program was a huge success, perhaps because the volunteers had relatively modest and limited duties, the newsletters were hand delivered, and the organization was decentralized and flexible. There was also a great deal of latitude with regard to the extent of participation as well as a largely diverse volunteer group. Perhaps most important of all, the program offered a chance to develop a social network among the elderly.

The profile of the typical volunteer is changing—from the middle-aged housewife to a more diverse selection, including college students, corporate executives, and senior citizens (Paxman, 1981). Lambert et al. (1964) found that older persons are willing to become involved in voluntary associations and that their abilities are needed in community service activities. A crucial quality seems to be a genuine concern for people and their problems as well as an interest in helping people solve their problems (Routh, 1972). This quality is more likely found in older volunteers—who are motivated by altruistic aims such as using their expertise to help the community— than in younger volunteers—who tend to have self-serving motives such as gaining experience for their careers (Frisch and Gerrard, 1981).

There are, however, a number of barriers that discourage agencies from using volunteers of any age. One factor that surfaced in the Lambert et al. (1964) study is the fact that the volunteer is a layperson—a problem for health agencies, for example, which are concerned with the confidentiality of records. Also, volunteers need concrete skills, not just a desire to help others (Rosenblatt, 1966). In this study by Rosenblatt, most volunteers did not possess the necessary skills to serve in high-level volunteer activities; all needed extensive training.

A second barrier Lambert et al. (1964) described is the stereotypic view of the elderly and their abilities. Most agency executives surveyed believed that the elderly are physically limited and dependent, that they have little to contribute, that they are financial and legal liabilities, that they will impinge negatively on civil service requirements, and that they require too much supervision. These barriers, of course, could apply to the use of volunteers of any age.

The elderly themselves hold certain stereotypic attitudes about volunteer work. In Harris's (1981) study of voluntarism, many elderly expressed a real reluctance to volunteer their time; if the job was valuable enough, they felt that they would be paid for doing it. This substantiates earlier findings by Carp (1968) who concluded that paid work had a higher value than volunteer work, not only because of the compensation involved, but also because pay denoted the work was worthwhile by societal standards.

Of course, many older people have no interest in volunteer work. In his study, Rosenblatt (1966) found that 75 percent of the people between the ages of 60 and 74 years old had no interest in pursuing either paid or volunteer employment. Still, for those elderly who choose to volunteer, their work can be a most rewarding and satisfying experience.

The 1970s saw a large number of studies concerning voluntarism and the elderly. The topics of these studies ranged from voluntary association membership through interest in volunteer activity to actual rates of participation in volunteer activities. The vast majority of these studies pointed to the emotional, physical and sometimes economic benefits of voluntarism. Whether they were involved in local or national activities, whether they were working in schools, hospitals, or the community, older volunteers tended to feel better about themselves because of what they were doing. In the words of one elderly volunteer, a retired businessman working in a Dade County, Florida school, "It gives you a purpose in life, something to do when you get up in the morning. Volunteering is better than having a regular job. Of course, when I want a raise, I don't get it, but on the other hand, when I want a vacation, I can take it." (Slack, 1978)

REFERENCES

ACTION News, *Older American Volunteer Programs Fact Sheet,* Washington, D.C.: 1982.

Adams, D.L. Correlates of satisfaction among the elderly. *Gerontologist,* 1971, 11:64–68.

Amis, W.D., and Stern, S.E. A critical examination of theory and functions of voluntary associations. *Journal of Voluntary Action Research,* 1974, 3:91–99.

Ashby, V.R. Foster grandparents teach Indian lore and language. *Children Today,* 1981, 10:16–17.

Babchuk, N., Peters, G., Hoyt, D., and Kaiser, M. The voluntary associations of the aged. *Journal of Gerontology,* 1979, 34:579–87.

Beverley, E.V. The double-barreled impact of volunteer service. *Geriatrics,* 1975, 30:132ff.

Blau, Z.S. *Old Age in a Changing Society.* New York: New Viewpoints, 1973.

Blumenfield, S. Counselor-assistants for a geriatric program in a community hospital. *Dissertation Abstracts International,* 1978, 38:1657A.

Bolton, C.R., and Dignum-Scott, J.E. Peer-group advocacy counseling for the elderly: a conceptual model. *Gerontological Society, 31st Annual Scientific Meeting,* (program abstracts) 1978, 18:51.

Bull, C.N., and Aucoin, J.B. Voluntary association participation and life satisfaction: a replication note. *Journal of Gerontology,* 1975, 30:73–76.

Butler, R.N., and Lewis, M.I. *Aging and Mental Illness.* St. Louis: C.V. Mosby, 1982, pp. 3–60.

Carp, F.M. Differences among older workers, volunteers, and persons who are neither. *Journal of Gerontology,* 1968, 23:497–501.

Clemente, F., Rexroad, P.A., and Hirsch, C. The participation of the black aged in voluntary associations. *Journal of Gerontology,* 1975, 30:469–72.

Cutler, S.J. Age differences in voluntary association memberships. *Social Forces,* 1976, 55:43–58.

Cutler, S.J. Age profiles of membership in sixteen types of voluntary associations. *Journal of Gerontology,* 1976, 31:462–70.

Cutler, S.J. Aging and voluntary association participation. *Journal of Gerontology,* 1977, 32:470–79.

Dye, D., Goodman, M., Roth, M., Bley, N., and Jensen, K. The older adult volunteer compared to the nonvolunteer. *Gerontologist,* 1973, 13:215–18.

Edwards, A.B. A community college model for training older volunteers in rendering human services. *Dissertation Abstracts International,* 1979, 40:3070-A.

Edwards, J.N., and Klemmack, D.L. Correlates of life satisfaction. *Journal of Gerontology,* 1973, 28:497–502.

Faulkner, A.O. The black aged as good neighbors: an experiment in volunteer services. *Gerontologist,* 1975, 15:554–59.

Friedman, S. The resident welcoming committee: institutionalized elderly in volunteer services to their peers. *Gerontologist,* 1975, 15:362–67.

Frisch, M.B., and Gerrard, M. Natural helping systems: a survey of Red Cross volunteers. *American Journal of Community Psychology,* 1981, 9:567–79.

Graney, M.J. Happiness and social participation in aging. *Journal of Gerontology,* 1975, 30:701.

Harris, L., and Associates: *The Myth and Reality of Aging in America: A Study for the National Council on the Aging, Inc.* Washington, D.C.: National Council on Aging, 1981.

Havighurst, R.J. The nature and value of meaningful free time activity. In Kleemeier, R.W. (Ed.), *Aging and Leisure,* New York: Oxford University Press, 1961, p. 317.

Heller, B.R., Walsh, F.J., and Wilson, K.M. Seniors helping seniors: training older adults as new personnel resources in home health care. *Journal of Gerontological Nursing,* 1981, 7:552–55.

Hendricks, J., and Hendricks, C.D. *Aging in a Mass Society: Myths and Realities,* Cambridge, Mass.: Winthrop, 1977, 299–301.

Hirsch, K., and Linn, M.W. How being helpful helps the elderly helper. *Gerontologist,* 1977, 17:75.

Kallan, F.K., and Leyendecker, G.T. Factors relating to retention of senior volunteers. *Resources in Education,* 1978, 13:ED 154 272.

Knoke, D., and Thomson, R. Voluntary association membership trends and the family life cycle. *Social Forces,* 1977, 56:48–65.

Lambert, C., Guberman, M., and Morris, R. Reopening doors to community participation for older people: How realistic? *Social Service Review,* 1964, 38:42–50.

Monk, A., and Cryns, A.G. Predictors of voluntaristic intent among the aged: an area study. *Gerontologist,* 1974, 14:425–29.

Morris, R., Lambert, C., and Guberman, M. *New Roles for the Elderly: A Report of a Study and Demonstration Program Conducted by Brandeis University under Contract (PH-86-62-40) with the Gerontology Branch, Division of Chronic Diseases, U.S. Public Health Service.* Waltham, Mass.: Brandeis University, 1964.

Paxman, C. A comparative study of formal volunteer programs in educational settings. *Dissertation Abstracts International,* 1981, 41:4549.

Payne, B.P., and Mazur, K.L. The older volunteer: social role continuity and development. *Gerontologist,* 1975, 15:68.

Peppers, L.G. Patterns of leisure and adjustment to retirement. *Gerontologist,* 1976, 16:441–46.

Pritchard, D.C., and Tomb, K. Emerging new service roles for older adults on college and university campuses. *Educational Gerontology,* 1981, 7:167–75.

Rath, S.F. Senior citizens as volunteers: a descriptive study of a group who chose to work with children and a group who chose to work with older adults. *Dissertation Abstracts International*, 1978, 39:2709-A.

Riessman, F. The "helper" therapy principle. *Social Work*, 1965, 10:27–32.

Rosenblatt, A. Interest of older persons in volunteer activities. *Social Work*, 1966, 11:87–94.

Routh, T.A. *The Volunteer and Community Agencies*. Springfield, Ill.: Charles C. Thomas, 1972, p. 35.

Ruffini, J.L., and Todd, H.F. A network model for leadership development among the elderly. *Gerontologist*, 1979, 19:158–162.

Sainer, J., and Zander, M. Guidelines for older person volunteers. *Gerontologist*, 1971, 11:201–204.

Schindler-Rainman, E., and Lippitt, R. *Volunteer Community: Creative Use of Human Resources, 2nd ed.* Fairfax, Va.: NTL Learning Resources, 1975, pp. 38–62.

Seligman, R. Elderly to elderly: a mutual aid program in Jerusalem. *Hadassah Magazine*, 1973, pp. 16–18.

Sheppard, N.A. Older Americans: an untapped resource. *Vocational Education*, 1981, 56:39–42.

Slack, G. Volunteering is in. *American Education*, 1978, 14:6–11.

Swartz, E.L. The older adult: creative use of leisure time. *Journal of Geriatric Psychiatry*, 1978, 11:85–88.

Tenenbaum, F. *Over 55 Is Not Illegal*. Boston: Houghton Mifflin, 1979, pp. 62–83.

Trela, J.E. Social class and association membership: an analysis of age-graded and nonage-graded voluntary participation. *Journal of Gerontology*, 1976, 31:198–203.

Wan, T.T.H., Odell, B.G., and Lewis, D.T. *Promoting the Well-being of the Elderly: A Community Diagnosis*. New York: Haworth Press, 1982, pp. 68–73.

Weiner, M.B., Brok, A.J., and Snadowsky, A.M. *Working with the Aged*. Englewood Cliffs, N.J.: Prentice-Hall, 1978, pp. 60–61.

Williams, J.A., Babchuk, N., and Johnson, D. Voluntary associations and minority status. *American Sociological Review*, 1973, 38:637–646.

13

Planning a Therapeutic Institutional Environment

Edith Kettel
G. Maureen Chaisson-Stewart

One can create an environment, as Van Gogh claimed he did in his painting "Night Café," where persons "can ruin . . . [themselves], go mad or commit a crime." "Night Café" is a scene dominated by repellent colors—kidney bean red and acid green—and patches of stark white and metallic yellow. (see Figure 13.1) There is too much space in it so that figures huddle together for intimacy. Uneven rows of acid green benches on thin black legs are lined up with small brown chairs against high, damp-looking walls. They face a mammoth dark brown billiard table with bulbous legs which stretches from one end of the vast hall to the other and appears to rest heavily on the bare wooden floor. Four round overhead lamps bombard every corner with searing yellow and white arcs of glaring light. There is no trace of shadow except for the muddy brown one cast by the grotesque billiard table; sunlight is absent. One hostile man in white shirt and trousers, hair gleaming with green reflections, stares moodily at the viewer. It is a place in which few would find delight or relaxation. The emotions aroused in the viewer are precisely what Van Gogh intended they should be—despair and alienation.

By creating a simulated environment with pigment on canvas, Van Gogh was able to elicit in the viewer the negative emotions he desired and a wish to flee the place. This painting reveals the profound impact that the elements of an environment—space, light, color, design, and accessories (a grab bag of furniture)—can have on the mood and behavior of the individual. The place defies anyone's ability to experience joy and satisfaction. Space, light, and color are stretched and repeated beyond the human's senses to grasp them or to experience them with pleasure. The

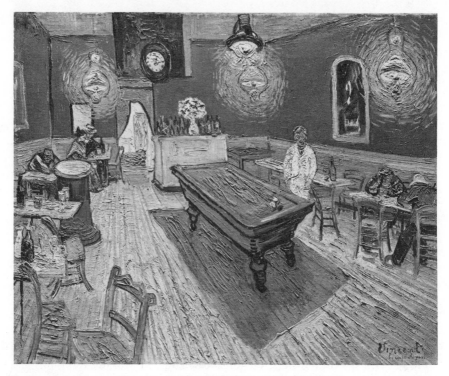

Figure 13.1 Vincent Van Gogh, *The Night Café,* 1888. (Yale University Art Gallery. Bequest of Stephen Carlton Clark, B.A. 1903.)

enormous boxlike design does not relate comfortably to the human size. Soothing stimulation is absent and, with it, satisfying emotions. It is a vivid illustration of an inhumane environment.

Environmental research, continually reaffirms the strong and intimate link between environmental factors and the individual's health, both mental and physical. The effect of the environment on a person's psyche is especially acute in institutional settings where there is no escape and few choices. In such settings efficiency is paramount. The factors that compose the environment often operate or are ordered to promote simplicity of function and design. This goal of simplification for the sake of efficiency helps to reduce costs in physical and human resources but, sadly, also promotes reduced psychic stimulation and personalization of surroundings and care. Efficient personnel who are frequently overstressed by incessant demands often seek to reduce the load by reverting to the least common and most manageable denominator—meeting the patient's physical needs. In so doing they sacrifice a rich and enriching person-to-person involvement with each unique resident, an involvement that may be perceived as complicating, time-consuming, or unmanageable. Efficiency in the building and its contents means reducing costs of construction, decoration, and maintenance with high utilization of space. The result is often a sleek, standardized structure and decor with the only available space for escape and solitude being in one's bed. Such settings breed depression. Also, if staff-patient interactions are routine and superficial, the resident is apt to lose a sense of self-esteem and hope for the future.

Whether the resident succumbs to such depression-inducing environmental factors will depend upon his or her ability to organize and regulate the intensity, complexity, and proportions of the environmental stimuli (Klein et al., 1967; Lawton, 1975a, 1977). This highly individualized form of coping or "personal style" is a product of the individual's past experiences, which are in turn influenced by heredity, culture, social, and intellectual history, and life-long habits (Neugarten, 1971). Although it is assumed that personal styles differ in the institutionalized elderly and that some clients are more adaptable than others, "little is known about the process or extent to which such personal coping efforts succeed in counteracting maladaptation" (Lawton, 1977) to the restricted environments of institutions.

Nevertheless, a holistic view of the old person recognizes that the person's physical self—eyes, ears, nose, mouth, skin, and muscles—transmits what they experience in their surroundings to their brains, which in turn process this information and stimulate a response, both physical and emotional. Thus, the environment influences clients' moods as well as their actions. This holistic perspective has been called an "ecological view of aging" (Fozard and Popkin, 1978).

In this chapter we will discuss the ecological view of aging, several methodologies for investigating the environment of the elderly, and, finally, the specific environmental factors, both living and nonliving, which either detract from or promote the well-being of the elderly.

ECOLOGICAL VIEW OF AGING

An enlightened view of aging is that it is a process that *continues in* and is *affected by* one's environment. This perspective, called an "ecological view of aging," states that "the optimum environment for the aging person promotes independence of activity and provides challenges to the individual not simply maximizing physical comfort and safety" (Fozard and Popkin, 1978; Lawton and Nahemow, 1973; Fozard and Rose, 1975; Fozard and Thomas, 1973). The ecological view of aging considers the effects on older persons of *all* elements in the surroundings and how they influence the elderly's psychosocial and physical health. The cause-and-effect relation between the person and his environment has been theorized to be a sensory feedback system.

The Sensory Feedback System

The sensory feedback system is a circular connection of environmental stimuli with the individual and, in return, of the individual with the environment. Within this system, the person's initial perception of a stimulus is highly individualized (Schooler, 1960; Selye, 1971; Wohwill, 1973). Repeated exposures to the same stimulus over time can either increase or decrease the intensity of the sensory response.

In explaining this phenomenon, psychologists theorize that the eye, "the transmitter of emotion" (Rogers, 1965), as well as the nose, ears, and muscles, work with the brain and memory to help the individual identify and organize the signs, odors, sounds, and dimensions in their surroundings. Even in the same setting identical stimuli can evoke a variety of moods and behaviors in the occupants, depending upon individualized perceptions of meaning and form. An example of a sensory feedback system at work is the anxiety many feel at the sight of a dentist's drill.

When the stimulus is extreme, either too much or too little, an individual may react with immobility, aggression, or flight. Such responses indicate that the person is unable or unwilling to adapt to some or all of the elements in the environment. But, in an environment that is balanced in sensory input, neither too bland nor too stimulating, the individual relaxes and behaves with interest, social awareness, and acceptable activity (Kahana, 1975).

Environmental stimuli play significant and continual roles in shaping individual behavioral and emotional states. In modern communities, especially in the man-made environments of the elderly, "one's unconscious picture of one's self—the minute to minute process of existence is constructed from the bits and pieces of sensory feedback in a largely manufactured environment" (Hall, 1966). It is not just the factors in the environment but each individual's perception of them as well that molds the mood and behavior of humans. When the environment is planned in consideration of human needs and perception it can be called humane.

A Humane Environment

A humane environment has been identified by professionals, researchers, and the elderly alike as one that satisfies the person's needs and desires for 1) privacy, 2) social interaction both inside and, when possible, beyond the borders of a restricted setting (Hammer and Chapin, 1972), 3) autonomy in decision making (Slover, 1972; Marlowe, 1973), 4) intellectual and sensory stimulation (Kahana, 1975), 5) cleanliness, safety, and security, and 6) adequate and appropriate health care and facilities.

In a humane environment, the aging resident is encouraged to maintain a personal support network of family and friends through regular visits, letters, and telephone calls. The residents are also encouraged to perform at a high level of independence by staff, who do not confuse physical caution with incompetence (Bengston, 1977). Instead, the staff urge residents to make new discoveries, to pursue learning as a lifetime activity, and to motivate themselves with meaningful personal and group goals.

When the environment is confined, it is especially important that caregivers encourage but do not push clients, lest the setting appear more like a prison than a home. Urging is most effective when it takes the form of a partnership in which the elderly residents join with family, friends, and caregivers to create a milieu in which they feel at home.

Planning Environmental Changes

Studies of environmental stress and the effects of institutionalization and transplantation on the elderly support the need for making changes to promote a therapeutic milieu. Many of the transitions, conflicts, and losses of the old which produce stress have been shown to be related to environmental factors (Holmes and Rahe, 1967; Mechanic, 1968; Carp, 1972; Nahemow and Lawton, 1973; Lowenthal, 1971; Lawton, 1975a). In addition, studies of disease liability (Selye, 1971; Levi, 1971), specifically, early hypertension and cardiovascular disease (Speith, 1965; Brod, 1971; Wolf, 1971; Forsyth, 1974) manifest similar individual-environment links at all ages.

In designing or remodeling an environment, the wishes of the aging residents ought to be considered. They know their own priorities best (Huttman, 1977). Sometimes the preferences of the elderly "may be at variance with those ordinarily considered important by the human factors engineer, architect and physician" (Chapanis, 1974). A comparison of the results of just three client and professional surveys illustrates these differences.

A report of 1,750 residents' responses to a questionnaire about their housing indicated that climate, location, privacy, access to public transportation, and environmental safety were important factors in selection and satisfaction with housing (Hamovitch and Peterson, 1969). When clients' preferences were compared with those of the staff members', the researchers reported the following findings. While 60 percent of the elderly rated proximity to shopping and laundry as important, professional personnel considered proximity to medical and religious personnel as important (Hamovitch and Peterson, 1969).

A Canadian survey of 262 residents in homes for the aging showed that 43.9 percent expressed dissatisfaction with housing design elements relating to "bedrooms, balconies, closets, light and noise" (Huttman, 1977). On the other hand, the staff members of a geriatric facility in Linn's (1974) survey mentioned the physical plant, residents' meals, and administrative policies. Comparing these results, it appears as if residents are extremely concerned with the details of their habitat, whereas staff members are concerned with an efficient, smooth-functioning health system.

In short, it appears that older persons tend to emphasize what professionals consider as extras, factors that promote their independence: shopping, laundry, public transportation, and architectural details. They seem secure in the knowledge that health facilities are available in their environment (Lawton, 1969), but their priorities appear to lie elsewhere—with the amenities.

Changes to improve the environment will be more attuned to the needs of the elderly if the residents are invited, along with staff, to become members of an environmental planning committee. Environment committees can also help to overcome residents' resistance to someone disturbing the nest, even when the nest is uncomfortable.

EVALUATING THE ENVIRONMENT'S QUALITY

One may accept the characteristics of a humane environment already described, but how does one evaluate a geriatric setting to determine if it is, in fact, a humane and stimulating one? Observation can help detect obvious defects such as faulty plumbing or gloomy corridors, but observation is not enough to assess clients' satisfaction with their surroundings.

Outcome Measures

One possible indicator of a negative cause-and-effect relation between the environment and the individual is mortality rate. Yet, residents' low mortality rates do not necessarily reveal milieu satisfaction nor a humane environment. Instead, they may only measure the older persons' successful use of their adaptation techniques represented by their individual "personal styles".

> With all the study of institutions, no dependable quality criterion has yet been defined. Most institutions for the aged are one-way streets, where death rates (or length of remaining life) is the only possible ultimate criterion. Given the wide variation among residents in their input characteristics, remaining life span is, at present, an almost totally useless criterion for comparing one institution to another (Lawton, 1977).

Presumed qualities (Lawton, 1977) such as the presence of adequate health facilities and personnel, efficient management, or nutritious meals have also been utilized as measures of the quality of the environment. However, if the institution meets the standards for numbers of staff on duty but the staff administer health care mechanically *or* if the management designs social programs that are impervious to residents' preferences *or* if the menu includes nutritious meals but they are served in a noisy, colorless, windowless hall, the quality of the environment falls dramatically. Therefore, it seems that a truly thorough and accurate assessment of the environment must monitor the complex and interacting array of multiple variables. When operationalized, these variables usually demand a complex assortment of data collection methods from interview to pen-and-pencil instruments to on-site observations. One must identify the environment's physical, psychological, and social aspects and, at the same time, consider its effects on the residents' moods, behaviors, and health.

For example, what are the characteristics of an environment that prompts a client to respond to his circumstances with anger? Is the angry resident reacting to an environment that he perceives as too restricted because its programs do not permit him enough choices? Does he resent his dependence on others because the environment does not include sufficient compensation devices to allow him to exert more independent living? Or is his anger a response to overcrowding?

Research Methods

Most of the environmental research studies to date have been concerned with institutionalization, adaptation, or transfer. Although methodologies differ, there seem to be similar stages in the research design. First, certain elements (factors) in the environment which appear germane to the study are identified and listed by the investigators. Second, these elements are placed in several physical, psychological, or social categories, or environmental dimensions, and third, an attempt is made to correlate them with clients' responses. Last, from these environment/dimensions—resident/response correlations the researcher attempts to draw valid conclusions about the effect of the environment on the client. In effect, the investigators ask two questions: Do the clients' responses indicate a humane environment or an impoverished one? Do they simply measure clients' ability to *adapt* to whatever conditions surround them? Though the steps in the research process are similar, the theoretical framework and descriptive categories have differed considerably.

For example, Slover (1972) lists 189 environmental factors in physical, social, and service categories. Marlow (1973) uses a similar list. Linn (1974) uses a list of institutional care factors.

A brief summary of one method developed by Allen Pincus (1968) (see Table 13-1) illustrates the difficulties that are involved in any assessment of institutional environments for the older adult. He divides the environment into four dimensions and three shapers or aspects of the institutional setting.

The first environmental dimension is space, which is divided into private and public space. *Private space* consists of three interrelated parts: living,

TABLE 13.1

SOME EXAMPLES OF ASPECTS OF THE INSTITUTIONAL SETTING RELATED TO THE FOUR ENVIRONMENTAL DIMENSIONS

Aspects of the Institutional Setting	Public/Private	Structured/Unstructured	Resource Sparse Resource Rich	Integrated/Isolated
Physical plant	Proportion of single and double rooms Number of day rooms	Existence of signs displayed around the home reminding residents of rules and regulations	Availability of facilities where residents can cook a meal or prepare a snack Existence of a library	Distance from public transportation Distance from shopping area
Rules regulations, and program	Existence of rules requiring residents to keep the doors to their rooms open at all times	Existence of rules regulating residents' bedtime Provisions for residents to help in planning	Existence of regular jobs around the home performed by residents	Extent of restrictions placed on visiting Frequency with which residents are taken on trips outside the home
Staff behavior	Extent to which staff knock on doors before entering residents' rooms	Extent to which staff decide what programs are to be watched on TV Extent to which staff expect strict obedience from residents	Extent to which staff encourage residents to participate in activities	Extent to which staff assist residents who need help in making phone calls or writing letters

Source: Pincus, A. The definition and measurement of the institutional environment in homes for the aged. *Gerontologist,* Autumn 1968, 8:208.

social, and hygenic. *Public space* is all other institutional space. The remaining dimensions are structured versus unstructured, resource sparse versus resource rich, and integrated versus isolated. *Structured/unstructured* defines the degree of control exerted by staff and/or patients over the environment. *Resource sparse/resource rich* describes the resources in the environment that promote independence and stimulate interest, activity and creativity in residents. *Integrated/isolated* refers to the extent of inter-action with the surrounding heterogeneous population, including distances from public transportation and shopping as well as schedules of visiting hours and outside trips.

The "shapers" of the environment that interact with the dimensions described above are the physical plant itself, administrative rules and programs, and staff behavior. Environmental dimensions and shapers in combination compose the total psychosocial milieu and, according to Pincus, must be viewed as an interrelated whole in order to determine their total effect on the residents.

Lawton and Nahemow (1973) use a different perspective (see Figure 13.2). They correlate a range of low to high client competence (perform-ance) levels with weak to strong "environmental press" factors. Their purpose is to indicate "(clients') shifts in adaptation levels . . . at various (environmental) press strengths" (Lawton, 1977).

Competence, as defined by Lawton (1975a), is the individual's limits of abilities in health, perception, action, and cognition. *Environmental press* includes any aspect of the environment which motivates behavior. "Positive (behavior) outcomes fall within the shaded area [see Figure 13.2], where the individual's competence is adequate to deal with the press level at a given time" (Lawton, 1977). When competence or press strength changes, so does adaptation. From this viewpoint, an environment is regarded as stimulating when "press strengths" range above "adaptation level."

ELEMENTS IN THE ENVIRONMENT:
LIVING AND NONLIVING

For the purposes of this discussion we have categorized the elements in the environment of the elderly into two main categories: the living and the nonliving. In the living environment are staff, residents, animals, and plants. In the nonliving environment are architectural elements, space, color, light, and personal possessions.

Staff

Clients' high morale and milieu satisfaction exist in institutions where professionals use skilled assessments, careful prognosis and appropriate interventions as the basis of their health care programs. The accurate perception of a patient's abilities and performance can inspire in the

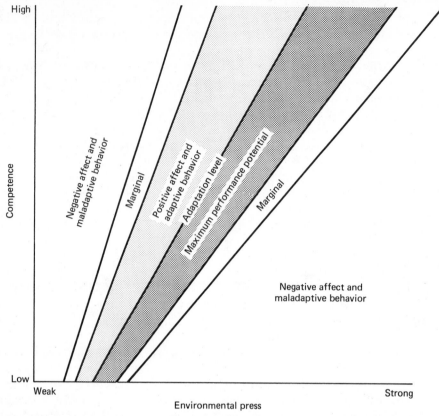

Figure 13.2 Diagrammatic representation of the behavioral and affective outcomes of person–environment transactions. (Lawton, M., and Nahemow, L. Ecology and the aging process. In E.C. Eisdorfer and M.P. Lawton, Eds., *The Psychology of Adult Development and Aging.* Copyright 1973 by the American Psychological Association. Reprinted by permission.)

elderly residents the desire to achieve new and valuable goals so necessary to a positive self-image as well as to high morale. Proper evaluations of each client can end the vicious circle by which low staff expectations influence failure in the older adult.

Also, staff members who provide daily services to the elderly should not underestimate their contributions to raising the level of their clients' psychosocial well-being in ways not directly related to the services they are hired to perform.

Staff members play a crucial role in institution morale because there is "a contagion of high morale in a well-motivated staff" (Goldfarb, 1969). Therapeutic personnel do not stand on the periphery of the elderly's environment—they are part of it. If they withdraw and behave like royal philosophers who are hired to perform tasks, and little else, for another species of man and womankind, they create an atmosphere that is both inhumane and emotionally impoverished. Personnel who collaborate with the elderly in shaping and enriching their shared milieu can fashion an environment that offers its aging residents support, rehabilitation, and stimulation.

Active staff-client communication is an important factor in a therapeutic environment (Moos and Houts, 1968; Slover, 1972).

> In general, institutional staffs have too little appreciation of their importance as psychotherapists and of the importance of their nonpsychiatric skills and duties as vehicles for psychotherapy. . . . Personnel on all levels need much instruction about the value of transference, rapport, "parentification," . . . in promoting self-sufficiency or optimal function . . . in the men and women in their charge (Goldfarb, 1969).

The interaction of individual personalities and behavior can make or break an environmental atmosphere. Also, it is known that "the differences in social climate and attitudes fostered in an environment may, in and of themselves, greatly affect the success of a treatment program" (Fozard and Popkin, 1978). Achieving and maintaining high morale through communication between the clients and their caregivers in a geriatric establishment is an intrinsic part of residents' therapy and milieu satisfaction.

Personnel, sensitive to the needs and wishes of the elderly, are also concerned with each client's personhood. They understand, for example, that when the elderly narrate their family histories they are experiencing the exhilarating sensation of being known as an individual. Verbalizing family histories allows older adults, as it does everyone, to feel that they are unique among all others and that they are no longer the stranger to be scorned or villified (Guttman, 1977).

> Attentive listening—accompanied by justifiable praise and admiration at critical points in the historical reporting, can be a very effective spontaneous process in accomplishing the goal of reinforcing the inherent and proven strengths of the client (Chaisson, 1981).

In altruistic Oriental and African cultures a narrator role is granted to the elderly as an age reward to which younger members of the tribe or community look forward as they age. However, in American society it is hot yet regarded as a symbol of prestige and is, therefore, a self-created role. The narrator must function without receptive younger audiences since America's cultural traditions have not yet developed in that direction. Narrators must choose their listeners where they can find them. Nevertheless, in a restricted environment, or in any place in which the older adult lives, he "needs someone to talk to about his life, to review it, make sense of it, and come to terms with his dying" (Butler, 1975). A sensitive staff member can be that someone.

The amounts of emotional support professionals offer their elderly client-consumers can be strengthened and extended when staff members encourage residents to form their own sharing-caring in-house network. Personnel can follow the principles of a therapeutic self-governing community as described by Maxwell Jones (1968). They can structure space to provide a variety of social communication areas for residents, such as game rooms, a cocktail lounge, or club room, where older adults can enjoy the rituals, ceremonies, and play so essential to a civilized life. The supportive friendships vital to mental health care can flourish with a glass of wine in a lounge area, over cards in a game room, or in a discussion of mutual concerns in a cozy alcove.

One Link in Staff-Client Collaboration: Laughter

Staff who can see humor in life and stimulate laughter in others can use this gift to reduce boredom and evoke positive mood states in the elderly. The best defense against boredom, of course, is work, but when the opportunity or ability to work is absent, laughter becomes a precious commodity in one's daily life. Furthermore, there is increasing evidence that laughter "increases circulation, respiration and the endorphin level in the blood" (Larsen, 1982). Its effects are like those derived from jogging in place (Fry, 1982). The possibilities laughter has in achieving and maintaining high morale among the institutionalized elderly should not be ignored.

Residents

The characteristics of the residents should be monitored closely in environmental research because the resident population itself also shapes the environment (Pincus, 1968). For example, while it may be assumed that limited resources are needed when there is a high proportion of disabled residents, this assumption may become a self-fulfilling prophecy. When personnel expect low performances from their clients, the clients, in turn, tend to live up to these low expectations. Therefore, in order to increase the validity of any study of an environment's quality, Pincus suggests that the researcher identify the characteristics of the clients as well as the characteristics of the environment.

Plants and Animals

Work in a garden or greenhouse has been credited with creating remarkable changes in withdrawn patients. The garden gives the withdrawn patient an emotional bridge to build relationships with other people. Estelle Douglas, director of the Department of Rehabilitation Activities of the Long Island Jewish–Hillside Medical Center, reports that patients who find other types of therapeutic programs unacceptable are often willing to work in a greenhouse. They feel peace among the plants. "Plants are alive, something to touch and handle, but also safe. They provide pleasure, hope, expectation. They even help bring acceptance of the workings of nature, for when a plant dies, you have to replace it and get on with raising the next plant," says Dr. Philip Goldberg, psychiatrist at Hillside.

The therapeutic value of animals as source of pleasure, comfort, love, and companionship has been documented in approximately a dozen research reports and also in a few dissertations. Pets can provide diversion, physical contact, and a sense of being needed (Spier, 1980).

NONLIVING ELEMENTS IN THE ENVIRONMENT

One's positive attitude is "the most vital ingredient" (Smith, 1977) one can bring to an extended life. But, how can anyone manage positive thoughts about or affection for a "private room" that is neither "private" nor comfortable as most understand the term? How can anyone love an environment that is awash with clinical echo chambers and indiscriminate fluorescent lighting? How can anyone enjoy or survive happily the killing effects of long corridors? Today's structures which house the elderly and which so obviously bear the mistakes and stigma of institutional housing must be reevaluated in order to correct the serious emotional consequences they create in their aging occupants (Hall, 1966).

The form, function, and construction of housing for the elderly should complement each other (Banham, 1975) as well as they do in a New England farmhouse or a monastery. These designs grew naturally from the clearly understood needs and desires of their residents. As a result, they are self-contained milieus in which their residents' chosen life-styles are supported and enhanced. Their simple, attractive designs and decorative details use imagination to serve the unique purposes of those who dwell in them.

Architecture and Interior Design

The architecture of every domicile, both institutional and private, is the stage on which life is lived; it determines the character of its residents' lives. As noted before, life satisfaction, mood, and behavior are greatly influenced by the variety and kinds of challenges and stimulation in one's surroundings. In institutions for the elderly, architectural design determines *how* the older adult lives and "How one lives can be far more important than how long" (Smith, 1977). Architecture and interior design in homes for the elderly ideally ought to be planned to provide physical comfort and stimulation, compensate for and prevent physical losses, prevent disorientation, promote bonding and laughter and minimize anger.

Providing Comfort and Stimulation

Architectural design and renovations for the communities of the aging must include visual and kinesthetic* comforts and stimulation because both are necessary to create an environment in which human dignity is preserved and a meaningful life is possible. It is the milieu's exterior architecture that can establish the humane atmosphere of a geriatric setting and it is its interior design and accessories that confirm it.

The setting's architectural features can be a source of delight or of depression, of milieu satisfaction or boredom. Its features can provide an array of visual and kinesthetic comforts *and* stimulation or they can limit them. Both the details and overall design of all architecture have the power to reassure the individual with physical comforts and conveniences and to stimulate by their beauty. Consequently, architecture's potential to provide a therapeutic milieu and sensory stimulation deserves more attention because architecture is "more than a commentary on the human condition . . . it *is* the human condition" (Giedion, 1958).

Building designs that relate to the human size and floor plans that are easily memorized are as essential to enjoyable living in an institutionalized home as they are in a private one. Windows that offer a variety of views to the outside from lying, sitting, and standing positions, and that let the sunlight in, can satisfy the human need for both sensory stimulation and relaxation. Color and wood or stone texture contrasts can solve the disorientation problems of residents and, at the same time, they can transform dull surroundings into exhilarating ones. Intimate scale, logical space plans, windows, color, and texture are some of the architectural elements that can provide physical and emotional comfort, as well as sensory stimulation, in a geriatric setting.

Compensating and Preventing Physical Losses

A humane architectural design for the elderly includes features that both *compensate* for their physical losses as well as *prevent* future losses. Adequate soundproofing can eliminate unpleasant sounds; four-foot-wide doorways and flat doorsills permit independent travel by wheelchair clients. Dutch doors on residents' bedrooms allow discrete client viewing by personnel and, at the same time, offer residents the opportunity to regulate

---

* *Kinesthesia* (noun); *kinesthetic* (adjective): The sensation of position, movement, and tension of parts of the body perceived through nerve and organs in muscles, tendons, and joints. (*Webster's New World Dictionary,* 1980.)

their own privacy. Clients' freedom to alter the amount of privacy in their personal living area can act as an incentive for them to begin and to continue their projects without frequent staff interruptions.

"An important need is to design interiors for people whose mental, physical and emotional powers may be reduced. The opportunities for sound constructive work in this direction are substantial" (Proppe, 1968). The permanent architectural fixtures in homes for the elderly are often designs created for the young and disabled. But there is a need for more innovative variations of these features that meet older persons' physical requirements. For example, lights that can be easily lit, adjusted in height, direction, or intensity by arthritic clients' fingers from a wheelchair or at bedside allow the elderly to conserve their strength and to manage their environment to suit their particular needs and desires.

Therefore, all architectural elements in homes for the elderly have two main functions: provision for physical comfort and sensory stimulation, and compensation for and prevention of physical losses. In addition, architecture and interior design can be planned to prevent disorientation and to promote bonding and laughter.

Preventing Disorientation

When the sense of self in space is lost, when individuals occupy space that is unfamiliar to them, they suffer disorientation and they are terrified. Persons must know that *this* space and no other, is where they exist *now;* they must know how they feel about it so that they can know how to act in it.

> Where am I . . . is one of the most poignant of human formulations. It speaks of an anxiety that is intense, recurrent and all but unbearable. Not to know where we are is torment, and not to have a sense of place [in space] is a most sinister deprivation (Russell, 1982).

Disorientation responses include depression, withdrawal, inactivity, pessimism, anxiety and, above all, a collapse of one's self-image. Disorientation causes emotional havoc in human beings which they cannot overcome without assistance; they become emotionally insecure both about themselves and their surroundings. Therefore, all orientation cues in environments for older persons must be regarded as more than geographic landmarks; they are vital parts of milieu therapy.

The value of on-site examination is perhaps demonstrated by a study that compared preparation for transfer in two groups of elderly. Both groups participated in family and staff conferences and examined slides and photographs of the new facility. In addition, one group was allowed to visit the new housing site four times; the other group made only one visit. After transfer, mortality rates for the members of the one-visit group were higher than the mortality rate for the four-visit group members. In short, although the purpose of the study was to compare clients' preparation for transfer (Bourestom and Pastalan, n.d.), the authors of this chapter suggest that advance on-site examination seemed to be a critical variable in the elderly's adjustment to their surroundings and, presumably, in their ultimate well-being and longevity.

From these study results, we can conclude that the elderly require, and should have, more first-hand information about their present or future surroundings rather than second-hand verbal descriptions, flat photographs, and rapid film sequences. Verbal and visual reproductions can be spatially confusing because they do not allow client-users to experience the atmosphere or the kinesthetic feel of the environment. Without this sensory input, the elderly cannot fully perceive the new environment or experience personal feelings about it. When the camera and the environment's spokesmen translate everything for them, the aging man and woman have but one option—persuasion by others or by the camera.

When on-site examination is impossible, a down-scaled three-dimensional model of the institution can act as a substitute. Architects consider the skyscraper replica as an essential selling tool in achieving the corporate or municipal building contract. The replica allows the eye to travel around the floor plan; it helps the client to locate his or her private space as well as to identify the location and variety of public spaces. A replica of a geriatric setting prepares the resident for its dimensions as well as the distances between rooms and health care units. This information is reinforced over time when it is placed in a permanent location and available for repeated examination as desired.

For the disoriented or wandering client a building in the round (Goldfarb, 1969) or one with segmented room clusters help residents to overcome their orientation fears. Such architectural designs encourage strolling without assistance and permit residents to visit other areas outside the narrow confines of their more familiar locales. They also reduce the need for humiliating mechanical restraints.

Long hallways that offer no clue to their destinations or to the units they serve waste the body strengths and vision of the aging man and woman. These sterile highways also numb the emotions because they repeat one design endlessly, reinforce noise, and offer no view to the outside. "Although . . . [their] efficiency in terms of economics and fire egress may not be directly questioned the [negative] effects of this 'psychological railroading' cannot be overstressed" (Proppe, 1968).

If long hallways must remain part of institutional designs, they can include soundproofing, windows, seating alcoves, and recessed doors in order to introduce into them comfortable acoustics, sunlight, occasional rest areas, and visual variety. Their distances can appear to shrink with color contrasts, abstract wall paintings and murals, or decorative art and woven wall hangings. Thus, the debilitating effects on the elderly of the long institutional hallway can be minimized by using foresight and imagination.

Promoting Bonds

When architecture adapts to the emotional, cultural, and social needs of its aging inhabitants, it becomes for them the *symbol* of their social, ceremonial, and community lives. As such it should encourage, through its design elements, cohesiveness among the diversified community of the old. The common bonds shared by residents of nursing homes sponsored by fraternal, cultural, religious, military, or labor union groups provide common ties to promote bonding. Cohesiveness occurs easily from their shared traditions, experiences, and value systems. These bonds are above and beyond the shared experience of being old. Although living in the same place with people in the same age cohort can encourage some affinity among members, there is such a variety in the prior life experience and abilities of the elderly that *old age alone is insufficient* to cause and sustain group cohesiveness.

Where this binding relationship does not exist, architectural design must provide the means for establishing new ones. Social interaction rooms and intimate group space can encourage the creation of new ties within the geriatric setting. Residents tend to develop these ties by sharing their personal histories until, at some point, a common meeting ground or partner-relationship is discovered.

Where the philosophic bond is not so great and the residents are individuals with diffuse goals, values and roles, the architectural environment must try harder to provide the cohesive and environmental [opportunities] . . . which would offset the lack of a binding social matrix. *And it is precisely in this crucial role that present architectural design is most often inadequate* [emphasis added]. (Proppe, 1968)

An effective exterior design, with one dominant, easily recognized architectural theme, such as English Tudor or Spanish villa, imparts an immediate feeling of unity, as well as pride, in its residents. The exterior design theme can be repeated inside with appropriate decoration that follows the outside pattern. For example, fabric with English garden or hunting scenes and some accessories in pewter reflect the English Tudor tradition. For the Spanish villa hanging plants, vivid color accents, and baskets unify the setting and give further clues to its cohesive theme.

In summary, when building designs reflect the physical and sensory needs of older persons, it is because the residents' needs are clearly understood. But, too often institutional architecture for the elderly seems created, first, to house health equipment and second, to house the bed patient. Although residents of life-care institutions comprise a

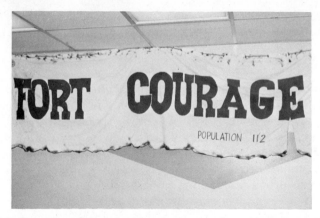

Figure 13.3 Shared traditions build cohesiveness in a Veterans Administration hospital. (Nursing Home Care Unit, Veterans Administration Medical Center, Phoenix, Arizona.)

population with a wide variety of abilities and interests, they all share the need for shelter that permits the continuation of a full and challenging life. Therefore, housing for the elderly must offer them designs that provide compensation for their physical losses, prevention of additional losses, and the sensory delights of an attractive home in which they can age comfortably.

Promoting Laughter

The gloom, frustration, and fatigue that inept architectural design produce in the aging man and woman is reinforced by interiors decorated without wit or imagination. Wit in interior design startles the spectator and provokes laughter because it is unexpected and often playful in effect.

Examples of the use of wit in design to startle and charm the viewer are a vegetable scale used as a hanging planter; a flag draped on a wall which bears the name of the nursing home for veterans, "Fort Courage" (see Figure 13.3).

With wit and imagination one can change or reduce the deplorable physical and psychological effects on clients of architectural errors. Hans Proppe, who develops architectural concepts for housing the old, bemoans the lack of wit and imagination in some homes for the elderly. He writes that too many lack imagination in design ideas and consequently they are residential environments that are both dismal and cold.

Lighting, color, corridors and spatial definition were segments of the design which were consistently of questionable application [lighting was unvaried or insufficient] . . . especially in areas of circulation or in common spaces [colors were often used] without purpose, without contrast and . . . blended too much for tired eyes.

Corridors were tunnel-like because of the lighting pattern. One row of lights down the middle of a wide corridor not only obscures the individual room openings but makes the entire journey a dark and dreary one. . . .

[Spatial definitions in one home] for some 150 people offered only two sizes of spaces; those spaces for the individual rooms and one very large space to accommodate all the residents—which was never used. . . . The ceiling height was 30 feet. (Proppe, 1968)

Such interior designs clearly lack imagination and stimulate sadness rather than joy.

Minimizing Anger

Anger, so unwelcome but so prevalent in the institutions for the older adult, can be a behavioral response to environmental factors. Some researchers believe it may be a survival asset. [Lieberman, (1973); Guttman, (1977), and Nardini's (1952) studies revealed anger as a survival tool in prison while depression led to sickness and death of Japanese prison camp inmates.

As a response, anger may appear useless and it may be habitual in some residents; but in displaying anger, the resident adopts "the paranoid position . . . [and] avoids the more lethal depressive position. Furthermore, by being vigilant and active he tunes up his cardiovascular system and he avoids the vegetative position that is perhaps prodromal to death" (Guttman, 1977).

If certain conflicts or frustrations within the environment are removed or lessened, this aggressive posture may change (Rosenman, 1974). However, the elements in the environment that produce these responses must be identified before they can be changed. This requires close observation of the client's mood and behavior as well as a sensitivity to the impact of certain identified environmental stimuli on the client. By this method the caregiver becomes increasingly aware of the subtle relationship between aging man or woman and the various elements in their surroundings. This relationship is obvious when the client complains of too much sunlight or too little heat, but the client-environment connection exists in other less noticeable situations. This is especially true when the individual is unable or unwilling to verbalize complaints and, as noted above, may simply erupt with anger.

Space

Human beings need enough private space to physically work through their personal problems and needs apart from the community. Insufficient livable, private space thwarts this need and promotes depression or aggression. At the very least, everyone needs enough space to avoid colliding with people or things in walking, sitting, and stretching positions.

On the other hand, too much interior space—width, length, and height—produces anxiety because people cannot see all of their surroundings or cannot mentally picture its limits. Huge interior spaces, such as theaters, sports arenas, or bus terminals, invite spectator activity, and discourage intimacy. Smaller spaces, such as lounges and porches, on the other hand, almost demand sociability and familiarity.

Space boundaries in life-care institutions must assure an adequate number of square feet for private space and more square feet for social space (Proppe, 1968). Private space, or the client's bedroom, should include a variety of space areas to accommodate the resident's body in bed, chair, wheelchair, and desk positions. It must be well-planned, providing enough space for traffic into and within the room as well as provide generous storage space for the client's personal possessions and a separate area for nurses' equipment. Ideally, both private and public space in homes for the elderly are large enough to permit clients in wheelchairs to turn them around without help, to pull up to a card table or bathroom sink, and to pass through doorways with ease (Lawton, 1975b).

Social or public space in institutions is all the space exclusive of the client's bedroom. It is space in which residents, personnel, or visitors congregate. It includes a variety of room sizes to provide choices among gatherings of various sizes and purpose. It is a mistake to regard social space in life-care institutions as one vast single hall, serving every social need, out of which are born so many unused waiting-for-something-to-happen rooms.

Persons do not always suddenly move from private space (one person) into another space with 20 or more people in it; they normally move gradually from private space into larger and larger social circles and back again to their private domains. Therefore, a realistic concept of institutional social (public) space is as a range of space sizes that fit the way persons normally arrange themselves for different reasons; it includes a different space size for the dining room and the visitors' lounge plus two or more different sizes for clients' other social activities.

Lorraine Hiatt Snyder (1978, p. 48) diagrams social space groups as shown below: two persons, three to six persons, seven to twenty persons, twenty-one to forty persons, and over forty persons. Readers can mentally visualize similar person-group sizes among their own family, friends, acquaintances, local neighborhoods, and communities.

A Continuum of Social Spaces Needed by Each Older Person

(1)	*(2)*	*(3–6)*	*(7–20)*	*(21–40)*	*(over 40)*
One-li-ness	Dyads	Family-sized groups	Neighborhoods	Community	Full assemblage

A floor plan that includes one private space for the individual and some variety of social space sizes for from 6 to over 40 persons allows the elderly resident 1) to mentally visualize and remember their locations and purposes, 2) to experience social space with pleasure because each fits the human need for small, medium, or large group size, and 3) to make choices among several social groups.

Space and Floor Plans

In a geriatric setting, the variety, size, and location of spaces begins with a person-oriented floor plan. It includes enough space for essential health, food, and hygenic facilities and equipment. It confines noise areas, such as kitchens and elevators to locations that are convenient to but distant from residents' rooms. When social areas are separate from living quarters, a bedroom truly becomes a peaceful haven for rest and renewal. But social areas need to be centrally located, because central social areas are used five times more than those peripherally located (Lawton, 1977). Two resident lounges, one located with a view to, but not encroaching upon, the nurses' station, and one near the elevator foyer or visitors' entrance are more stimulating sites than one secluded lounge adjacent to residents' rooms.

Spaces that evolve naturally from the chosen activities of the institution's population can be valuable social interaction points. For example, the mailroom and dining room foyer are often popular social areas because they attract residents by their activities and by their promise of pleasurable experiences (Butler, 1975; Huttman, 1977). In existing facilities, these areas may be enlarged to make room for comfortable chairs. In future design plans these spaces could replace one uninteresting lounge hall. Mail and food act as lures to these points and provide a natural incentive for clients' ambulation and socialization.

Sanctuaries, inside or outside, are person-oriented. The library, exclusively for reading and without a television, and a chapel or meditation room are sanctuaries that afford different kinds of privacy than does one's own bedroom. Intimate hall alcoves with chairs set beside a window, or hall junctions with inviting, comfortable conversation corners, provide additional spaces for solitary or selected group conversation and activities. Outside, a grotto or partially secluded portion of the patio, offer residents the opportunity to distance themselves, occasionally, from active social circles (Hiatt Snyder, 1978).

Floor plans that are designed to provide comfortable living space for client-users also include generous storage space. A bedroom closet subtracts some bedroom space; therefore, it must be considered as a separate portion of space in the bedroom's initial floor plan. When the bedroom closet is not large enough to hold a client's personal possessions it becomes a source of constant irritation and frustration (Huttman, 1977). The same initial plans for storage areas are necessary to hold therapy, exercise, hobby, and kitchen equipment. Adequate storage space for unused items prevents disordered and cluttered surroundings which can confuse and depress residents.

Seating Arrangements

Although "few formal research explorations have been done thus far on space and behavior in institutions" (Lawton, 1977), the experiments of Osmond (1966) and Sommer and Ross (1958) demonstrate the value of cross-corner seating (in space) as a spur to conversation. Rows of chairs lined up against the walls are appropriate for bus terminals or train stations but not for persons' homes. U-shaped or L-shaped seating patterns (Lawton, 1975b) are preferable for people who wish to enjoy each others' conversation. Furniture on swivel casters, keeping in mind their possible safety hazards, allow convenient groupings especially after the invasion of cleaning personnel. High tables, around which wheelchair clients may group (Hiatt Snyder, 1981) are also natural focal points that can eliminate those haphazard groups that form in remote corners of the room or at its center.

The same principle for cluster seating can be employed outdoors. Benches with backs in permanent U-shaped or L-shaped patterns, in addition to winding footpaths with benches and some crossovers, create serendipitous meetings among clients.

Open and Outdoor Space

Outdoor green spaces, cherished by many, provide them with opportunities to use their senses in order to enhance sedentary and active pleasures. Whether sitting, strolling, or gardening, they can experience the delights of fresh air and sunlight amid the colorful evidences of nature's seasonal changes. This proximity to nature's constant renewal can offer solace to men and women who have learned that their days "at the most are a hundred years: as a drop of water of the sea are esteemed, as a pebble of the sand, so are a few years compared to eternity" (Ecclesiasticus, 18).

The Japanese, masters in the imaginative uses of space, extend and beautify space by stimulating the senses. Through creative design they stimulate humans to perceive space configurations, textures, and the natural elements when, or where, they do not exist. Huge screens and hanging scrolls with scenes of colorful and spacious landscapes bring the natural elements—sky, land, and water—into their homes. A mixture of wood textures on their unadorned walls in both horizontal and vertical lines give the illusion of added space.

Free or unused space is more aesthetically pleasing and appreciated by the Japanese than it is by Western man. They use optical tricks to create the sense of space and texture. *Trompe l'oeil,** creates similar spatial and textural effects. A *trompe l'oeil* painting or wall mural merges with the wall and architectural design of a room and gives the illusion of space and real objects. Subjects for murals may be landscapes or seascapes or festival views. In paintings, hunters' gear and dead prey or musical instruments appear authentic and seem to hang, with uncanny realism, directly on the room's wall. The genuine sense of space and objects and the emotional impact that results from experiencing these tricks on the eye are no less because they are not "true."

Outdoors, the Japanese tea-garden "is an important part of our habitation," writes Noritake Tsuda (1976), a lecturer on fine arts. "It gives us rest and comfort and has an influence upon our life." The garden's purpose is to create an atmosphere of natural beauty in which persons can experience serenity and far-reaching space: Flowers, shrubs, stepping stones, and a stone basin or lantern on the island of a small pond all invite strolling. Both its natural and man-made elements soothe the senses.

The Japanese also stimulate the ears and nose with sounds and odors to give the illusion of expanded space. Tinkling wind chimes and the delicate sounds of moving water achieve multiple sensory effects both inside and outside the Japanese home; the odors of incense, blossoms, and herbs do the same. Odors, furthermore, evoke more memories than do either sights or sounds (Hall, 1966). In a drab institutional setting the scent of new baked bread or cookies or of simmering goulash can transport residents back to childhood so that they can reexperience some of the sensations of family celebrations. In addition, odors, as well as sounds, can provide seductive distractions and happy nostalgia in any humdrum day.

In summary, an architectural design that is therapeutic or healing permits its inhabitants the opportunity to enjoy as full and as normal a life as possible. It conforms to human behavior principles (Lawton, 1970b) which include the human need for and responses to adequate private space, choices among social spaces, views of the natural elements outside, and the aesthetic pleasures of design details, color, and texture (see Figure 13.4). The purpose of its overall design is to create the particular conditions in which its client-users may enjoy an extended life not merely as patients but as maturing individuals as well.

---

* *Trompe l'œil.* French term meaning "deceive the eye," applied to paintings in which objects in still-life arrangement are depicted with such clever mimicry of their counterparts in nature as to confuse the spectator. Probably the best modern examples of *trompe l'oeil* are to be found in the work of the nineteenth-century American painter William Harnett (*McGraw Hill Dictionary of Art*).

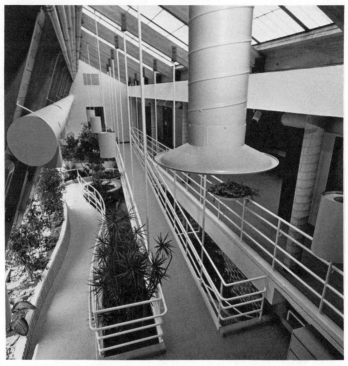

Figure 13.4 Space, air and light combined to bring the outdoors inside. (Girl Scout Council of St. Croix Valley and B. W. B. R. Architects, St. Paul, Minnesota.)

COLOR

Depending upon how it is perceived, color can modify behavior, change the weight and volume of architecture, and visually add distance from the spectator. One environmental psychologist proposes the use of gold, plum, and deep red in a gambling casino "to create an environment that relaxes the morality of people" (Morin, 1983) because those colors are associated with royalty and wealth, both strong attractions for the tourist and gambler.

A building's exterior color can change "the exterior volume of architecture, its sensitive weight, its distance" for the viewer (Giedion, 1958). Concrete that bears a rosy glow, for example, appears less intimidating and more lightweight than a massive structure in stark white. Frank Lloyd Wright employed a shimmery rose for the mammoth Gammage Center in Tempe, Arizona and, as a result, it seems to float above the landscape. Differing responses to a building's size, weight, and distance occur due to perception of color and the emotional impact of color.

Color in daylight is perceived differently than it is under artificial light. Therefore, when choosing any color for an institutional environment it is necessary, first, to see it under both conditions. Colored tiles, issued by paint manufacturers, make this previewing possible; they are more reliable as the basis for color choices than are the named favorites of residents or personnel. Coral, mauve, yellow, and blue, for example, are not perceived by everyone as the same . . . by daylight or by lamplight. Purple and violet produce after images (Hiatt Snyder, 1980) under any conditions and are better used as color accents.

Color is a symbol of life and love; it is a lively addition to an environment. Wall color or the colors in a painting can alter surroundings dramatically especially if they are changed from time to time. Paintings should be circulated around the institution frequently in order to allow clients to perceive their different effects in different locations. If they remain in one place too long they merge with the surroundings and, as a result, they are no longer noticed. Also, changes in wall color, by occasional repainting, is a stimulating renewal of the environment.

> Color changes can be most exciting; they bring new faces to a unit or building and the attention of staffs and visitors alike. In fact, one of the most therapeutic aspects of painting may be . . . the social attention . . . [it brings] to the . . . occupants of the [repainted] area. (Hiatt Snyder, 1981)

Colors have both a physical and emotional influence on persons. Because they emit light they affect the body as well as the eye. They produce stimulating effects on "the vascular system, pulse, blood pressure [and] muscular tension" (Birren, 1978). Although all colors are potentially therapeutic because they allow individuals to transcend their mundane surroundings (Birren, 1978), some have predictably satisfying effects whereas others are controversial.

Color's effect on the body was demonstrated by Kurt Goldstein in the 1940s, when he compared the effects of green and red on body balance. The study suggests that red may disturb the body's equilibrium but green does not. Therefore Birren (1978) concludes, "persons suffering from tremors and twitching may find such (balance) distortions relieved if green glasses are worn."

Physical problems of the aging eye itself make certain colors unsuitable. The lens tend to yellow with age, which means colors are viewed through a yellow-tinted filter, a fact that can be disastrous to certain colors such as blues, particularly pale blues, which will appear dull and grayed. Colors such as yellow and those containing yellow are far more suitable, because they tend to remain constant and not become dulled or depressing. Focusing also is impaired with age, very small and fussy wallpaper patterns should be avoided as they can become disturbingly blurred (Edwards, 1979).

Tints or shades of orange (but not pure orange) may be considered to replace the ubiquitous institutional beiges or off-whites. Pale orange, mixed with white to reduce its shock value, is known to have a tranquilizing effect on people (Ertel, 1978); orange shades mixed with brown or black can do the same. Orange-tinted walls and upholstery are frequently used in airplane cabins for their restful effects on passengers.

Pink also appears to have a soothing effect. It was used experimentally in one penitentiary to reduce agitation among inmates. A room decorated in soft pink also complements the complexions of everyone in it; robes and gowns of pink or rosy hue are a popular choice among chic matrons and its use among the institutionalized aging women can lift their morale.

Some colors appear to have an effect on the intelligence quotient. Again as a result of Ertel's experiments, light blue, yellow, yellow green, and orange seem to increase the IQ, whereas white, black, and brown decrease it (Birren, 1978). White and off-white (except for ceilings) are intolerable for social areas; no one seeks out a place where he will be surrounded with cold, light-reflecting glacial walls. Black and brown, of course, are accent colors. While they are useful for landmark symbols, such as in dark wood sculpture, when they are used in large proportions they become oppressive. Bright, fresh colors such as yellow and pale orange should be considered for institutional environments to stimulate and mentally revitalize residents.

"Too much of the same [color], whether it is light, bright, or white is an invitation to boredom" (Hiatt Snyder, 1981). Colors, and their tints and shades, should be chosen to contrast or harmonize with other colors. Choosing different colors (and their tints and shades) for different corridors is better than using one color repeatedly. Long walls broken up into wide color bands or abstract designs in two or three shades or tints of the original color make a journey seem shorter because it is more visually interesting.

Color also serves as an orientation device for residents, staff members, and visitors alike. Broad color bands on floors are not universally accepted as orientation cues because they may be visually deceiving to some persons and, if so, they become safety hazards when they are perceived as steps or stairs. More useful may be narrow-colored bands that run along the floor at the base of the wall. However, if color bands are used as direction finders to units, the color and unit name can be color-connected. For example, use a gold band for the association to "gold for the X-ray unit" or an orange band for the association "orange for the dining room." These title and color combinations offer clear directions and serve to recall locations. The same approach to color as a destination and location clue functions when there is a different color for each floor in the building especially near elevators (Donahue, 1969).

Additional color orientation devices may take the form of one abstract design or silhouette in bold color, on a contrasting color background, like those used for directions and cautions to guide international travelers. These abstract designs or silhouettes can extend outward from the door to distinguish offices from other rooms.

Printed signs in large and simple lettering, on a colored background, may be useful for some residents but they may be difficult to perceive by the visually impaired. They may perceive the letters as meaningless columns and curves. The same difficulty in perception may confuse the non-English-reading client. A survey of the residents' opinions, and observations of their nonverbal physical responses, can reveal such difficulties.

Color coding can also be a technique for identifying the client with his ethnic background and personal taste. Miniature national flags when placed on the bedroom's door frame personalize both the room and its occupant. Small fabric banners on the door which repeat the patterns chosen by the clients for their drapes and upholstery can be used to distinguish each room as unique, different from every other room. When selected by occupants, flags and banners, or any other distinctive and colorful emblem such as metal knockers or porcelain knobs on a bedroom door can increase personal pride and feelings of ownership.

LIGHT

The implications of the effects of artificial light on the institutionalized elderly is a tantalizing subject for further research. Present studies of age-related changes in biological (Circadian) rhythms indicate that when the light rhythm is disturbed, mood and performance changes (Birren and Renner, 1977). Circadian rhythms follow both a 24-hour, daytime-night-time cycle, as well as a seasonal one that varies with the winter versus the summer duration of sunlight. In one study, a manic-depressive's winter depression "remitted after several winter days were extended with bright artificial light" (Lewy et al., 1982).

On the other hand, another study of the elderly's ability to absorb calcium under artificial light,

> found that a control group of elderly residents of a nursing home who lived under conventional fluorescent lights absorbed calcium less efficiently than the test group who lived under special fluorescent bulbs which more closely replicated the spectral range [color wave lengths] of natural sunlight even though the diet of both groups was the same in calcium content (Filler, 1983).

Fluorescent lights have also been used at the National Institute of Mental Health to reduce depression. Researchers found that when depressed, patients were exposed to eight fluorescent bulbs for several hours morning and night, their depression decreased. And at the Veteran's Administration Hospital in San Diego, researchers found that even one hour of exposure to intense fluorescent light can briefly relieve a depressed patient's condition (*New York Post.* December 21, 1983). These two examples among the many studies of artificial light and its effects illustrate the exciting potential for the therapeutic use of light. It is a topic deserving of more attention.

The reduced ability of the lens of the aging eye to adapt to darkness (Carotenuto and Bullock, 1980) means that the elderly need higher intensity, focused light in order to see. Reduced night and peripheral vision makes unlit paths from bed to bathroom at night, and poorly lit hallways and stairwells, frightening accident hazards.

At present, the wholesale use of fluorescent lighting to illuminate every space and every task in the life-care institutions for the older adult remains controversial. Fluorescent lighting is used with far more discrimination in private homes than it is in the public institutions for the elderly. Lighting, whether subdued or intensified, should match the need it serves. Certain tasks and hallways require more intense light than do conversation areas. And adjustable track lighting, decorative ceiling lights and wall fixtures create a homier atmosphere than do fluorescent tubes. These examples among the many studies of artificial light and its effects illustrate the exciting potential for the therapeutic use of light.

PERSONAL POSSESSIONS

Personal possessions are symbols of the individual's identity. Perla Korosec-Serfaty, a French psychologist, researched the implications for pleasure which personal articles have for the old. In a study of the items stored in the cellars and attics of France she found that their owners regarded them as precious relics of their forebears.

> People would say that an empty attic is not a real attic. They would say, "Oh, you don't want to look up there; there's nothing up there," and, of course, there were many, many things up there, things that their grandfather had made, or a doll, or a coin collection. These things were not worth anything, they were not even looked at or used, but to throw them away would be to violate the continuity, the affiliation with ancestors and offspring. . . . Continuity was the value, the reverence for the objects of continuity (Carroll, 1982).

These symbolic and historic links with the past establish a distinct identity for the individual—a unique image in communal space that is clearly the individual's own. They can create for clients a sense of self-worth because the jewelry, pictures, and souvenirs are visible emblems of their family, religious, social, and cultural memberships. While personal trinkets and momentoes may appear as clutter or dust collectors to the caregivers in an institutional setting, to the older person, whose home and current identity is wrapped up in the institution, personal possessions provide a sense of security—a touch of class status—in an otherwise equalizing environment.

In conclusion, when older adults perceive a congenial environment, which reflects both their physical and emotional needs, they will invariably feel at home in it, provided other and more strong feelings do not inhibit that perception. Furthermore, if life is worth living healthfully it should also be a life "sensorially worth experiencing" (Proppe, 1968). Among the essential elements in a stimulating environment, beyond adequate and appropriate health care, are the opportunities it offers its residents for privacy, autonomy and choices among a variety of resources both within and outside the confines of its institutional space. The setting's capacity to bestow on its residents a sense of security and pleasure can create a psychosocial milieu that permits and encourages their ability to age successfully. There are

> numerous demonstration projects [which] have shown that when the environment is more stimulating, residents who were previously assumed to be physically and mentally incapacitated and apathetic often became much more active and involved in the world around them (Pincus, 1968).

Thus far, person-environment interaction studies reveal that a geriatric environment that is indifferent to residents' needs for sensory and intellectual stimulation exerts a devastating, and unrelieved, emotional impact on them. While the degree of the elderly's responses to their environment may decline with advanced age or illness, surroundings continue to play a crucial role in their daily lives. If the environment is without stimulation, it magnifies the twin fears that in aging "social death may precede biological death" (Neugarten, 1982) and that institutionalization is a prelude to death (Smith, 1977). As a result, the aging man and woman, cut off from any pleasurable stimulation, reacts with rage or depression.

Few have described better the depressing effects on the elderly of an impoverished environment than George L. Maddox, Duke University's Director of the Center for Study of Aging and Human Development, who writes,

> Impoverished environments mask the unused potential of older persons. Most people go through life with more energy, more intellectual capacity and more emotional resources than they need most of the time. Reserve capacity diminishes in late life, but, for the

most part older people have as much capacity as they need for daily living and certainly greater capacity than society encourages them to express (Maddox, 1977).

Clearly we need to change such environments, but we also need to monitor the effects of changes for such studies are in short supply.

REFERENCES

Alexander, S.T.M. Chairperson, *A Guide to the 1981 White House Conference on Aging.* Washington, D.C.: U.S. Department of Health and Human Services, 1981.

Banham, R. *Age of the Masters.* New York: Harper & Row, 1975.

Bates, J. Future of aging/impact of Jarvis-Gann. Committee publication No. 95-168. Hearing before the Subcommittee on Human Services of the Select Committee on Aging, House of Representatives, San Diego, July 5, 1978.

Bengston, V.L., Kasschau, P.L., and Ragan, P.K. The impact of social structure on aging individuals. In Birren, J.E., and Schaie, K.W. (Eds.), *The Handbook of the Psychology of Aging.* New York: Van Nostrand Reinhold, 1977.

Birren, F. *Color and Human Response.* New York: Van Nostrand Reinhold, 1978.

Bourestom, M., and Pastalan, L. *Death and Survival.* Relocation Report No. 2. Ann Arbor: University of Michigan, Institute of Gerontology, n.d.

Brod, J. The influence of higher nervous processes induced by psychosocial environment on the development of essential hypertension. In Levi, L. (Ed.), *Society, Stress and Disease.* London: Oxford University Press, 1971.

Butler, R. *Why Survive? Being Old in America.* New York: Harper & Row, 1975.

Carotenuto, R., and Bullock, J. *Physical Assessment of the Gerontologic Client.* Philadelphia: F.A. Davis, 1980.

Carp, F.M. (Ed) *Retirement.* New York: Behavioral Publications, 1972.

Carroll, J. Alienating environments. *Psychology Today,* July 1982.

Chaisson, G.M. Depression in the elderly. In Bauwens, E., and Anderson, S. (Eds.), *Chronic Illness: Concepts and Application.* St. Louis: C.V. Mosby, 1981.

Chapanis, A. Human engineering environments for the aged. *Gerontologist,* June 1974.

Dickman, I.R. *Ageism: Discrimination Against Older People.* Public Affairs Pamphlet. New York: Public Affairs Committee, 1979.

Donahue, W. Rehabilitation of the Aged Mental Patient. Paper presented at Eighth Annual Governors' Conference on Aging, New York, May 2, 1969.

Edwards, K. The environment inside the hospital. *The Practitioner,* June 1979, 222:746–51.

Ertel, H. In Birren, F. *Color and Human Response.* New York: Van Nostrand Reinhold, 1978.

Filler, M. Living color. *TWA Ambassador,* January 1983.

Forsyth, R.P. Mechanisms of the cardiovascular responses to environmental stressors. In Obrist, P., Black A.H., Brener, J., and DiCara, L.V. (Eds.), *Cardiovascular Psychophysiology.* Chicago: Aldine, 1974.

Fozard, J.L., and Popkin, S.J. Optimizing adult development: ends and means of an applied psychology of aging. *American Psychologist,* November 1978.

Fozard, J.L., and Rose, C.L. A systems approach to applications of human factors engineering to problems of aging. Paper presented at the meeting of the Human Factors Society, Dallas, 1975.

Fozard, J.L., and Thomas, J.C. Why aging engineering psychologists ought to get interested in aging. Paper presented at the meeting of the American Psychological Association, September 1973.

Frederiksen, N. Toward a taxonomy of situations. *American Psychologist,* February 1972.

Fry, W. *Newsday,* October 5, 1982.

Giedion, S. *Architecture You and Me.* Cambridge, Mass.: Harvard University Press, 1958.

Goldberg, Philip, *Arizona Republic,* February 5, 1984, p. 512.

Goldfarb, A.I. Institutional care. In Buse, E.W., and Pfeiffer, E. (Eds.), *Behavior and Adaptation in Late Life.* Boston: Little, Brown, 1969.

Gropius, W. In Anshen, R.N. (Ed.), *Scope of Total Architecture.* New York: Harper & Row, 1955.

Guttman, D. The cross-cultural perspective: notes toward a comparative psychology of aging. In Birren, J.E. and Schaie, K.W. (Eds.), *The Handbook of the Psychology of Aging.* New York: Van Nostrand Reinhold, 1977.

Hall, E.T. *The Hidden Dimension.* Garden City, N.Y.: Doubleday, 1966.

Hammer, P.G., and Chapin, F.S. *Human Time Allocation: A Case Study of Washington, D.C.* Chapel Hill, N.C.: University of North Carolina, Center for Urban Regional Studies.

Hamovitch, M.B., and Peterson, J.E. Housing needs and satisfactions of the elderly. *Gerontologist,* Spring 1969.

Hiatt Snyder, L.G. Architecture for the aged: design for living. *Inland Architect,* November–December 1978.

Hiatt Snyder, L.G. Disorientation is more than a state of mind. *Nursing Homes,* July/August 1980.

Hiatt Snyder, L.G. The color and use of color in environments for older people. *Nursing Homes,* May/June 1981.

Holmes, T.S., and Rahe, R.H. The social readjustment rating scale. *Journal of Psychosomatic Research,* April 1967.

Huttman, E.D. Housing and social services for the elderly. *Social Policy Trends.* New York: Praeger Publishers, 1977.

Jones, M. *Beyond the Therapeutic Community: Social Learning and Social Psychiatry.* New Haven, Conn: Yale University Press, 1968.

Kahana, E. A congruence model of person-environment interaction. In Windley, P.G., and Ernst, G. (Eds.), *Theory Development in Environment and Aging.* Washington, D.C.: Gerontological Society, 1975.

Kleemeier, R.W. The use and meaning of time in special settings. In Kleemeier, R.W. (Ed.), *Aging and Leisure.* New York: Oxford University Press, 1961.

Klein, G.S., Barr, H.L., and Wolitsky, D.L. *Personality.* In Farnsworth, P.R., McNemar, O., McNemar, Q. (Eds.), *Annual Review of Psychology.* Palo Alto, Calif.: Annual Reviews, 1967.

Kruger Smith, B. *The Pursuit of Dignity.* Boston: Beacon Press, 1977.

Larsen, D. To stay in good health, try to keep your funny side up. *Newsday,* December 27, 1982.

Lawton, M.P. Supportive services in the context of the housing environment. *Gerontologist,* Spring 1969.

Lawton, M.P. *Planning and Managing Housing for the Elderly.* New York: Wiley-Interscience, 1975.

Lawton, M.P. Competence, environmental press, and the adaptation of older people. In Windley, P.G., and Ernst, G. (Eds.), *Theory Development in Environment and Aging.* Washington, D.C.: Gerontological Society, 1975.

Lawton, M.P. The impact of the environment on aging and behavior. In Birren, J.E. and Schaie, K.W. (Eds.), *Handbook of the Psychology of Aging.* New York: Van Nostrand Reinhold, 1977.

Lawton, M.P., and Nahemow, L. Ecology and the aging process. In Eisdorfer, E.C., and Lawton, M.P. (Eds.), *The Psychology of Adult Development and Aging.* Washington, D.C.: American Psychological Association, 1973.

Levi, L. (Ed.) *Society, Stress and Disease.* London: Oxford University Press, 1971.

Lewy, A., Kern, H.A., Rosenthal, N.E., and Wehr, T.A. Bright artificial light treatment of a manic-depressive patient with a seasonal mood cycle. *American Journal of Psychiatry,* November 1982.

Lieberman, M. Grouchiness: a survival asset. *University of Chicago Alumni Magazine,* April 1973.

Linn, M.W. Predicting quality of patient care in nursing homes. *Gerontologist,* June 1974.

Lowenthal, M.F. Toward a sociological theory of change in adulthood and old age. In Birren, J.E., and Schaie, K.W. (Eds.), *The Handbook of the Psychology of Aging.* New York: Van Nostrand Reinhold, 1977.

Maddox, G.L. Introduction: options for the aging. In Smith, B.K. (Ed.), *The Pursuit of Dignity.* Boston: Beacon Press, 1977.

Marlowe, R.A. Effects of environment on elderly state hospital relocatees. Paper presented at annual meeting of the Pacific Sociological Association, Scottsdale, Ariz., May 1973.

Mechanic, D. *Medical Sociology.* New York: The Free Press, 1968.

Moos, R., and Houts, P. The assessment of the social atmosphere of psychiatric wards. *Journal of Abnormal Psychology,* February 1968.

Morin, S.P. Interior designer sets out to make casino that relaxes your morality. *The Wall Street Journal,* January 10, 1983.

Nahemow, L., and Lawton, M.P. Toward an ecological theory of adaptation and aging. In Preiser, W.F.E. (Ed.), *Environmental Design Research,* vol. 1, Strouds-burg, Pa.: Dowden, Hutchinson, and Ross, 1973.

Nardini, J. Survival factors in American prisoners of war of the Japanese. *American Journal of Psychiatry,* October 1952.

Neugarten, B.L. Let's treat the elderly as individuals. *Newsday,* September 16, 1982.

New York Post. MDs throw light on winter blues. December 12, 1983.

Nisbet, R. *Prejudices: A Philosophical Dictionary.* Cambridge, Mass.: Harvard University Press, 1982.

Osmond, H., cited by Hall, E.T. in *The Hidden Dimension.* New York: Doubleday, 1966.

Peter, L.J., and Dana, B. *The Laughter Prescription.* New York: Ballantine Books, 1982.

Pfeiffer, E. Psychopathology and social pathology. In *Birren, J.E., and Schaie, K.W. (Eds.), The Handbook of the Psychology of Aging.* New York: Van Nostrand Reinhold, 1977.

Pincus, A. The definition and measurement of institutional environment in homes for the aged. *Gerontologist,* Autumn 1968.

Proppe, H. Housing for the retired and the aged in Southern California: an architectural commentary. *Gerontologist,* Autumn 1968.

Rogers, W.B. *What's up in Architecture? A Look at Modern Buildings.* New York: Harcourt, Brace and World, 1965.

Rosenman, R.H. The role of behavior patterns and neurogenic factors in the pathogenesis of coronary heart disease. In Eliot, R.W., (Ed.), *Stress and the Heart.* New York: Futura, 1974.

Russell, J. How art makes us feel at home in the world. *New York Times,* September 12, 1981.

Schooler, K.K. Response of the elderly to environment: a stress-theoretic perspective. In Windley, P.G., and Ernst, G. (Eds.), *Theory Development in Environment and Aging.* Washington, D.C.: Gerontological Society, 1975.

Sells, S.B. (Ed). *Stimulus Determinants of Behavior.* New York: Ronald, 1962.

Selye, H. The evolution of the stress concept—stress and cardiovascular disease. In Levi, L. (Ed), *Society, Stress and Disease.* London: Oxford University Press, 1971.

Slover, D. Relocation for therapeutic purposes of aged mental hospital patients. Paper presented at annual meeting of Gerontological Society, San Juan, Puerto Rico, 1972.

Snyder, L.H. Environmental changes for socialization. *Journal of Nursing Administration,* January 1978.

Sommer, R., and Ross, H. Social interaction in a geriatrics ward. *International Journal of Social Psychiatry,* Autumn 1958.

Sonnenfeld, J. Diagram of nested set of environments. In Saarinen, T.F., *Perception of Environment,* Resource Paper #5. Washington, D.C.: Association of American Geographers, 1969.

Spier, B.E. The nursing process as applied to the developmental tasks of the aged. In Yurik, A.G., et al. (Eds.), *The Aged Person and the Nursing Process.* New York: Appleton, Century and Crofts, 1980.

Spieth, W. Slowness of task performance and cardiovascular diseases. In Welford, A.T., and Birren, J.E. (Eds.), *Behavior, Aging and the Nervous System.* Springfield, Ill.: Charles C. Thomas, 1965.

Stanford, E.P., and Toseland, R. Future of aging: impact of Jarvis-Gann. Committee Publication No. 95-168. Hearing before the Subcommittee on Human Services of the Select Committee on Aging, House of Representatives, San Diego, July 5, 1978.

Thomae, H. Theory of aging and cognitive theory of personality. In *Human Development,* vol. 13. Basel and New York: S. Karger Publishers, 1970.

Tsuda, N. *Handbook of Japanese Art.* Vermont and Tokyo, Japan: Charles E. Tuttle, 1976.

Wohwill, J.F. *The Study of Behavioral Development.* New York: Academic Press, 1973.

Wolf, S. Psychosocial forces in myocardial infarction and sudden death. In Levi, L. (Ed.), *Society, Stress and Disease.* London: Oxford University Press, 1971.

Index